# Respiratory Medicine

Respiratory Medicine offers clinical and research-oriented resources for pulmonologists and other practitioners and researchers interested in respiratory care. Spanning a broad range of clinical and research issues in respiratory medicine, the series covers such topics as COPD, asthma and allergy, pulmonary problems in pregnancy, molecular basis of lung disease, sleep disordered breathing, and others.

The series editors are Sharon Rounds, MD, Professor of Medicine and of Pathology and Laboratory Medicine at the Alpert Medical School at Brown University, Anne Dixon, MD, Professor of Medicine and Director of the Division of Pulmonary and Critical Care at Robert Larner, MD College of Medicine at the University of Vermont, and Lynn M. Schnapp, MD, George R. And Elaine Love Professor and Chair of Medicine at the University of Wisconsin-Madison School of Medicine and Public Health.

Bridget F. Collins • Sydney B. Montesi
Editors

# Precision Medicine in Interstitial Lung Disease

Humana Press

*Editors*
Bridget F. Collins
Kirkland, WA, USA

Sydney B. Montesi
Boston, MA, USA

ISSN 2197-7372 ISSN 2197-7380 (electronic)
Respiratory Medicine
ISBN 978-3-031-87182-5 ISBN 978-3-031-87183-2 (eBook)
https://doi.org/10.1007/978-3-031-87183-2



This Humana imprint is published by the registered company Springer Nature Switzerland AG
The registered company address is: Gewerbestrasse 11, 6330 Cham, Switzerland

# Introduction: Precision Medicine in Interstitial Lung Disease

The interstitial lung diseases (ILDs) are a large and diverse family of conditions due to inflammation and/or scarring in the lungs. ILD diagnosis is often a complex and multi-step process. Idiopathic pulmonary fibrosis (IPF) is the best studied among the fibrotic ILDs. IPF is a uniformly progressive fibrotic lung disease of unknown cause with median survival 3–5 years from time of diagnosis [1, 2]. Despite poor prognosis and progressive disease, diagnosis of IPF and other fibrotic lung diseases is often delayed. Registry data has shown that greater than 50% of patients diagnosed with IPF were not diagnosed until at least 1 year after symptom onset [3, 4]. IPF and other progressive fibrotic lung diseases are not curable without lung transplantation. Antifibrotic medications reduce the rate of decline in lung function over time, but do not reverse fibrosis or clearly improve symptoms [5–7]. With this background, there has been increasing interest in employing precision medicine to aid in earlier, timely diagnosis and more targeted treatments for progressive fibrotic lung disease. This book highlights various aspects of precision medicine in the field of ILD.

Precision medicine has been defined as tailoring medical treatment based on individual patient characteristics and classifying people into subpopulations based on susceptibility to a specific disease or treatment response [8]. A primary goal of precision medicine is to objectively direct preventative and therapeutic interventions to those individuals most likely to benefit. Precision medicine aims to increase quality of care and reduce costs by avoiding unnecessary diagnostic tests and ineffective treatments [8, 9]. Over the past 10–15 years, there has been an explosion of studies of various biomarkers and technologic advances that have the potential to transform ILD diagnosis and treatment. A goal of this book is to describe various aspects of precision medicine in ILD in their current form. Additional studies are needed to validate and streamline precision medicine in ILD clinical care with consideration to cost and equity before such approaches will be ready for use in general pulmonary clinical practice. In Chap. 1, Dr. Neuringer highlights lessons learned from implementation of precision medicine in other lung diseases, specifically Cystic Fibrosis.

Early precision medicine efforts in ILD focused broadly on disease behavior and radiologic pattern on high-resolution computed tomography (HRCT) imaging. In

2001, the American Thoracic Society (ATS) and European Respiratory Society (ERS) published a multidisciplinary consensus statement to describe and categorize idiopathic interstitial pneumonias (IIPs) based on clinical, radiologic, and pathologic features, which was updated in 2013 [10, 11]. This allowed relatively standardized diagnostic criteria to be applied in clinical practice and in research, emphasizing a dynamic diagnostic approach with input from providers across specialties [10]. The ATS/ERS/JRS/ALAT 2011 evidence-based guideline for diagnosis and management of IPF defined clinical, radiologic, and histologic features supporting or refuting an IPF diagnosis, with multiple updates since [1]. The clinico-radiographic patterns generated by these statements could be considered biomarkers, defined by the National Institutes of Health as "characteristics that can be objectively measured and used as an indicator of normal biological processes, disease processes, or pharmacologic responses to a therapy" [12].

Twenty percent of pulmonary fibrosis patients are estimated to have familial disease [13]. Familial cohorts have been an essential cornerstone in shaping precision medicine in ILD, particularly in our understanding of genetics. There is still much to learn as only 20–30% of patients with familial pulmonary fibrosis (FPF), defined as having two or more first degree relatives with pulmonary fibrosis, have an identifiable causative genetic variant [13, 14]. Furthermore, even among individuals with known FPF, genetic testing is not uniformly available or applied, even at expert centers [13, 15]. In Chap. 2, Pearmain, Finn and Rivera-Ortega describe the role of precision medicine in screening and disease course prediction among those with familial ILD.

Over time, biomarkers have become increasingly precise, focusing on genetics, molecular markers, and transcriptomics. A signature of blood-based protein biomarkers recently has been shown to confer important prognostic information in IPF that outperformed clinically derived information [16]. Given increasing elucidation of both common and rare genetic variants contributing to the risk for pulmonary fibrosis, the presence of individual genetic variants may help quantify disease risk in an at-risk individual. However, advances in incorporation of genetic information to clinical care hinge on expanded access of genetic testing and a better understanding of genetic variants associated with pulmonary fibrosis in diverse ethnic populations. Zhang and Newton discuss Genetic Biomarkers for Interstitial Lung Disease in Chap. 3, while Zanini, Faverio, and Luppi review Molecular Biomarkers in Interstitial Lung Disease in Chap. 4.

Biomarker identification is only a first step in precision medicine. Once a potential biomarker is discovered, it must be further studied and validated with standardization and consistency of measurement. Even after a biomarker is validated, the scientific and medical community must determine how valuable such a marker will be both in terms of its role in clinical practice/patient care and from a cost-effectiveness standpoint. Once these steps are completed, awareness must be increased among academic and community providers to allow adoption into clinical practice. It is likely that different biomarkers will be needed for different components of clinical care, for example, risk stratification vs. assessment of treatment response. It is critical that equity and accessibility are considerations in development of precision medicine biomarkers. Most biomarker studies, such as genetic studies, have been conducted using cohorts of individuals of European ancestry with limited validation done in more diverse cohorts. Additionally, complex biomarker assessments are unlikely to be widely available, especially in rural areas or resource limited settings. Figure 1 shows a three-tiered approach from conceptualization to implementation in precision medicine [17].

The use of bronchoscopy in the management of patients with pulmonary fibrosis has expanded beyond assessment of bronchoalveolar lavage fluid cell profile and microbiology to assess for alternative diagnoses and now routinely includes tissue sampling for pathological characterization due to advances in bronchoscopy techniques. The expansion of cryobiopsy to parenchymal lung diseases provides the opportunity to less invasively (in comparison to surgical lung biopsy) diagnose the underlying ILD subtype with high confidence [18]. Additionally, a genomic classifier performed on tissue obtained from a trans-bronchial lung biopsy is now in clinical use as a diagnostic tool for usual interstitial pneumonia with high specificity [19]. This represents a major step in the application of precision medicine to pulmonary fibrosis via bronchoscopy as discussed in Chap. 5 by Abdelghani, Pyarali, and Kheir.

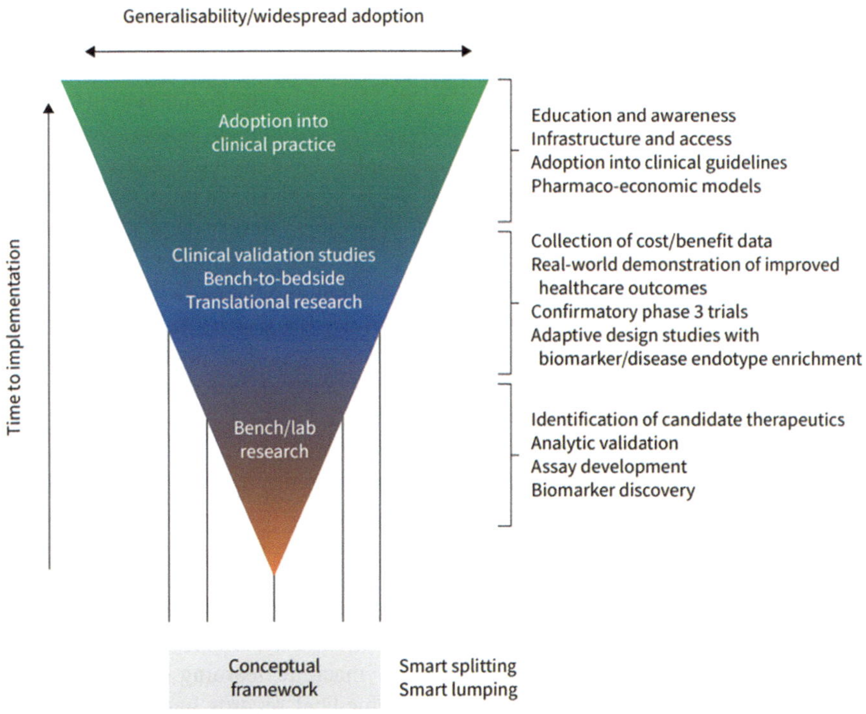


**Fig. 1** Three-tiered approach to the advancement of precision medicine in interstitial lung disease. (Reproduced with permission from: Maher et al. [17])

Alongside these advances, we have improved understanding of how environmental factors may interact with or compound risk from underlying genetic factors. Air pollution exposure has been associated with increased incidence of ILD including IPF and Hypersensitivity Pneumonitis (HP) as well as increased risk of acute exacerbations in IPF [20–23]. There is accumulating evidence that PM2.5 levels and other pollutants have epigenomic impacts affecting DNA methylation and telomerase activity [22, 24, 25]. This will likely become increasingly relevant as air pollution levels continue to rise. Barnes and Barber review this and other data in depth in Chap. 6. It is also critical to note that in the United States, PM2.5 associated deaths are increased among non-Hispanic Black or African American individuals and those who are socioeconomically disadvantaged [26]. Furthermore, individuals with pulmonary fibrosis who are racial and ethnic minorities, particularly Black individuals, have earlier disease onset and higher rates of hospitalization, yet lower rates of lung transplantation compared to White individuals [27]. Ferraro and Morisset discuss the influence of race and ethnicity in precision ILD diagnosis and treatment in Chap. 7.

Ideally, precision medicine can be achieved with as little individual risk as possible. For instance, HRCT biomarkers and assessment of CT with deep machine learning are useful, but one must consider minimizing risks associated with repeated radiation exposure. There is increasing interest in detecting markers in exhaled breath, which can be easily obtained from an individual without invasive testing or radiation risk and unlike serum biomarkers, provide lung-specific information. However, factors in the surrounding environment that might influence testing must be considered. Standardization and accessibility are additional challenges. Jeong, Kim, and Im provide an in-depth summary of exhaled breath biomarkers in ILD in Chap. 8.

Advancements in precision medicine hinge on ongoing mechanistic discoveries in animal models. To date most preclinical studies have been conducted using the bleomycin mouse model. While it is purported to be a model of pulmonary fibrosis, there are notable differences from human pulmonary fibrosis. These differences combined with other model factors may explain in part the number of promising preclinical therapeutic studies that did not translate into improved clinical outcomes when studied in human participants [28]. There is increasing appreciation of the need for improved animal models that more closely capture features of pulmonary fibrosis present in humans [29]. Newer models such as *Sftpc* mouse models are primed to enable a precision medicine investigation of the pathways driving fibrogenesis as detailed in Chap. 9 by Katzen and Knipe.

With advances in technology and artificial intelligence, big data can now be utilized to better understand real-world patient characteristics, disease outcomes, and prescribing patterns. While big data is often equated with "omic" analyses, health system data can be leveraged to provide insights on a larger scale. For example, using a large claims database, it was found that treatment with metformin in individuals with concurrent IPF and diabetes mellitus was associated with reduced hospitalizations and all-cause mortality [30]. A machine learning algorithm using comorbidity signatures applied to electronic medical records has been shown to have good test characteristics at predicting a diagnosis of IPF [31]. Further uses of big data to facilitate precision medicine are discussed in Chap. 10 by Kaul, Collard, and Petersen.

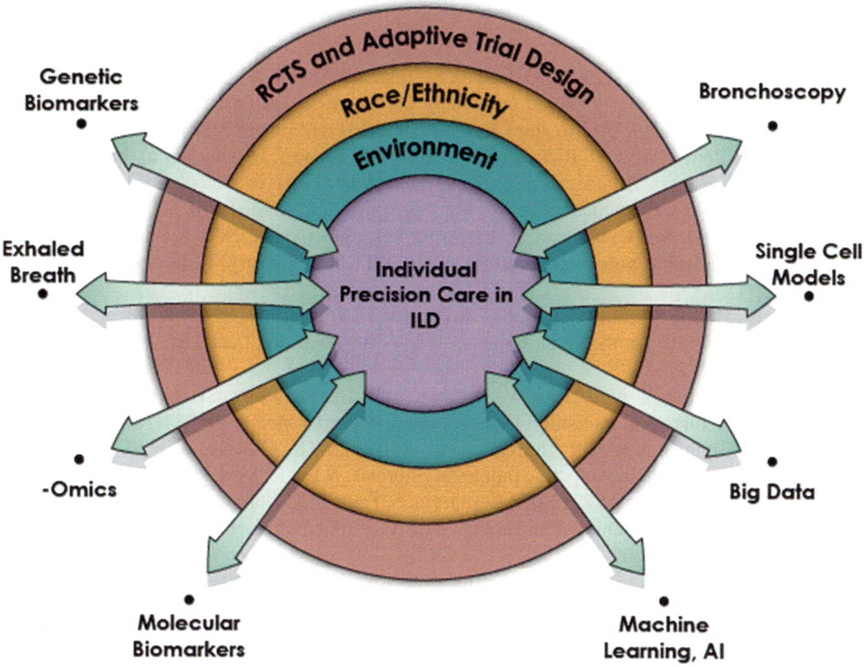


**Fig. 2** Aspects of precision medicine influencing individual patient precision care in interstitial lung disease. Abbreviations: *RCT* randomized controlled trials, *ILD* interstitial lung disease, *AI* artificial intelligence. (Figure render courtesy of Sean McLaughlin, B.F.A)

The application of precision medicine to pulmonary fibrosis is poised to make great advances to the field especially pertaining to earlier diagnosis, improved disease course prediction, and determination of treatment response. Chapter 11 authored by Adams, Patel, and Gulati summarizes the future of precision medicine in ILD. As additional therapeutics are developed for treatment of pulmonary fibrosis, precision medicine approaches with ongoing bidirectional feedback will become essential to identifying the most effective therapy for an individual patient (Fig. 2). A precision medicine approach has revolutionized the treatment of lung cancers and other pulmonary diseases such as cystic fibrosis, and it is our hope that it will do the same for individuals living with pulmonary fibrosis in the coming years.

Center for Interstitial Lung Diseases, Division of Pulmonary, Critical Care and Sleep Medicine, University of Washington Medical Center, Seattle, WA, USA — Bridget F. Collins

Division of Pulmonary and Critical Care Medicine, Massachusetts General Hospital, Boston, MA, USA — Sydney B. Montesi

## References


1. Raghu G, Collard HR, Egan JJ, Martinez FJ, Behr J, Brown KK, et al. An official ATS/ERS/JRS/ALAT statement: idiopathic pulmonary fibrosis: evidence-based guidelines for diagnosis and management. Am J Respir Crit Care Med. 2011;183(6):788–824.
2. Raghu G, Remy-Jardin M, Richeldi L, Thomson CC, Inoue Y, Johkoh T, et al. Idiopathic pulmonary fibrosis (an update) and progressive pulmonary fibrosis in adults: an official ATS/ERS/JRS/ALAT clinical practice guideline. Am J Respir Crit Care Med. 2022;205(9):e18–e47.
3. Snyder LD, Mosher C, Holtze CH, Lancaster LH, Flaherty KR, Noth I, et al. Time to diagnosis of idiopathic pulmonary fibrosis in the IPF-PRO Registry. BMJ Open Respir Res. 2020;7(1).
4. Herberts MB, Teague TT, Thao V, Sangaralingham LR, Henk HJ, Hovde KT, et al. Idiopathic pulmonary fibrosis in the United States: time to diagnosis and treatment. BMC Pulm Med. 2023;23(1):281.
5. Flaherty KR, Wells AU, Cottin V, Devaraj A, Walsh SLF, Inoue Y, et al. Nintedanib in Progressive Fibrosing Interstitial Lung Diseases. N Engl J Med. 2019;381(18):1718–27.
6. Richeldi L, du Bois RM, Raghu G, Azuma A, Brown KK, Costabel U, et al. Efficacy and safety of nintedanib in idiopathic pulmonary fibrosis. N Engl J Med. 2014;370(22):2071–82.
7. King TE, Jr., Bradford WZ, Castro-Bernardini S, Fagan EA, Glaspole I, Glassberg MK, et al. A phase 3 trial of pirfenidone in patients with idiopathic pulmonary fibrosis. N Engl J Med. 2014;370(22):2083–92.
8. National Research Council Committee on AFfDaNToD. The National Academies Collection: Reports funded by National Institutes of Health. Toward Precision Medicine: Building a Knowledge Network for Biomedical Research and a New Taxonomy of Disease. Washington (DC): National Academies Press (US). Copyright © 2011, National Academy of Sciences; 2011.
9. Ginsburg GS, Phillips KA. Precision medicine: from science to value. Health Aff (Millwood). 2018;37(5):694–701.
10. American Thoracic Society/European Respiratory Society International Multidisciplinary Consensus Classification of the Idiopathic Interstitial Pneumonias. This joint statement of the American Thoracic Society (ATS), and the European Respiratory Society (ERS) was adopted by the ATS board of directors, June 2001 and by the ERS Executive Committee, June 2001. Am J Respir Crit Care Med. 2002;165(2):277–304.
11. Travis WD, Costabel U, Hansell DM, King TE, Jr., Lynch DA, Nicholson AG, et al. An official American Thoracic Society/European Respiratory Society statement: update of the international multidisciplinary classification of the idiopathic interstitial pneumonias. Am J Respir Crit Care Med. 2013;188(6):733–48.
12. U.S. Department of Human Services NIoH, National Center for Advancing Translational Sciences. Understand Translational Research Tools 2024 [cited 2024 November 1]. Available from: https://toolkit.ncats.nih.gov/module/discovery/developing-translational-research-tools/biomarkers/
13. Newton CA, Oldham JM, Applegate C, Carmichael N, Powell K, Dilling D, et al. The Role of genetic testing in pulmonary fibrosis: a perspective from the pulmonary fibrosis foundation genetic testing work group. Chest. 2022;162(2):394–405.
14. Kropski JA, Young LR, Cogan JD, Mitchell DB, Lancaster LH, Worrell JA, et al. Genetic evaluation and testing of patients and families with idiopathic pulmonary fibrosis. Am J Respir Crit Care Med. 2017;195(11):1423–8.
15. Terwiel M, Borie R, Crestani B, Galvin L, Bonella F, Fabre A, et al. Genetic testing in interstitial lung disease: an international survey. Respirology. 2022;27(9):747–57.
16. Oldham JM, Huang Y, Bose S, Ma SF, Kim JS, Schwab A, et al. Proteomic biomarkers of survival in idiopathic pulmonary fibrosis. Am J Respir Crit Care Med. 2024;209(9):1111–20.
17. Maher TM, Nambiar AM, Wells AU. The role of precision medicine in interstitial lung disease. Eur Respir J. 2022;60(3).

18. Troy LK, Grainge C, Corte TJ, Williamson JP, Vallely MP, Cooper WA, et al. Diagnostic accuracy of transbronchial lung cryobiopsy for interstitial lung disease diagnosis (COLDICE): a prospective, comparative study. Lancet Respir Med. 2020;8(2):171–81.
19. Kheir F, Uribe Becerra JP, Bissell B, Ghazipura M, Herman D, Hon SM, et al. Use of a genomic classifier in patients with interstitial lung disease: a systematic review and meta-Analysis. Ann Am Thorac Soc. 2022;19(5):827–32.
20. Cui F, Sun Y, Xie J, Li D, Wu M, Song L, et al. Air pollutants, genetic susceptibility and risk of incident idiopathic pulmonary fibrosis. Eur Respir J. 2023;61(2).
21. Sesé L, Nunes H, Cottin V, Sanyal S, Didier M, Carton Z, et al. Role of atmospheric pollution on the natural history of idiopathic pulmonary fibrosis. Thorax. 2018;73(2):145–50.
22. Goobie GC, Nouraie M, Zhang Y, Kass DJ, Ryerson CJ, Carlsten C, et al. Air pollution and interstitial lung diseases: defining epigenomic effects. Am J Respir Crit Care Med. 2020;202(9):1217–24.
23. Singh S, Collins BF, Bairwa M, Joshi JM, Talwar D, Singh N, et al. Hypersensitivity pneumonitis and its correlation with ambient air pollution in urban India. Eur Respir J. 2019;53(2).
24. Chang-Chien J, Huang JL, Tsai HJ, Wang SL, Kuo ML, Yao TC. Particulate matter causes telomere shortening and increase in cellular senescence markers in human lung epithelial cells. Ecotoxicol Environ Saf. 2021;222:112484.
25. Goobie GC, Li X, Ryerson CJ, Carlsten C, Johannson KA, Fabisiak JP, et al. PM(2.5) and constituent component impacts on global DNA methylation in patients with idiopathic pulmonary fibrosis. Environ Pollut. 2023;318:120942.
26. Bowe B, Xie Y, Yan Y, Al-Aly Z. Burden of cause-specific mortality associated with PM2.5 air pollution in the United States. JAMA Netw Open. 2019;2(11):e1915834.
27. Adegunsoye A, Freiheit E, White EN, Kaul B, Newton CA, Oldham JM, et al. Evaluation of pulmonary fibrosis outcomes by race and ethnicity in US adults. JAMA Netw Open. 2023;6(3):e232427.
28. Yanagihara T, Chong SG, Vierhout M, Hirota JA, Ask K, Kolb M. Current models of pulmonary fibrosis for future drug discovery efforts. Expert Opin Drug Discov. 2020;15(8):931–41.
29. Montesi SB, Gomez CR, Beers M, Brown R, Chattopadhyay I, Flaherty KR, et al. Pulmonary fibrosis stakeholder summit: a joint NHLBI, three lakes foundation, and pulmonary fibrosis foundation workshop report. Am J Respir Crit Care Med. 2024;209(4):362–73.
30. Teague TT, Payne SR, Kelly BT, Dempsey TM, McCoy RG, Sangaralingham LR, et al. Evaluation for clinical benefit of metformin in patients with idiopathic pulmonary fibrosis and type 2 diabetes mellitus: a national claims-based cohort analysis. Respir Res. 2022;23(1):91.
31. Onishchenko D, Marlowe RJ, Ngufor CG, Faust LJ, Limper AH, Hunninghake GM, et al. Screening for idiopathic pulmonary fibrosis using comorbidity signatures in electronic health records. Nat Med. 2022;28(10):2107–16.

# Contents

# Contributors

**Ramsy Abdelghani** Division of Pulmonary Diseases, Critical Care and Environmental Medicine, Tulane University Health Sciences Center, New Orleans, LA, USA

**Traci N. Adams** Division of Pulmonary and Critical Care Medicine, University of Texas Southwestern Medical Center, Dallas, TX, USA

**Christopher Barber** Centre for Workplace Health, Science Division, Health and Safety Executive, Buxton, UK
Department of Respiratory Medicine, Northern General Hospital, Sheffield, UK

**Hayley Barnes** Department of Respiratory Medicine, Alfred Health, Melbourne, Australia
Monash Centre for Occupational and Environmental Health, Monash University, Melbourne, Australia
School of Translational Medicine, Monash University, Melbourne, Australia

**Harold R. Collard** University of California San Francisco, San Francisco, CA, USA

**Jack Callum** Respiratory Consultant, Homerton University Hospital NHS Foundation Trust, London, UK

**Paola Faverio** University of Milano-Bicocca, Fondazione IRCCS "San Gerardo dei Tintori", Monza, Italy

**Vincent Ferraro** Département de Médecine, Centre Hospitalier de L'Université de Montréal (CHUM), Montreal, QC, Canada

**Mridu Gulati** Yale Occupational Medicine and Environmental Medicine, Yale School of Medicine, New Haven, CT, USA

**Hyungsoon Im** Center for Systems Biology, Massachusetts General Hospital, Boston, MA, USA
Department of Radiology, Massachusetts General Hospital, Boston, MA, USA

**Mi Ho Jeong** Center for Systems Biology, Massachusetts General Hospital, Boston, MA, USA

**Jeremy Katzen** Division of Pulmonary, Allergy, and Critical Care Medicine, University of Pennsylvania Perelman School of Medicine and Penn-CHOP Lung Biology Institute, Philadelphia, PA, USA

**Bhavika Kaul** Baylor College of Medicine, Houston, TX, USA
Center for Innovations in Quality, Effectiveness and Safety, Department of Veterans Affairs, Houston, TX, USA

**Fayez Kheir** Division of Pulmonary and Critical Care Medicine, Massachusetts General Hospital, Harvard Medical School, Boston, MA, USA

**Joong-Yub Kim** Division of Pulmonary and Critical Care Medicine, Department of Internal Medicine, Seoul National University Hospital, Seoul National University College of Medicine, Seoul, South Korea

**Rachel Knipe** Division of Pulmonary and Critical Care Medicine and Center for Immunology and Inflammatory Diseases, Massachusetts General Hospital and Harvard Medical School, Boston, MA, USA

**Fabrizio Luppi** University of Milano-Bicocca, Fondazione IRCCS "San Gerardo dei Tintori", Monza, Italy

**Julie Morisset** Département de Médecine, Centre Hospitalier de L'Université de Montréal (CHUM), Montreal, QC, Canada

**Isabel Neuringer** MGH Adult Cystic Fibrosis Center, Pulmonary Division, Massachusetts General Hospital, Boston, MA, USA

**Chad A. Newton** Department of Internal Medicine, University of Texas Southwestern Medical Center, Dallas, TX, USA

**Chandni Patel** Division of Pulmonary and Critical Care Medicine, University of Texas Southwestern Medical Center, Dallas, TX, USA

**Laurence Pearmain** Respiratory NIHR Clinical Lecturer, University of Manchester, Manchester, UK
Respiratory Specialist Registrar, Wythenshawe Hospital, Manchester University NHS Foundation Trust, Manchester, UK

**Laura A. Petersen** Baylor College of Medicine, Houston, TX, USA
Center for Innovations in Quality, Effectiveness and Safety, Department of Veterans Affairs, Houston, TX, USA

**Fahim Pyarali** Division of Pulmonary and Critical Care Medicine, Massachusetts General Hospital, Harvard Medical School, Boston, MA, USA

**Pilar Rivera-Ortega** Interstitial Lung Disease Unit, Wythenshawe Hospital, Manchester University NHS Foundation Trust, Manchester, UK

**Stefan Stanel** Interstitial Lung Disease Unit, Wythenshawe Hospital, Manchester University NHS Foundation Trust, Manchester, UK

**Umberto Zanini** University of Milano-Bicocca, Fondazione IRCCS "San Gerardo dei Tintori", Monza, Italy

**David Zhang** Department of Medicine, Columbia University Irving Medical Center, New York, NY, USA

# Chapter 1
# Lessons Learned from Precision Medicine in Other Lung Diseases

**Isabel Neuringer**

## Cystic Fibrosis: Introduction

CF is autosomal recessive disorder causing variable degrees of CFTR chloride ion channel dysfunction, abrogation of ion transport across epithelial cell surfaces, with a net result of inspissated, thick, mucous along the airways and digestive organs, predominantly. In 1938, Dorothy Andersen and colleagues reviewed the anatomy of 49 children who had died from possible celiac disease and noted cystic changes of the pancreas as well as mucosal edema in the lungs, thus characterizing the clinical manifestations of CF disease [1]. In general, cystic fibrosis occurs in about 1 in 3500 births in the USA, Europe, and Australia, affecting about 35,000 persons in the USA [2]. CF affects an estimated 188,000 patients worldwide, a significant percent undiagnosed; and access to state-of-the-art CFTR modulator therapies is disparate across the world [3, 4]. People with CF (pwCF) may present with meconium ileus or respiratory insufficiency at birth, or in early childhood, and historically developed bronchiectasis, inflammation of the respiratory tract, and many pwCF succumbed to an early death from respiratory failure. Since the initial description of CF, interventions aimed at restoring optimal digestion with pancreatic enzymes supplementation, intensive physical therapy, and antibiotic treatment for pulmonary exacerbations. Other complications include sinusitis, pancreatic exocrine and endocrine insufficiency, suboptimal bone health, gastrointestinal disease affecting the foregut to the colon and rectum (GERD, gastroparesis, distal intestinal obstruction, malabsorption), liver and biliary system dysfunction, pancreatic insufficiency, and pancreatitis, to reproductive organ involvement [5]. The average life expectancy in 1960 for a CF child was <10 years of age and approached ~20 s during the 1990s.

I. Neuringer (✉)
MGH Adult Cystic Fibrosis Center, Pulmonary Division, Massachusetts General Hospital, Boston, MA, USA
e-mail: INEURINGER@mgh.harvard.edu



B. F. Collins, S. B. Montesi (eds.), *Precision Medicine in Interstitial Lung Disease*, Respiratory Medicine, https://doi.org/10.1007/978-3-031-87183-2_1

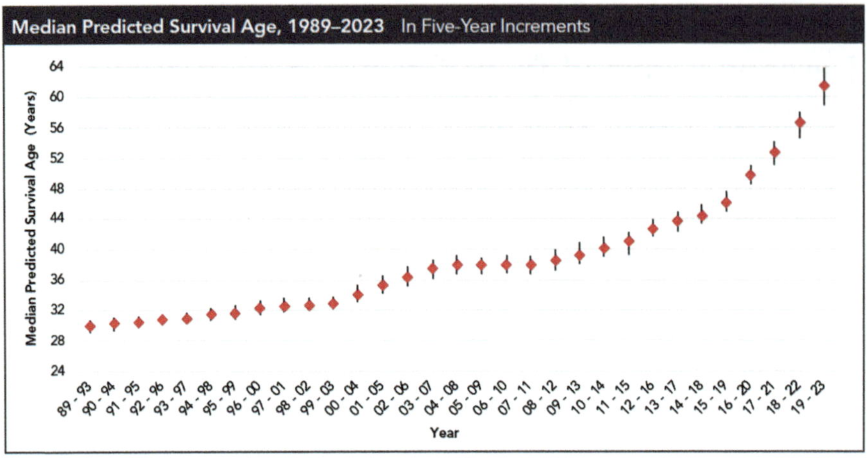


**Fig. 1.1** The median predicted survival age of an individual born with CF in 2023 [6]

Significant progress has been made in understanding the CFTR gene, classes of CFTR mutations, and identification of over 2000 CFTR mutations, which have subsequently led to the recent development of mutation-specific, customized precision therapeutics aimed at correcting and potentiating protein misfolding and chloride channel gating at the epithelial cell surface [5].

Since Dr. Andersen first characterized the clinical manifestations of CF, significant progress has been made to provide personalized therapy for pwCF, mutation-specific therapies including CFTR modulators, analytical tools to study CFTR function and phenotype, and novel therapies aimed at restoring CFTR function though gene addition, gene editing, cell-based, mRNA, and oligonucleotide therapies. Per the most recent CFF Registry report, the predicted survival age of a pwCF born in 2023 was 68.0 years (Fig. 1.1). For those born 2019–2023, the predicted survival age was 61.4 years. Annual mortality rate has also decreased, averaging 0.7 deaths per 100 individuals with CF in the Registry [6].

## Discovery of the CF Gene/CFTR Structure

Observations of profound salt loss after a heat wave in NY in the 1940s led to the hypothesis of salt depletion as the critical physiologic abnormality in CF, leading to further focus upon how ion channels are regulated, and the development of the sweat chloride iontophoresis [7].

In 1989, John Riordan, Lap-Cee Tsui, Francis Collins, and colleagues identified complementary DNA clones on chromosome 7, coding for putative CFTR protein, consisting of 6500 nucleotides, forming the CFTR protein with membrane-binding and intracellular ATP-binding properties. Structurally, the CFTR protein forms a chloride ion channel, is able to promote absorption of chloride and bicarbonate across the apical epithelial surface, and, if dysfunctional, impedes mucociliary transport [8]. CFTR function correlates with healthy physiology of the epithelial sodium channel (ENaC), alternative chloride, and calcium channels [9–11]. Transport of chloride and bicarbonate occurs across organs including the sweat glands, respiratory and gastrointestinal tracts, pancreas, and vas deferens. The airway surface within the lung becomes dehydrated, due to impaired CFTR function, resulting in failed chloride secretion and sodium hyper-absorption. Clinically, this manifests as accumulation of secretions along the airways, reduced mucociliary clearance, and a cycle of bacterial colonization, inflammation, and anatomical destruction of the airways. Bicarbonate secretion impacts pH of pancreatic ducts, with altered CFTR function leading to loss of function of pancreatic enzymes, protein malabsorption, damage to ducts, and fibrosis. Effects across the luminal parts of the GI tract include distal intestinal obstruction, cholestasis, and ductal fibrosis within the hepatobiliary system [12, 13].

Over 2000 mutations have been recognized in the CFTR gene. A patient with two pathogenic CFTR mutations and a sweat chloride level greater than 60 mEq/L qualifies as CF. Homozygous mutations indicate two of the same CFTR mutations, while heterozygous status means two different CFTR mutations. The CFTR gene contains 27 exons spreading over 250 kb of chromosome 7 (7q31) and encodes an mRNA of 6.5 kb. The CFTR protein contains a single chain of 1480 amino acids which spans the cell membrane. The CFTR protein consists of five functional regions called domains. Two transmembrane domains (TMD1 and TMD2) span the cell surface, and two nucleotide-binding domains (NBD1 and NBD2) and a regulatory (R) domain are situated within the cell. The membrane spanning domains form the chloride channel, and the two nucleotide-binding domains within the cell bind ATP resulting in phosphorylation of PKA/PKC within the regulatory domain, permitting opening of the channel [14, 15], as depicted in Fig. 1.2 [16]. The most common CFTR mutation affecting 85% of all pwCF, deltaF508, is the deletion of three nucleotides resulting in the loss of phenylalanine at amino acid position 508. CFTR mutations which occur after the regulatory domain, amino acid 838, are associated with less severe disease [9]. While exons hold the information for cDNA and protein translation, intron mutations may play a role as identified though whole genome sequencing [17].

The Cystic Fibrosis Mutation Database (CFTR2) tracks CFTR mutations. As of the most recent update of September 24, 2024, 1167 variants are annotated on the CFTR2 website, CF-causing 1085, variants of varying clinical consequence 55, and non-CF-causing 27. An estimated 40% are missense mutations, and many variants remain ill-defined, may not impact mRNA creation or protein production, and may form a complex allele in cis with unpredictable phenotype [18]. Models capable of predicting possible pathogenic CFTR mutations may fill the gaps in knowledge of as yet uncharacterized CFTR variants [19].

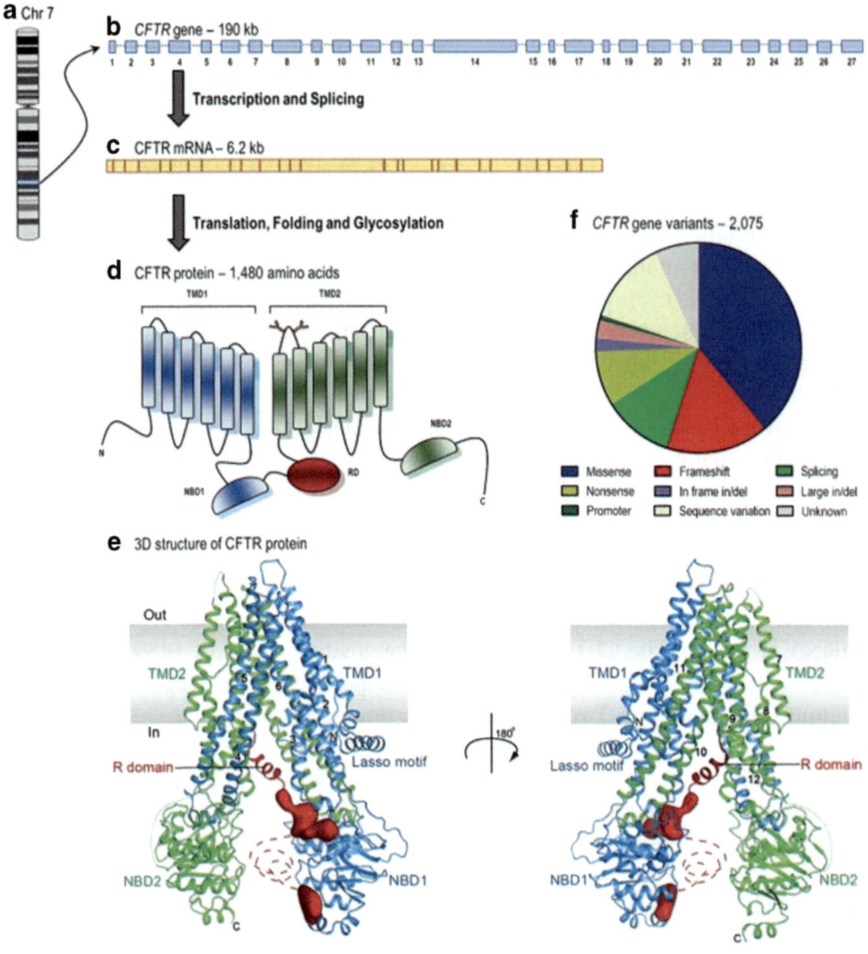


**Fig. 1.2** CFTR gene and protein structure [16]

## CFTR Mutation Classes

CFTR mutations generally fall within six types of mutations, related to the degree of protein expression. Class I mutations produce little to no CFTR protein, may result from a nonsense mutation causing a premature stop codon in the mRNA, as well as frameshift and splicing mutations. Mutations such as G542X and W1282X, occurring in pwCF at 4.5% and 1–2% frequency, respectively. Protein processing mutations are class II, the prototypical deltaF508 present in 85% of CF patients, which undergoes premature degradation due to protein misfolding within the endoplasmic reticulum. Class III mutations constitute gating mutations resulting in impaired opening of the chloride channel at the apical cell surface and reduced probability of channel opening and include G551D, which occurs in 2–5% of pwCF. In class IV mutations, the conductance of the chloride channel is abnormal resulting in impaired chloride secretion to a milder degree, with preserved pancreatic exocrine function, the R117H mutation being a typical nutation in this class. Class V mutations result in less protein but again cause a milder disease phenotype and include 3849 + 10kbC > T, 2789 + 5G > A, and A455E mutations and often retain residual CFTR function or may present later in life. Lastly, class VI mutations have reduced CFTR stability, resulting in reduced half-life at the cell surface, but also retain residual function [5, 20, 21]. Many mutations may not fall along classic predicted mutation class but may be better characterized according to theratype, based upon a predicted CFTR therapeutic response to CFTR modulator therapy [22].

CFTR mutation classes are characterized in Fig. 1.3 [5].

## Discovery of Mechanisms of Protein Misfolding and Mutational Defects

Once the mechanism of CFTR misfolding was elucidated, efforts by the CFF, CFF Therapeutics lab, CFTR Folding Consortium, and in partnership with biotech and academic labs promoted high-throughput screening of small-molecule correctors [23, 24]. Class II CFTR mutations such as deltaF508 which undergoes protein misfolding and premature degradation [22] are stabilized by CFTR modulators. CFTR as an ATP-binding cassette transporter (ABC transporter) consists of transmembrane domains (TMD 1 and 2), nucleoside-binding domains (NBD1 and 2), and a regulatory domain. The transmembrane domains contain 12 transmembrane helices (TH) spanning the membrane, each two helices forming intracellular hairpins connected to the nucleoside-binding domain, and extracellular transmembrane domain. Small-molecule correctors bind to the transmembrane domains at different transmembrane hairpin locations. ETI, elexacaftor/tezacaftor/ivacaftor, is composed of two correctors, VX-661 and VX-445, and the potentiator VX-770. Type 1 correctors include VX-809 and VX-661 which stabilize the TMD1/NBD1 conformation. Type II correctors are not commercially approved but stabilize NBD2. Lastly, type III correctors include VX-445 connects at transmembrane helix 10-11 (TH10-11) and lasso motif, Fig. 1.4, showing chemical structures of CFTR modulators, and location of binding sites for VX-770, VX-661, and VX-445 [22].

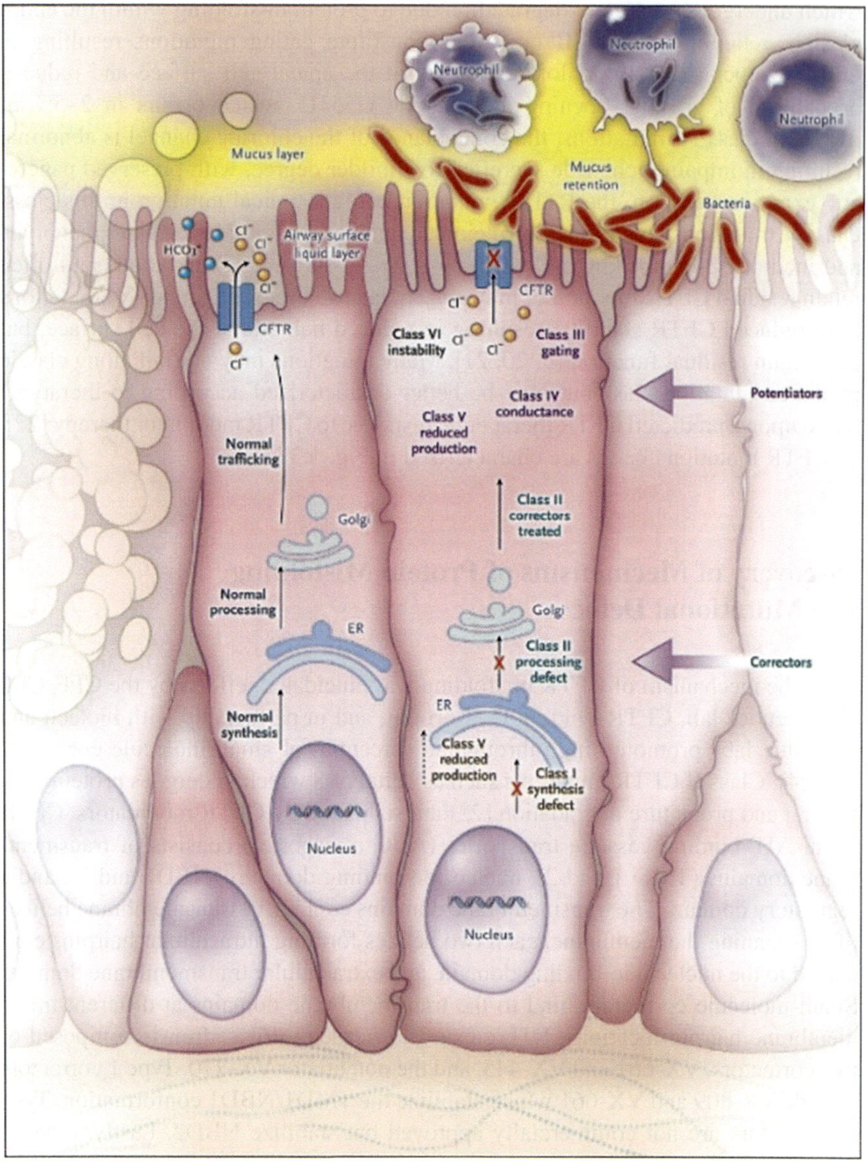


**Fig. 1.3** CFTR mutation classes [5]

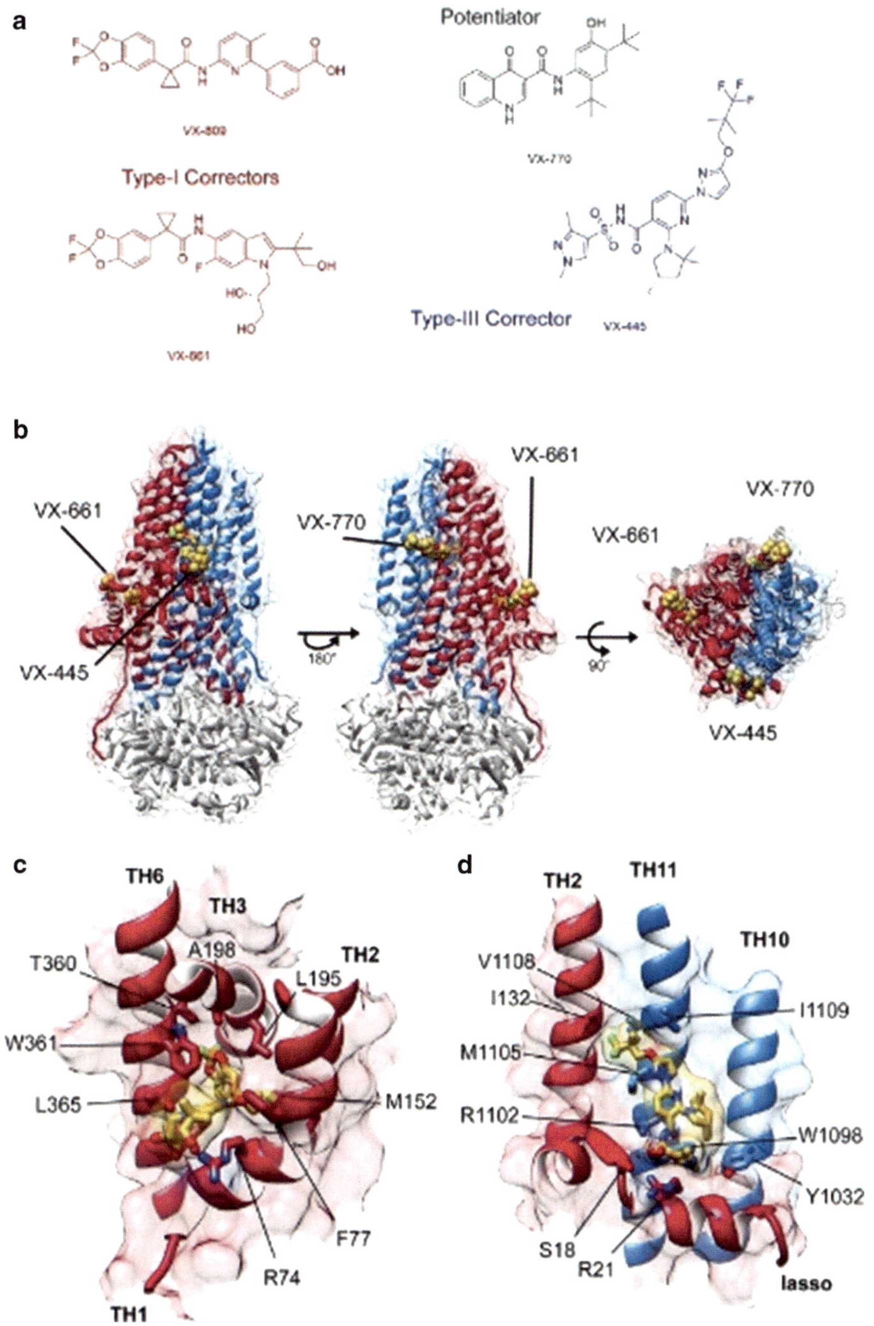


**Fig. 1.4** Chemical structure and binding sites of CFTR modulators [22]

## Toward Mutation-Specific Therapies: Clinical Development of CFTR Modulators: Ivacaftor, Lumicaftor, Tezacaftor, and Elexacaftor

Once the folded structure of the CFTR protein was elucidated and small-corrector molecules screened by high-throughput screening, multiple candidate potentiators and correctors were identified. Potentiators function to open the chloride channel gate, while correctors work to improve intracellular protein folding and trafficking. The first target was improving gating function present in class III CFTR mutation, G551D. Ivacaftor, or VX-770, was developed in 2012, and functions as a potentiator, increasing the probability of channel opening at the apical epithelial cell surface [25]. Clinical trials began in 2010, initially included approval for G551D in 2012, and subsequently approved for additional gating mutations, G1244E, G1349D, G178R, G551S, S1251N, S1255P, S549N, and S549R, in 2014. Outcome measures demonstrated a decrease in nasal potential difference and sweat chloride ~59 mmol per liter and improved FEV 1 ~ 8.7% above baseline. A randomized double blind clinical trial led by Ramsey and colleagues of VX-770 over 48 weeks, published in 2011, confirmed improvement of FEV 1 by 10.6%, decrease in pulmonary exacerbations by 55%, improved respiratory scores, decrease in sweat chloride by ~55 mmol per liter, and weight gain of 2.7 kg [26–31]. Follow-up over 5 years of pwCF treated with ivacaftor in US and UK registries demonstrated preserved lung function with a drop of only 0.7% in contrast to matched controls who experienced a drop of 8.3%, average BMI improved by 2.4 kg/m2 in the those on ivacaftor compared to 1.6 kg/m2 in matched controls, frequency of having >1 CF exacerbation decreased from 37.5% to 25.7%, but rose in the matched control group from 33.1% to 44.0%, CFRD was lower in the ivacaftor cohort, and lastly, pseudomonas colonization decreased in the ivacaftor group [32]. Similar real-world outcomes were shown in pwCF on ivacaftor from the CF Registry in Ireland, in terms of improved FEV 1, weight gain, decrease in need for IV, and oral antibiotic therapy [33]. Despite studies proving that ivacaftor was a highly effective modulator (HEMT) for gating mutations, additional efforts to rescue misfolded CFTR protein in the endoplasmic reticulum were needed to treat the 85% of pwCF harboring a deltaF508 mutation. Eventually, the concept of combining potentiators and correctors to work in tandem developed, originally studied in vitro [34, 35]. Optimally, in order to correct deltaF508, stabilizing both NBDs as elucidated from structural studies would prove most effective [36–38]. The first trials using both potentiator and corrector involved two phase 3 trials of the lumacaftor–ivacaftor (VX-809-VX-770) combination in deltaF508 homozygotes (TRAFFIC, TRANSPORT) [39, 40]. The study found improvement in FEV 1 of 2.6 to 4.0% in the lumacaftor-ivacaftor group, and a reduction in rate of pulmonary exacerbations by 30–39%, resulting in a lower rate of need for IV antibiotics. Adverse events more commonly in the lumacaftor-ivacaftor group included dyspnea and chest tightness, rash, and elevation of CPK, AST, and ALT levels. The next corrector, tezacaftor, VX-661, was combined with ivacaftor in the EVOLVE study, which examined tezacaftor-ivacaftor in deltaF508 homozygotes. In the tezacaftor-ivacaftor study group, the absolute and relative improvements in FEV 1 were 4% and 6%, respectively, compared to placebo. Those who received tezacaftor-ivacaftor experienced a 35% reduction in exacerbations and had similar adverse events between the study groups. Overall, those treated with tezacaftor-ivacaftor had fewer respiratory adverse events compared to the lumacaftor-ivacaftor groups. The EXPAND study was then performed in pwCF with deltaF508 and residual function mutations such as 2789 + 5G → A, 3849 + 10kbC → T, 3272-26A → G, and 711 + 3A → G, and missense mutations including most commonly P67L, L206W, R347H, A455E, D1152H, and S945L. In the tezacaftor-ivacaftor group, FEV 1 improved 6.8%, and respiratory measures improved [41–43]. Taken together, these pivotal trials proved that directed small-molecule correctors had the potential to stabilize CFTR and improve clinical outcomes, albeit with modest improvements in FEV 1 for deltaF508 homozygotes, and a low level of drug discontinuation for adverse events. However, pwCF harboring deltaF508 and minimal function mutations as well as pwCF with progressive lung disease did not see any benefit nor stabilization of lung function [44].

Major advancement of modulator therapy occurred with the addition of elexacaftor, a next-generation corrector, to the tezacaftor-ivacaftor combination, termed ETI. Elexacaftor qualifies as a type III corrector, due to beneficial effects with type 1 (NBD1:TMD1/2) and type II (NBD2) correctors on CFTR processing defects [45, 46]. The pivotal clinical trials of ETI in pwCF who were deltaFF508 homozygotes or deltaF508 and a minimal function mutation offered dramatic improvements in FEV1 of 10% and 13.8% at 4 weeks, respectively [47, 48]. DeltaF508 homozygotes experienced a drop in sweat chloride of 45.1 mmol/Lit and improved CFQ-R RD score. pwCF with a deltaF508 and minimal function mutations experienced 63% fewer exacerbations, improved patient reported respiratory symptoms score, and a decline in sweat chloride by 41.8 mmol/Lit (Fig. 1.5) [47, 48]. Subsequently, pwCF with deltaF508 and a gating or residual function mutation received approval for ETI.

Open-label extension and post-approval real-world studies confirmed ETI benefit [49–51], as well as ETI benefit for CF advanced lung disease and those listed for lung transplant [52]. ETI delayed the need for lung transplant and improved survival, and in the study by Martin and colleagues, 61/65 CF patients originally undergoing listing for lung transplant no longer needed lung transplant. Need for IV antibiotic therapy declined by 86%, oxygen use by 59%, and noninvasive ventilation by 62% [53]. This substantial improvement in survival for those with advanced CF lung disease is reflected in the CF Registry database; 61 registry participants were reported as receiving a lung transplant in 2023, compared with ~250 performed in 2019, prior to widespread availability of ETI [6]. As clinical trials for lumacaftor-ivacaftor, tezacaftor-ivacaftor, and ETI were initially trialed in the >12-year-old population initially, studies examined the pediatric population, finding similar benefits, and currently ETI is approved for all pwCF >2 years of age [54, 55].

Recently, a phase 2 clinical trial of a once-a-day CFTR modulator, vanzacaftor-tezacaftor-deuticaftor, demonstrated equal to slightly better clinical effectiveness than ETI on the basis of changes in FEV 1, CF respiratory symptom scores, and sweat chloride reduction [56]. Subsequently, two randomized, double-blind,

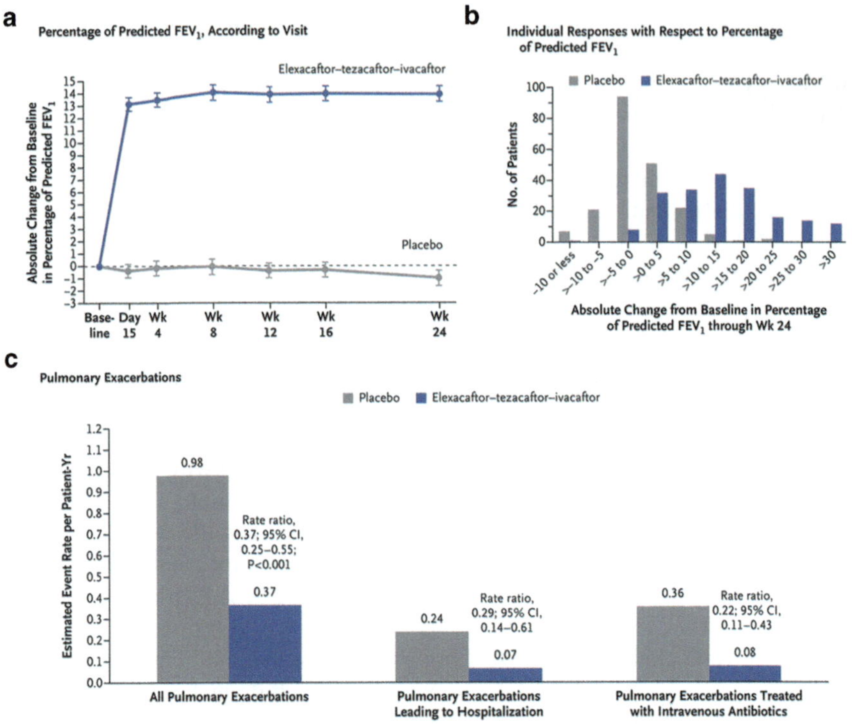


**Fig. 1.5** Improvement in FEV 1 and reduction in pulmonary exacerbations in deltaF508/minimal function CFTR mutation [48]

active-controlled, 52-week phase 3 trials for this triple combination, SKYLINE 102 and 103, reported positive results in early 2024, noting a significant reduction in sweat chloride compared to ETI. Toward the end of 2024, the vanzacaftor-tezacaftor-deuticaftor triple combination was approved by the FDA for pwCF aged 6 years and older with at least one *F508del* mutation or another responsive mutation in the CFTR gene.

Clinical trials of CFTR modulators provided the proof and basis for widespread FDA approval in pwCF and also initiated a new paradigm for subsequent CFTR mutation FDA approvals for modulators through in vitro testing. Starting with FDA approval of an additional 23 CFTR mutations for ivacaftor in 2017, the term theratyping may apply to predictions of how CF cells transfected with CFTR mutations respond to CFTR modulators in vitro [57]. Bihler and colleagues evaluated 655 CFTR variants using transfected Fisher rat thyroid cells, finding clinical responsiveness to ETI in 292 previously unapproved variants with minimal to low-level baseline CFTR function [58]. These results may ultimately provide evidence for FDA approval for these rare variants.

## Models of Precision Medicine

The understanding the CFTR protein structure as a chloride and bicarbonate anion channel at the apical membrane of epithelial tissues led to the development of small-molecule correctors able to bind to the protein and stabilize processing, ultimately tested in clinical trials for proof of efficacy. Understanding a monogenic disease like CF with variable phenotype-genotype manifestations, related in part to underlying genotype but also subject to gene modifiers and environmental factors, yields variable predictions about disease-causing CFTR mutations. Up to 2000 CFTR variants exist, thus, approximately ~10–12% of pwCF in the USA are not eligible for CFTR modulator therapy. Identifying personalized therapy for each and every variant may require individual theratyping or testing of patient-derived cells for response to modulators and other CF therapies.

Patient-derived samples for in vitro modeling may include primary nasal, bronchial epithelial, intestinal/rectal organoid structures, and induced pluripotent (iPSC) stem cells. Human nasal epithelial cells (HNE) derived from patient nasal brushings, differentiated to air-liquid-interface (ALI) cell monolayers in vitro, demonstrate CFTR modulator drug testing responsiveness and can form structural organoids for testing of CFTR activity [59–63]. Human bronchial epithelial cells (HBE) from pwCF most often derived from explanted donor lungs or a bronchial brush under bronchoscopy and grown at ALI demonstrate properties of CFTR channel activity and have been used to test CFTR modulator responsiveness [25, 34, 64]. Functional assays which may be used on HNE and HBE cultures include testing channel conductance, Ussing chambers, and evaluation of mucociliary clearance. These models may be limited for large-scale testing of cultures, as well as difficulty obtaining cells from rare variants [65, 66].

Intestinal organoids may develop 3D structures amenable to testing of CFTR functionality. Self-renewing stem cells within intestinal and rectal crypt cells positioned with apical direction toward a centered lumen with the basal layer situated within a matrix compound may mimic CFTR activity. Lumenal size may grow with stimulants of CFTR activity such as forskolin, which activates adenyl cyclase and increases intracellular concentration of cAMP; drives chloride secretion, resulting in organoid swelling; and serves as a biomarker of CFTR activity [67–69]. Patient-derived intestinal tissue can thus be studied to test CFTR modulator effects as well and can track with clinical outcome measures such as FEV 1 and sweat chloride [67–71]. Figure 1.6 highlights the schematics of these culture systems to study individual CFTR variants.

These models for translational determination of CFTR functionality are increasingly becoming standard tools in the diagnosis of CF and prediction of clinical phenotype. Recent multicenter validation of the forskolin-induced welling assay (FIS) was undertaken demonstrating excellent reproducibility and repeatability across four European centers, thus standardizing the technique for testing rare CF patient variants and advancing precision medicine for pwCF [72]. Similarly, the application of HNE culture systems for testing sweat chloride changes and CFTR

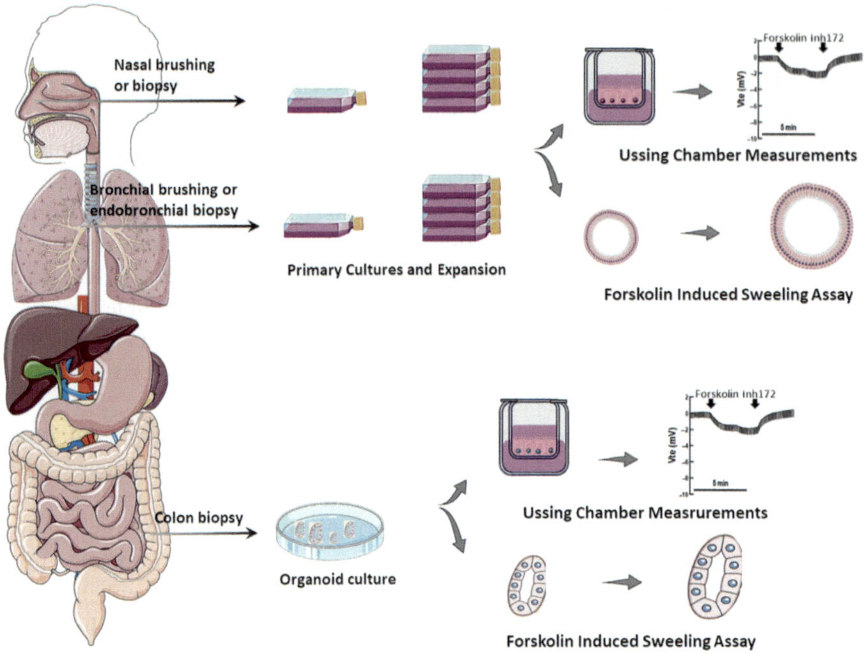


**Fig. 1.6** Models to study CFTR function in patient-derived tissue [66]

responsiveness to modulators can guide precision therapeutics, aid in diagnosis of mild CF, characterize CFTR function in rare spice mutations, and function as a tool for clinical CF diagnosis [73].

Lastly, although still at a preclinical level, induced pluripotent stem cells may recapitulate lung, intestine, and ductal structures are amenable to bioelectric and functional assays, and offer scalable models for high-throughput testing. iPSCs are programmed from somatic cells such as fibroblasts, by genes which direct their terminal differentiation, including c-Myc, Oct4, Sox2, and Kfl4. CFTR modulators have successfully corrected iPSC-derived airway cells expressing deltaF508, nonsense mutations such as W1282X, and splicing mutations [74–77].

## Future Therapies: Gene Addition, RNA, Antisense Oligonucleotides, Gene Editing

The progress in elucidating the structure of CFTR, development of correctors, and potentiators based upon knowledge of CFTR protein binding, genotype-phenotype characteristics of a multitude of CF variants, and availability of research tools for clinical diagnosis and evaluation of therapeutics has advanced precision medicine in pwCF. However, approximately 10–15% of pwCF are ineligible or intolerant of

CFTR modulator therapy. Emerging genetic therapies on the horizon include gene addition through viral and nonviral delivery systems, RNA-based strategies, antisense oligonucleotides, and gene editing including cell-based approaches using iPSCs with gene editing. Mutation agnostic therapies include gene addition and mRNA therapies, while mutation-specific include antisense oligonucleotides, gene editing, and cell based. Lastly, read-through agents and tRNA therapies may address nonsense mutations [78].

Gene addition may involve a viral vector delivery system, with low integration within the genome such as adeno-associated virus (AAV), or integration within the genome such as with lentivirus. Adeno-associated virus and lentivirus delivery systems are integrated into dividing and non-diving cells and exhibit moderate to high level of expression and low degrees of immunogenicity. Adenoviral vectors were initially trialed due to natural attachment to airway epithelium; however, early trials were limited by inflammation and lack of sustained expression. These barriers have been better optimized with adeno-associated viral vectors, although packaging of genetic material is limited, and some immune responses persist. Overall, AAVs carry a favorable risk-benefit profile and carry minimal risk for oncogenic potential due to low genome integration. A current phase I/II trial, 4D-710, uses an AAV vector in adults with CF who are ineligible for, or unable to tolerate, CFTR modulator therapy (NCT05248230) [79–81]. Lentiviral vectors used for gene delivery have been trialed in nonhuman primates with CFTR transgene detected. Lentiviral vectors are integrated into the genome, offering prolonged expression after single dosing; can carry the full-length CFTR; have minimal inflammatory side effects; but raise the unpredictable possibility of mutagenesis. Further techniques to reduce oncogenesis related to lentiviruses include self-inactivating vectors lacking the transcriptionally active long terminal repeat elements [82]. Lastly, HSV viral vectors are similar to AAV, in that they are not integrated into the genome, have low inflammatory profile, and a larger packaging capability. A phase II/IIa clinical trial KB407 using an HSV-1 viral vector is currently in clinical trials [83]. Figure 1.7 highlights approaches for CFTR gene addition [84].

Nonviral vectors are not integrated into the genome, can carry full-length DNA or mRNA CFTR, have minimal oncogenic potential, and carry low risk for inflammatory effects. Mechanisms of delivery include liposomes, lipid nanoparticles, extracellular vesicles, and polymeric nanoparticles. The first major trial performed in the UK was a phase 2b trial of nebulized pGM169/GL67A gene-liposome complex monthly vs. placebo, which proved to stabilize lung function compared to placebo [85]. Currently three clinical trials are underway, RCT2100 (NCT06237335), ARCT-032 (NCT06747858), and VX-522 (NCT05668741), delivering mRNA via repeated inhaled nebulized therapies. BEACON-CF, or VX-522, is a phase 1/II study in pwCF who is not responsive to CFTR modulator therapy. It delivers an inhaled messenger RNA (mRNA) therapy using a lipid nanoparticle. The 28-week, single-ascending dose portion was completed, and the 12-week multiple-ascending dosing phase is underway [86–89].

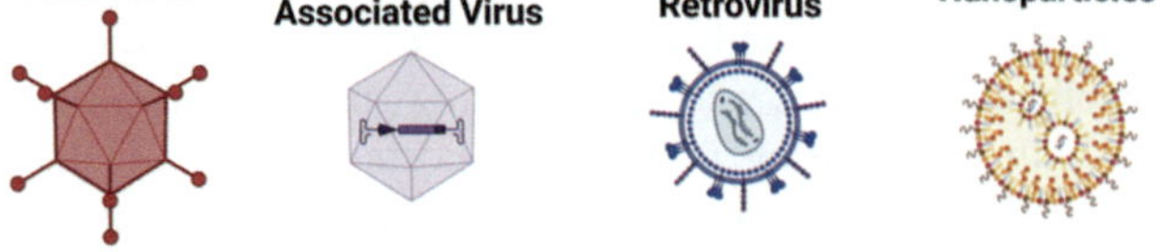

| | Adenovirus | Adeno Associated Virus | Lentivirus & Retrovirus | Nanoparticles |
|---|---|---|---|---|
| ① Expression & Genomic integration | High level<br>Long-term expression<br>Transient expression<br>No genomic integration | Moderate level<br>Long-term expression<br>Transient expression<br>No genomic integration | High level<br>Long-term expression<br>Stable gene expression<br>Genomic integration | High level<br>Short-term expression<br>Transient expression<br>No genomic integration |
| ② Transduction & Packaging capacity | Dividing and non-dividing cells<br>4-5 kb | Dividing and non-dividing cells<br>5kb | Dividing cells (Retrovirus)<br>Dividing and non-dividing cells (Lentivirus)<br>8kb | Dividing and non-dividing cells<br>> 10 kb |
| ③ Immunogenicity | High Immunogenicity | Moderate Immunogenicity | Moderate Immunogenicity | Low Immunogenicity |
| Clinical trial | Yes | Yes | No | Yes |

**Fig. 1.7** Approaches to CFTR gene addition [84]

Antisense oligonucleotides (ASO) and gene editing offer mutation-specific precision therapy for CF. The ASOs consist of customized single-stranded nucleotides designed to bind to mutant CFTR mRNA and to correct mRNA, forwarding read-through of mRNA, or repairing splice mutations or [90]. A phase I study of SPL84 containing an ASO for pwCF with at least one 3849 + 10kbC → T mutation was completed [91] with phase II in process. Gene editing uses the principle of DNA repair to respond to a break in the DNA induced by CRISPR (clustered regularly interspaced short palindromic repeats), Cas (CRISPR-associated proteins), and non-CRISPR techniques, at a desired site of a CFTR mutation. CRISPR/Cas9 functions through RNA directed at DNA sequences, which are subsequently cleaved by Cas9 endonuclease. Although still in preclinical development, CRSIPR/Cas9 has been used to correct CFTR in deltaF508 intestinal organoids [92], deltaF508 iPSCs which when corrected demonstrated chloride transport [93], and variants with premature stop codons [94]. As a technique to correct all CFTR mutations, CRSPR/Cas9 has been used to insert full-length CFTR into airway stem cells [95]. Non-CRISPR approaches include zinc finger nuclease-(ZFN-) and transcription activator-like effector nuclease- (TALEN-), optimized to work with AAV delivery systems. The latest technique involves peptide nucleic acid (PNA) gene editing which can be delivered using polymer nanoparticles [96, 97].

Current treatment for CF has evolved to a highly personalized approach, originating from the initial timeline of CFTR protein characterization, subsequent methodical development of small molecule correctors, and current comprehensive clinical trials proving significant benefit of CFTR modulators. Yet greater than 2000 CF variants are known, and many remain difficult to characterize genotype-phenotype connections. Treatment remains elusive for some pwCF, including those ineligible and intolerant of CFTR modulators, as well as those with preexisting advanced lung disease. Approaches to achieve precision medicine for all will include strategies aimed at better characterization of individual variants to predict clinical response to medication, mutation agnostic and mutation-specific approaches, gene editing, and cell-based therapies [65, 78, 97–99].

## References


1. Andersen DH. Cystic fibrosis of the pancreas and its relation to celiac disease – a clinical and pathological study. Am J Dis Child. 1938;56:344–99.
2. Stephenson AL, Swaleh S, Sykes J, et al. Contemporary cystic fibrosis incidence rates in Canada and the United States. J Cyst Fibros. 2023;22:443–9. https://doi.org/10.1016/j.jcf.2022.10.008. Epub 2022 Nov 10
3. Guo J, Garratt A, Hill A. Worldwide rates of diagnosis and effective treatment for cystic fibrosis. J Cyst Fibros. 2022;21(3):456–62. https://doi.org/10.1016/j.jcf.2022.01.009. Epub 2022 Feb 4
4. Guo J, King I, Hill A. International disparities in diagnosis and treatment access for cystic fibrosis. Pediatr Pulmonol. 2024;59(6):1622–30. https://doi.org/10.1002/ppul.26954. Epub 2024 Apr 1
5. Grasemann H, Ratjen F. Cystic fibrosis. N Engl J Med. 2023;389(18):1693–707. https://doi.org/10.1056/NEJMra2216474.
6. Cromwell EA, Ostrenga JS, Todd JV, Elbert A, Brown AW, Faro A, Goss CH, Marshall BC. Cystic fibrosis prevalence in the United States and participation in the Cystic Fibrosis Foundation Patient Registry in 2020. J Cyst Fibros. 2023;22(3):436–42.
7. di Sant'Agnese PA, et al. Abnormal electrolyte composition of sweat in cystic fibrosis of the pancreas; clinical significance and relationship to the disease. Pediatrics. 1953;12(5):549–63.
8. Riordan JR, Rommens JM, Kerem BS, et al. Identification of the cystic fibrosis gene: cloning and characterization of complementary DNA. Science. 1989;245(4922):1066–73.
9. Liou TG. The clinical biology of cystic fibrosis transmembrane regulator protein. Its role and function in extrapulmonary disease. Chest. 2019;155(3):605–16. https://doi.org/10.1016/j.chest.2018.10.006. Epub 2018 Oct
10. Stutts MJ, Canessa CM, Olsen JC, et al. CFTR as a cAMP-dependent regulator of sodium channels. Science. 1995;269(5225):847–50.
11. Mall MA. Role of the amiloride-sensitive epithelial Na+ channel in the pathogenesis and as a therapeutic target for cystic fibrosis lung disease. Exp Physiol. 2009;94(2):171–4.
12. Shteinberg M, Haq IJ, Polineni D, Davies JC. Cystic fibrosis. Lancet. 2021;397(10290):2195–211. https://doi.org/10.1016/S0140-6736(20)32542-3.
13. Mall MA, Burgel PR, Castellani C, et al. Cystic fibrosis. Nat Rev Dis Primers. 2024;10(1):53. https://doi.org/10.1038/s41572-024-00538-6.
14. Zhang Z, Liu F, Chen J. Conformational changes of CFTR upon phosphorylation and ATP binding. Cell. 2017;170(3):483–491.e8. https://doi.org/10.1016/j.cell.2017.06.041. Epub 2017 Jul 20
15. Sheppard DN, Welsh MJ. Structure and function of the CFTR chloride channel. Physiol Rev. 1999;79(1 Suppl):S23–45. https://doi.org/10.1152/physrev.1999.79.1.S23.
16. Lopes-Pacheco M. CFTR modulators: the changing face of cystic fibrosis in the era of precision medicine. Front Pharmacol. 2020;10:1662. https://doi.org/10.3389/fphar.2019.01662. eCollection 2019
17. Morris-Rosendahl DJ, Edwards M, et al. Whole-gene sequencing of CFTR reveals a high prevalence of the Intronic Variant c.3874-4522A>G in cystic fibrosis. Am J Respir Crit Care Med. 2020;201(11):1438–41. https://doi.org/10.1164/rccm.201908-1541LE.

18. Michels M, Matte U, Fraga LR, et al. Determining the pathogenicity of *CFTR* missense variants: multiple comparisons of *in silico* predictors and variant annotation databases. Genet Mol Biol. 2019;42(3):560–70. https://doi.org/10.1590/1678-4685-GMB-2018-0148. Epub 2019 Nov 14
19. McDonald E, Oliver KE, Schlebach JP, et al. Benchmarking AlphaMissense pathogenicity predictions against cystic fibrosis variants. PLoS One. 2024;19(1) https://doi.org/10.1371/journal.pone.0297560.
20. Marson FAL, Bertuzzo CS, Ribeiro JD. Classification of CFTR mutation classes. Lancet Respir Med. 2016;4(8):e37–8. https://doi.org/10.1016/S2213-2600(16)30188-6. Epub 2016 Jul 1
21. Mall MA, Mayer-Hamblett N, Rowe SM. Cystic fibrosis: emergence of highly effective targeted therapeutics and potential clinical implications. Am J Respir Crit Care Med. 2020;201(10):1193–208. https://doi.org/10.1164/rccm.201910-1943SO.
22. McDonald EF, Meiler J, Plate L. CFTR folding: from structure and proteostasis to cystic fibrosis personalized medicine. ACS Chem Biol. 2023;18(10):2128–43. https://doi.org/10.1021/acschembio.3c00310. Epub 2023 Sep 20
23. Pedemonte N, Lukacs GL, Du K, et al. Small-molecule correctors of defective ΔF508-CFTR cellular processing identified by high-throughput screening. J Clin Invest. 2005;115(9):2564–71. https://doi.org/10.1172/JCI24898. Epub 2005 Aug 25
24. Peters KW, Okiyoneda T, Balch WE, et al. CFTR folding consortium: methods available for studies of CFTR folding and correction. Methods Mol Biol. 2011;742:335–53. https://doi.org/10.1007/978-1-61779-120-8_20.
25. Van Goor F, Hadida S, Grootenhuis PD, et al. Rescue of CF airway epithelial cell function in vitro by a CFTR potentiator, VX-770. Proc Natl Acad Sci USA. 2009;106(44):18825–30. https://doi.org/10.1073/pnas.0904709106. Epub 2009 Oct 21
26. Accurso FJ, Rowe SM, Clancy JP, et al. Effect of VX-770 in persons with cystic fibrosis and the G551D-CFTR mutation. N Engl J Med. 2010;363(21):1991–2003. https://doi.org/10.1056/NEJMoa0909825.
27. Ramsey BW, Davies J, McElvaney NG, et al. A CFTR potentiator in patients with cystic fibrosis and the G551D mutation. N Engl J Med. 2011;365(18):1663–72. https://doi.org/10.1056/NEJMoa1105185.
28. Rowe SM, Heltshe SL, Gonska T, et al. GOAL investigators of the cystic fibrosis foundation therapeutics development network. Clinical mechanism of the cystic fibrosis transmembrane conductance regulator potentiator ivacaftor in G551D-mediated cystic fibrosis. Am J Respir Crit Care Med. 2014;190(02):175–84. https://doi.org/10.1164/rccm.201404-0703OC.
29. Davies JC, Wainwright CE, Canny GJ, et al. Efficacy and safety of ivacaftor in patients aged 6 to 11 years with cystic fibrosis with a G551D mutation. Am J Respir Crit Care Med. 2013;187(11):1219–25. https://doi.org/10.1164/rccm.201301-0153OC.
30. De Boeck K, Munck A, Walker S, et al. Efficacy and safety of ivacaftor in patients with cystic fibrosis and a non-G551D gating mutation. J Cyst Fibros. 2014;13(06):674–80. https://doi.org/10.1016/j.jcf.2014.09.005. Epub 2014 Sep 26
31. Moss RB, Flume PA, Elborn JS, et al. Efficacy and safety of ivacaftor in patients with cystic fibrosis who have an Arg117His-CFTR mutation: a doubleblind, randomised controlled trial. Lancet Respir Med. 2015;3(07):524–33. https://doi.org/10.1016/S2213-2600(15)00201-5. Epub 2015 Jun 9
32. Volkova N, Moy K, Evans J. Disease progression in patients with cystic fibrosis treated with ivacaftor: Data from national US and UK registries. J Cyst Fibros. 2020;19(1):68–79. https://doi.org/10.1016/j.jcf.2019.05.015.
33. Kirwan L, Fletcher G, Harrington M, et al. Longitudinal trends in real-world outcomes after initiation of ivacaftor. A cohort study from the cystic fibrosis registry of Ireland. Ann Am Thorac Soc. 2019;16(02):209–16. https://doi.org/10.1513/AnnalsATS.201802-149OC.
34. Van Goor F, Hadida S, Grootenhuis PD, et al. Correction of the F508del-CFTR protein processing defect in vitro by the investigational drug VX-809. Proc Natl Acad Sci USA. 2011;108:18843–8. https://doi.org/10.1073/pnas.1105787108. Epub 2011 Oct 5

35. Kopeikin Z, Yuksek Z, Yang HY, et al. Combined effects of VX-770 and VX-809 on several functional abnormalities of F508del-CFTR channels. J Cyst Fibros. 2014;13:508–14. https://doi.org/10.1016/j.jcf.2014.04.003. Epub 2014 May 3
36. Rabeh WM, Bossard F, Xu H, et al. Correction of both NBD1 energetics and domain interface is required to restore DF508 CFTR folding and function. Cell. 2012;148:150–63. https://doi.org/10.1016/j.cell.2011.11.024.
37. Mendoza JL, Schmidt A, Li Q, et al. Requirements for efficient correction of DF508 CFTR revealed by analyses of evolved sequences. Cell. 2012;148:164–74. https://doi.org/10.1016/j.cell.2011.11.023.
38. Okiyoneda T, Veit G, Dekkers JF, et al. Mechanism-based corrector combination restores ΔF508-CFTR folding and function. Nat Chem Biol. 2013;9(7):444–54. https://doi.org/10.1038/nchembio.1253. Epub 2013 May 12
39. Wainwright CE, Elborn JS, Ramsey BW. Lumacaftor-ivacaftor in patients with cystic fibrosis homozygous for Phe508del CFTR. N Engl J Med. 2015;373:1783–4. https://doi.org/10.1056/NEJMc1510466.
40. Hubert D, Chiron R, Camara B, et al. Real-life initiation of lumacaftor/ivacaftor combination in adults with cystic fibrosis homozygous for the Phe508del *CFTR* mutation and severe lung disease. J Cyst Fibros. 2017;16:388–91. https://doi.org/10.1016/j.jcf.2017.03.003. Epub 2017 Mar 18
41. Taylor-Cousar JL, Munck A, McKone EF, et al. Tezacaftor–ivacaftor in patients with cystic fibrosis homozygous for Phe508del. N Engl J Med. 2017;377:2013–23. https://doi.org/10.1056/NEJMoa1709846. Epub 2017 Nov 3
42. Rowe SM, Daines C, Ringshausen FC, et al. Tezacaftor–ivacaftor in residual-function heterozygotes with cystic fibrosis. N Engl J Med. 2017;377:2024–35. https://doi.org/10.1056/NEJMoa1709847. Epub 2017 Nov 3
43. Donaldson SH, Pilewski JM, Griese M, et al. Tezacaftor/ivacaftor in subjects with cystic fibrosis and F508del/F508del-CFTR or F508del/F508del-CFTR. Am J Respir Crit Care Med. 2018;197:214–24. https://doi.org/10.1164/rccm.201704-0717OC.
44. Munck A, Kerem E, Ellemunter H, et al. Tezacaftor/ivacaftor in people with cystic fibrosis heterozygous for minimal function CFTR mutations. J Cyst Fibros. 2020;19(06):962–8. https://doi.org/10.1016/j.jcf.2020.04.015. Epub 2020 Jun 13
45. Veit G, Roldan A, Hancock MA, et al. Allosteric folding correction of F508del and rare CFTR mutants by elexacaftor-tezacaftor-ivacaftor (Trikafta) combination. JCI Insight. 2020;5(18):e139983. https://doi.org/10.1172/jci.insight.139983.
46. Keating D, Marigowda G, Burr L, et al. VX-445-tezacaftorivacaftor in patients with cystic fibrosis and one or two Phe508del alleles. N Engl J Med. 2018;379:1612–20. https://doi.org/10.1056/NEJMoa1807120. Epub 2018 Oct 18
47. Heijerman HGM, McKone EF, Downey DG, et al. Efficacy and safety of the elexacaftor plus tezacaftor plus ivacaftor combination regimen in people with cystic fibrosis homozygous for the F508del mutation: a double-blind, randomised, phase 3 trial. Lancet. 2019;394(10212):1940–8. https://doi.org/10.1016/S0140-6736(19)32597-8. Epub 2019 Oct 31
48. Middleton PG, Mall MA, Dřevínek P, et al. Elexacaftor–Tezacaftor–Ivacaftor for cystic fibrosis with a single Phe508del Allele. N Engl J Med. 2019;381:1809–19. https://doi.org/10.1056/NEJMoa1908639. Epub 2019 Oct 31
49. Griese M, Costa S, Linnemann RW, et al. Safety and efficacy of elexacaftor/tezacaftor/ivacaftor for 24 weeks or longer in people with cystic fibrosis and one or more F508del alleles: interim results of an open-label phase 3 clinical trial. Am J Respir Crit Care Med. 2021;203(03):381–5. https://doi.org/10.1164/rccm.202008-3176LE.
50. Sutharsan S, McKone EF, Downey DG, et al. VX18-445-109 study group. Efficacy and safety of elexacaftor plus tezacaftor plus ivacaftor versus tezacaftor plus ivacaftor in people with cystic fibrosis homozygous for F508del-CFTR: a 24-week, multicentre, randomised, double-blind, active-controlled, phase 3b trial. Lancet Respir Med. 2022;10(03):267–77. https://doi.org/10.1016/S2213-2600(21)00454-9. Epub 2021 Dec 20

51. Nichols DP, Paynter AC, Heltshe SL, et al. PROMISE Study group. Clinical effectiveness of elexacaftor/tezacaftor/ivacaftor in people with cystic fibrosis: a clinical trial. Am J Respir Crit Care Med. 2022;205(05):529–39. https://doi.org/10.1164/rccm.202108-1986OC.
52. Burgel PR, Durieu I, Chiron R, et al. Rapid improvement after starting elexacaftor-tezacaftor-ivacaftor in patients with cystic fibrosis and advanced pulmonary disease. Am J Respir Crit Care Med. 2021;204(01):64–73. https://doi.org/10.1164/rccm.202011-4153OC.
53. Martin C, Reynaud-Gaubert M, Hamidfar R, et al. Sustained effectiveness of elexacaftor-tezacaftor-ivacaftor in lung transplant candidates with cystic fibrosis. J Cyst Fibros. 2022;21(03):489–96. https://doi.org/10.1016/j.jcf.2022.01.012. Epub 2022 Feb 2
54. Regard L, Martin C, Da Silva J, et al. CFTR modulators: current status and evolving knowledge. Semin Respir Crit Care Med. 2023;44(2):186–95. https://doi.org/10.1055/s-0042-1758851. Epub 2022 Dec 19
55. Taylor-Cousar JL, Robinson PD, Shteinberg M, et al. CFTR modulator therapy: transforming the landscape of clinical care in cystic fibrosis. Lancet. 2023;402(10408):1171–84. https://doi.org/10.1016/S0140-6736(23)01609-4. Epub 2023 Sep 9
56. Uluer AZ, MacGregor G, Azevedo P, et al. Safety and efficacy of vanzacaftor-tezacaftor-deutivacaftor in adults with cystic fibrosis: randomised, double-blind, controlled, phase 2 trials. Lancet Respir Med. 2023;11(6):550–62. https://doi.org/10.1016/S2213-2600(22)00504-5. Epub 2023 Feb 23
57. Ratner M. FDA deems in vitro data on mutations sufficient to expand cystic fibrosis drug label. Nat Biotechnol. 2017;35(7):606. https://doi.org/10.1038/nbt0717-606.
58. Bihler H, Sivachenko A, Millen L, et al. In vitro modulator responsiveness of 655 CFTR variants found in people with cystic fibrosis. J Cyst Fibros. 2024;23(4):664–75. https://doi.org/10.1016/j.jcf.2024.02.006. Epub 2024 Feb 22
59. Pranke IM, Hatton A, Simonin J, et al. Correction of CFTR function in nasal epithelial cells from cystic fibrosis patients predicts improvement of respiratory function by CFTR modulators. Sci Rep. 2017;7(1):7375. https://doi.org/10.1038/s41598-017-07504-1.
60. Brewington JJ, Filbrandt ET, LaRosa FJ, et al. Brushed nasal epithelial cells are a surrogate for bronchial epithelial CFTR studies. JCI Insight. 2018;3(13):e99385. https://doi.org/10.1172/jci.insight.99385.
61. Pranke I, Hatton A, Masson A, et al. Might brushed nasal cells be a surrogate for CFTR modulator clinical response? Am J Respir Crit Care Med. 2019;199(1):123–6. https://doi.org/10.1164/rccm.201808-1436LE.
62. Liu Z, Anderson JD, Deng L, et al. Human nasal epithelial organoids for therapeutic development in cystic fibrosis. Genes (Basel). 2020;11(6) https://doi.org/10.3390/genes11060603.
63. Anderson JD, Liu Z, Odom LV, et al. CFTR function and clinical response to modulators parallel nasal epithelial organoid swelling. Am J Physiol Lung Cell Mol Physiol. 2021;321(1):L119–L29. https://doi.org/10.1152/ajplung.00639.2020. Epub 2021 May 19
64. Randell SH, Fulcher ML, O'Neal W, et al. Primary epithelial cell models for cystic fibrosis research. Methods Mol Biol. 2011;742:285–310. https://doi.org/10.1007/978-1-61779-120-8_18.
65. Dumas MP, Xia S, Bear CE, et al. Perspectives on the translation of *in-vitro* studies to precision medicine in cystic fibrosis. EBioMedicine. 2021;73:103660. https://doi.org/10.1016/j.ebiom.2021.103660. Epub 2021 Oct 28
66. Bacalhau M, Camargo M, Lopes-Pacheco M. Laboratory tools to predict CFTR modulator therapy effectiveness and to monitor disease severity in cystic fibrosis. J Pers Med. 2024;14(1):93. https://doi.org/10.3390/jpm14010093.
67. Dekkers JF, Wiegerinck CL, de Jonge HR, et al. A functional CFTR assay using primary cystic fibrosis intestinal organoids. Nat Med. 2013;19(7):939–45. https://doi.org/10.1038/nm.3201. Epub 2013 Jun 2
68. de Winter-de Groot, K. M., Berkers, G., Marck-van der Wilt, R. E. et al. Forskolin-induced swelling of intestinal organoids correlates with disease severity in adults with cystic fibrosis and homozygous F508del mutations. J Cyst Fibros 2019. doi: https://doi.org/10.1016/j.jcf.2019.10.022. Epub 2019 Nov 15.

69. Dekkers R, Vijftigschild LA, Vonk AM, et al. A bioassay using intestinal organoids to measure CFTR modulators in human plasma. J Cyst Fibros. 2015;14(2):178–81. https://doi.org/10.1016/j.jcf.2014.10.007. Epub 2014 Nov 6
70. Oliver KE, Carlon MS, Pedemonte N, et al. The revolution of personalized pharmacotherapies for cystic fibrosis: what does the future hold? Expert Opin Pharmacother. 2023;24:1545–65. https://doi.org/10.1080/14656566.2023.2230129. Epub 2023 Jul 3
71. Clancy JP, Cotton CU, Donaldson SH, et al. CFTR modulator theratyping: current status, gaps and future directions. J Cyst Fibros. 2019;18:22–34. https://doi.org/10.1016/j.jcf.2018.05.004. Epub 2018 Jun 20
72. Bierlaagh MC, Ramalho AS, Silva IAL, et al. Repeatability and reproducibility of the Forskolin-induced swelling (FIS) assay on intestinal organoids from people with cystic fibrosis. J Cyst Fibros. 2024;23(4):693–702. https://doi.org/10.1016/j.jcf.2024.04.014. Epub 2024 May 14
73. Pion A, Kavanagh E, Joynt AT, et al. Investigation of CFTR function in human nasal epithelial cells informs personalized medicine. Am J Respir Cell Mol Biol. 2024;71(5):577–88. https://doi.org/10.1165/rcmb.2023-0398OC.
74. Wong AP, Bear CE, Chi S, et al. Directed differentiation of human pluripotent stem cells into mature airway epithelia expressing functional CFTR protein. Nat Biotechnol. 2012;30:876–82. https://doi.org/10.1038/nbt.2328.
75. Jiang JX, Wellhauser L, Laselva O, et al. A new platform for high-throughput therapy testing on iPSC-derived lung progenitor cells from cystic fibrosis patients. Stem Cell Rep. 2021;16:2825–37. https://doi.org/10.1016/j.stemcr.2021.09.020. Epub 2021 Oct 21
76. Berical A, Lee RE, Lu J, et al. A multimodal iPSC platform for cystic fibrosis drug testing. Nat Commun. 2022;13(1):4270. https://doi.org/10.1038/s41467-022-31854-8.
77. Silva IAL, Laselva O, Lopes-Pacheco M. Advances in preclinical in vitro models for the translation of precision medicine for cystic fibrosis. J Pers Med. 2022;12(8):1321. https://doi.org/10.3390/jpm12081321.
78. Egan ME. Non-modulator therapies: developing a therapy for every cystic fibrosis patient. Clin Chest Med. 2022;43(4):717–25.
79. McLachlan G, Alton E, Boyd AC, et al. Progress in respiratory gene therapy. Hum Gene Ther. 2022;33:893–912. https://doi.org/10.1089/hum.2022.172.
80. Taylor-Cousar JL, Boyd AC, Alton E, et al. Genetic therapies in cystic fibrosis. Curr Opin Pulm Med. 2023;29:615–20. https://doi.org/10.1097/MCP.0000000000001019. Epub 2023 Sep 12
81. ClinicalTrials.gov. 4D-710 in adult patients with cystic fibrosis (CF). 2022. Available from: https://classic.clinicaltrials.gov/ct2/show/NCT05248230
82. Davies JC, Polineni D, Boyd AC, et al. Lentiviral gene therapy for cystic fibrosis: a promising approach and first-in-human trial. Am J Respir Crit Care Med. 2024;210(12):1398–408. https://doi.org/10.1164/rccm.202402-0389CI.
83. ClinicalTrials.gov. A study assessing KB407 for the treatment of cystic fibrosis. 2022. Available from: https://classic.clinicaltrials.gov/ct2/show/NCT05504837
84. Bisserier M, Sun XQ, Fazal S, et al. Novel insights into the therapeutic potential of lung-targeted gene transfer in the most common respiratory diseases. Cells. 2022;11(6):984. https://doi.org/10.3390/cells11060984.
85. Alton EWFW, Armstrong DK, Ashby D, et al. Repeated nebulisation of non-viral CFTR gene therapy in patients with cystic fibrosis: a randomised, double-blind, placebo-controlled, phase 2b trial. Lancet Respir Med. 2015;3(9):684–91. https://doi.org/10.1016/S2213-2600(15)00245-3. Epub 2015 Jul 3
86. ClinicalTrials.gov. A phase 1 study evaluating safety and tolerability of RCT2100 in healthy participants. 2024. Available from: https://classic.clinicaltrials.gov/ct2/show/NCT06237335
87. ClinicalTrials.gov. Safety, tolerability, and pharmacokinetics of ARCT-032 in healthy adult subjects. 2023. Available from: https://classic.clinicaltrials.gov/ct2/show/NCT05712538
88. ClinicalTrials.gov. A phase 1/2 study of VX-522 in participants with cystic fibrosis (CF). 2022. Available from: https://classic.clinicaltrials.gov/ct2/show/NCT05668741

89. Plasschaert LW, MacDonald KD, Moffit JS. Current landscape of cystic fibrosis gene therapy. Front Pharmacol. 2024;15:1476331. https://doi.org/10.3389/fphar.2024.1476331. eCollection 2024
90. Kim YJ, Krainer AR. Antisense oligonucleotide therapeutics for cystic fibrosis: recent developments and perspectives. Mol Cells. 2023;46:10–20. https://doi.org/10.14348/molcells.2023.2172.
91. Caraco Y, Wanounou M, Blotnick S, et al. A phase I study assessing the safety and tolerability of SPL84, an inhaled antisense oligonucleotide for treatment of cystic fibrosis patients with the 3849 +10kb C->T. J Cyst Fibros. 2024;S1569-1993(24):01798–3. https://doi.org/10.1016/j.jcf.2024.10.004.
92. Schwank G, Koo BK, Sasselli V, et al. Functional repair of CFTR by CRISPR/Cas9 in intestinal stem cell organoids of cystic fibrosis patients. Cell Stem Cell. 2013;13:653–8. https://doi.org/10.1016/j.stem.2013.11.002.
93. Firth AL, Menon T, Parker GS, et al. Functional gene correction for cystic fibrosis in lung epithelial cells generated from patient iPSCs. Cell Rep. 2015;12:1385–90. https://doi.org/10.1016/j.celrep.2015.07.062. Epub 2015 Aug 20
94. Sanz DJ, Hollywood JA, Scallan MF, et al. Cas9/gRNA targeted excision of cystic fibrosis-causing deep-intronic splicing mutations restores normal splicing of CFTR mRNA. PLoS One. 2017;12:e0184009. https://doi.org/10.1371/journal.pone.0184009. eCollection 2017
95. Gupta A, Barone C, Quijano E. Next generation triplex-forming PNAs for site-specific genome editing of the F508del CFTR mutation. J Cyst Fibros. 2024;S1569-1993(24):00795–1. https://doi.org/10.1016/j.jcf.2024.07.009.
96. Vaidyanathan S, Baik R, Chen L, et al. Targeted replacement of full-length CFTR in human airway stem cells by CRISPR-Cas9 for pan-mutation correction in the endogenous locus. Mol Ther. 2022;30:223–37. https://doi.org/10.1016/j.ymthe.2021.03.023. Epub 2021 Mar 29
97. Wang G. Genome editing for cystic fibrosis. Cells. 2023;12(12):1555. https://doi.org/10.3390/cells12121555.
98. Somerville L, Borish L, Noth I, et al. Modulator-refractory cystic fibrosis: defining the scope and challenges of an emerging at-risk population. Ther Adv Respir Dis. 2024;18:17534666241297877. https://doi.org/10.1177/17534666241297877.
99. Allen L, Allen L, Carr SB, et al. Future therapies for cystic fibrosis. Nat Commun. 2023;14(1):693. https://doi.org/10.1038/s41467-023-36244-2.

# Chapter 2
# All in the Family: Role for Precision Medicine in Screening and Disease Course Prediction

**Laurence Pearmain, Jack Callum, Stefan Stanel, and Pilar Rivera-Ortega**

## Familial Pulmonary Fibrosis

### *Introduction*

Interstitial lung disease (ILD) describes more than 200 different diseases and has a progressively rising prevalence, currently affecting approximately 4.71 million people globally [1]. Many of these cases are sporadic, though some demonstrate a clear genetic predisposition with cases running through families. Familial pulmonary fibrosis (FPF) refers either to [1] a case of fibrotic ILD with one or more relatives (first or second degree) affected, or [2] a sporadic case with a pathogenic genetic variant in a gene known to be related to FPF [2]. Young age (less than 50 years) at symptom onset is also often used as an additional FPF criteria. This is due to difficulties ascertaining historical diagnoses of family members and unrecognized extrapulmonary disease in family members (e.g., telomere biology disorders) but also due to incomplete knowledge of pathogenicity [2].

The current weight of evidence indicates FPF is primarily a monogenic disorder, with the majority of mutations in genes coding regions related to telomeres or surfactant homeostasis [2–4]. FPF is a rapidly developing field, and in 2017, France was the first country to recommend genetic sequencing for FPF [5]. Several other

The original version of the chapter has been revised. A correction to this chapter can be found at https://doi.org/10.1007/978-3-031-87183-2_12

L. Pearmain
Respiratory NIHR Clinical Lecturer, University of Manchester, Manchester, UK

Respiratory Specialist Registrar, Wythenshawe Hospital, Manchester University NHS Foundation Trust, Manchester, UK

J. Callum
Respiratory Consultant, Homerton University Hospital NHS Foundation Trust, London, UK

S. Stanel · P. Rivera-Ortega (✉)
Interstitial Lung Disease Unit, Wythenshawe Hospital,
Manchester University NHS Foundation Trust, Manchester, UK



B. F. Collins, S. B. Montesi (eds.), *Precision Medicine in Interstitial Lung Disease*, Respiratory Medicine, https://doi.org/10.1007/978-3-031-87183-2_2

countries have subsequently followed suit [5]. Despite these efforts, the majority of FPF patients do not currently have a monogenetic cause recorded, in part due to both limitations in both tests and access to testing. Greater use of genetic testing may improve the power of future studies to identify additional pathogenic rare variants.

This chapter examines the most important genetic mutations in FPF, their clinical presentations, diagnosis, and management.

## Pathobiology of Telomere Dysfunction

Telomeres are repeating noncoding DNA protective caps (TTAGGG) at the end of chromosomes which shorten with each cell division. The ribonucleoprotein (RNP) telomerase complex counteracts this shortening by adding telomeric repeats [6]. The pathogenic variants most frequently found in FPF exacerbate this shortening by affecting proteins in the RNP telomerase complex such as telomere reverse transcriptase (encoded by TERT) and telomerase RNA component (encoded by TERC) [6]. TERT and TERC variants were the first mutations to be associated with FPF, and subsequent research has linked excessive telomere shortening itself with the development of progressive pulmonary fibrosis (PPF) [6, 7].

TERT pathogenic variants are the most common monogenic cause for FPF and found in 15–22% of FPF patients followed by pathogenic variants of other telomere-related genes (TRGs) including RTEL1 (5–10%) and TERC (2–5%) [2]. Other rarer gene mutations include DKC1 and TINF2 followed by the ultra-rare mutations to NOP10, NHP2, ACD, NAF1, ZCCHC8, RPA, and POT1 [2, 8]. All TRG variants are inherited in an autosomal dominant manner except for DKC1 which is x-linked [2, 8]. Telomere length, an independent risk factor for FPF, can also be inherited by subsequent generations even without the transmission of the TRG thought to be responsible [9, 10]. Telomere shortening may cause disease at progressively younger ages in subsequent generations, the phenomenon of genetic anticipation [9, 10].

## Pathobiology of Surfactant Dysfunction

Surfactant is a substance that coats alveoli to reduce surface tension and facilitate lung expansion. It is secreted by type II alveolar epithelial cells and is composed of 90% lipids and 10% proteins [11]. These proteins play key roles in lung defense (proteins SP-A and SP-D) as well as surfactant function (proteins SP-B & SP-C) and are encoded by the genes SFTPA, SFTPD, SFTPB, and SFTPC, respectively [11]. SFTPA and SFTPC pathogenic variants are both linked to FPF, while SFTPA is also heavily linked with lung cancer [12–16].

Two other genes which can lead to ILD include ABCA3 and NKX2.1. ABCA3 encodes ATP bindings cassette family A, member 3 protein which transports surfactant lipids into lamellar bodies, while NKX2.1 encodes thyroid transcription factor 1 (TTF1) which regulates surfactant protein and ABCA3 gene transcription [17, 18]. As TTF1 is also found in thyroid and CNS tissue, NKX2.1 pathogenic variants can present with widespread neurological disease and hypothyroidism [19, 20]. ABCA3 pathogenic variants on the other hand lead to ILD mostly in the case of residual function mutations as biallelic null mutations lead to death in infancy [21, 22].

Overall surfactant-related gene (SRG) mutations are rare and make up <5% of ILD cases with the most common SRGs being SFTPA1, SFTPA2, and SFTPC [2]. SRGs, excepting ABCA3, are autosomal dominant in inheritance pattern, although de novo mutations may explain 50% of SFTPC mutations [12–16, 23–27].

## *Polymorphisms (Common Genetic Variants)*

Polymorphisms represent mutations with uncertain functional consequences and common allele frequency (i.e., found in >1% of the population). The most well-known of these is the rs35705950 MUC5B promoter gene polymorphism which codes a protein constituent of respiratory mucous leading to increased expression in terminal bronchioles [28, 29]. Due to low penetrance and high prevalence, it is not standard for FPF investigations. The minor allele is found in 10% of European populations and while significantly more common in idiopathic pulmonary fibrosis (IPF) & FPF (34–38%), its causal relationship with pulmonary fibrosis (PF) is unclear [30, 31]. Risk of PF from individual polymorphisms may be low, but multiple polymorphisms may be present. Polygenic risk scores (PRS) have been shown to account for up to 28% of sporadic IPF (sIPF) disease risk [32].

PRS scores use genome-wide association studies (GWAS) of IPF patients compared to a random sample of individuals as a reference panel. Elastic net-based penalized regression algorithms are then used to shrink GWAS effect size estimates to construct PRSs with high predictive values [32]. These scoring systems can then be used to predict ILD and interstitial lung abnormalities (ILA). A study across 24 common diseases demonstrated that polygenic risk is an independent variable from family history and can contribute complementary information [33]. Thus, polygenic risk scores may contribute to understanding of FPF; however, studies to date focus exclusively on sporadic pulmonary fibrosis (sPF) [32].

## *Clinical Features*

The initial presentation of FPF is similar to sPF with dyspnea, cough, inspiratory crackles on auscultation, and occasionally clubbing. The main distinction is that FPF patients often present far younger and are more likely to have progressive disease with limited survival [34–37].

The mean age of presentation depends very much on the pathogenic variant. Patients with SRG mutations generally present earlier than those with TRG mutations. The median age of diagnosis of ILD in patients with an SRG variant is 45 years compared to 62 years for TRG variants, though in some SRG variants, the average can be as low as 37 [13]. There has been no sex predominance identified for SRG variants, though a male predominance is seen in TRG variants [13, 38].

Beyond ILD, participants with TRG pathogenic variants and short telomere syndrome can present with a myriad of extrapulmonary features. Mucocutaneous features are common, and patients can present with buccal leukoplakia, nail dystrophy, premature hair greying, and abnormal pigmentation [6]. Hematological manifestations are also common with anemia seen in 17–27%, macrocytosis in 24–51%, thrombocytopenia in 8–54%, and even myelodysplasia or acute leukemia [39–43]. These are more common in DKC1, TINF2, and TERC mutation compared to TERT, PARN, or RTEL1 [40]. Liver enzyme derangement is also common (5–27%) and can range from asymptomatic to cryptogenic cirrhosis with portal hypertension [9, 39, 40, 44, 45]. Finally, patients can present with osteoporosis, primary immunodeficiency, retinal disorders, or dyskeratosis congenital (Table 2.1) [40].

**Table 2.1** Demographics, clinical features, and key genetic studies of rare variants

| | TERT | TERC | RTEL1 | PARN | SFTPA | SFTPC | NKX2.1 |
|---|---|---|---|---|---|---|---|
| Frequency | 15–22% | 2–5% | 5–10% | 1–5% | <5% | <5% | <5% |
| Age at presentation | Adults | Adults | Adults | Adults | Adults | Children | Children |
| Non-ILD feature | Premature graying, aplastic anemia, and hematolgoical abnormalities, osteoporosis, deranged liver enzymes, nail dystrophy, and buccal leukoplakia | | | | Lung cancer | | Chorea, hypothyroidism |
| References and total study size | Number of participants with rare variants within referenced studies | | | | | | |
| Borie [39]: $n = 237$ | 26 | 5 | | | | | |
| Chad [40]: $n = 115$ | 75 | 7 | 14 | 19 | | | |
| Legendre [12]: $n = 28$ | | | | | 28 | | |
| Borie [46]: $n = 252$ | 34 | 6 | 35 | | | | |
| Armanios [7]: $n = 73$ | 16 | | | | | | |
| Nathan [15]: $n = 22$ | | | | | 12 | | |
| Van Moorsel [16]: $n = 157$ | | | | | 4 | | |
| Stuart [47]: $n = 151$ | | | 5 | 6 | | | |
| Tsakiri [48]: $n = 88$ | 18 | 2 | | | | | |
| van der Vis [49]: $n = 2492$ | 13 | | | | | | |

(continued)

**Table 2.1** (continued)

| | TERT | TERC | RTEL1 | PARN | SFTPA | SFTPC | NKX2.1 |
|---|---|---|---|---|---|---|---|
| Cogan [50]: $n = 54$ | | | 40 | | | | |
| Kannengiesser [51]: $n = 47$ | | | 7 | | | | |
| Philippot [52]: $n = 31$ | | | | 31 | | | |
| Kropski [53]: $n = 188$ | | | | 36 | | | |
| van Moorsel [3]: $n = 229$ | | | | | | 40 | |
| Nattes [19]: $n = 20$ | | | | | | | 17 |

## Genetic Screening

### *Telomere Length Measurement*

Telomere length is typically measured in peripheral blood and may be expressed as an absolute number (kb) or as a relative length compared to a control population and corrected for age [2]. Comparison with an age-matched reference population allows comparison of telomere length between individuals of different ages. When compared with this reference population, a measurement below the tenth percentile of a normal distribution is considered as a severe reduction in telomere length [54]. Peripheral blood leukocyte telomere length correlates with lung tissue telomere length [55]. There are several different methods for measuring telomere length, each with their own advantages and drawbacks [56]. Quantitative polymerase chain reaction (qPCR) and flow-fluorescence in situ hybridization (flow-FISH) being the two more widely available techniques with Flow-FISH reported as the more reproducible and the gold standard [2].

Short telomere length in peripheral blood mononuclear cells is linked to pathogenic telomere-related gene variants [57, 58]. However, telomere length within normal values is frequently observed in families with pulmonary fibrosis, and telomere length yields insufficient information to exclude the presence of a short telomere syndrome or the risk of pulmonary disease, especially in subjects aged >60 years [40, 59–63]. Some telomere-related gene variants may not affect telomere length but rather telomere function, with similar clinical consequences [64].

In FPF patients without an identified mutation, a short telomere length may identify patients with a mutation in an unknown telomere-related gene or a phenocopy, where patients inherited very short telomere from their parents [2, 65].

## *Gene Sequencing*

Gene sequencing includes the detailed assessment of genomic DNA code extracted from cells within blood, saliva, buccal swabs, or skin biopsies. Multiple gene sequencing technologies are available to clinicians, including whole genome, whole exome, and gene panel testing [66]. Although whole genome and exome sequencing assess the entire genome or exome of the patient, gene panel testing sequences only the subset of genes that have been implicated previously in FPF and has a quicker turnaround time and lower cost [66].

Gene variants identified through gene sequencing are reported according to standards outlined by the American College of Medical Genetics, which include pathogenic, likely pathogenic, variant of uncertain significance (VUS), likely benign, and benign descriptions [67, 68]. These designations are derived by assimilating known information about the specific variant in question, including the functional consequence, variant prevalence within the population, previous associations, or cosegregation with disease [69]. Within this context, a result that explains the patient's condition (pathogenic or likely pathogenic variant in a gene previously implicated in FPF) can be found in up to 30% of patients with FPF. In contrast, uncertain or benign results are the more common finding, indicating that the patient does not have a causative genetic variant in the genes tested but still may harbor a causative variant that is yet to be identified. Rarely, negative results may be the consequence of technological limitations such as variants located deep within introns [66].

## *Wider Health Screening Implications*

Although genetic testing may provide high-yield results in the appropriate clinical setting, widespread genetic testing is not yet justified for all patients with pulmonary fibrosis, because the relevance of such results remains unclear in many settings [66]. Genetic testing is generally not recommended in sporadic PF patients, unless they or their family members display features suggestive of a genetic syndrome or are less than 50 years of age [2]. Nor is genetic testing recommended in unaffected relatives if the affected proband has either not undergone genetic testing or genetic sequencing has not found a pathogenic or likely pathogenic variant.

Genetic testing is considered for patients with FPF when the results [66]:

- Would influence patient-specific disease management.
- Would inform individual risk stratification.
- Would provide context for extrapulmonary disease manifestation.
- Would provide relevant information for the patient or their relatives, or a combination thereof.

## *Genetic Testing Considerations*

Genetic counseling is the process of helping people understand and adapt to the medical, psychological, and familial implications of genetic contributions to disease and should be offered to all individuals before undergoing genetic testing [70]. Genetic counselors are healthcare professionals with specialized training in both medical genetics and psychosocial counseling. In addition to helping patients understand the risks and benefits of genetic testing, genetic counselors can help clinicians to identify the appropriate testing method, can help to facilitate testing, and can assist in the interpretation of the results [66].

The cost of genetic testing varies significantly based on the number of genes tested, the technology used, and the specific laboratory selected. For instance, in the United States, the out-of-pocket cost to the patient (cost may range from zero to several thousand dollars) will depend on the list price for the test, insurance coverage, and whether preauthorization is required [66]. In some countries with universal access to equal health care, such as the United Kingdom, a gene panel is offered to ILD patients who meet the National Genomic Testing criteria (Table 2.2) [71].

## *Genetic Discrimination*

Patients often inquire if positive genetic test results could impact their ability to obtain health insurance. In the United States, although each state may have their own laws, the Genetic Information Nondiscrimination Act of 2008 is a federal law that prohibits health insurers from discriminating based on genetic information, including family history, and prohibits employers from using genetic information in employment decisions. However, the Genetic Information Nondiscrimination Act does not extend these protections to staff of companies within fewer than 15 employees. For this reason, it is not recommended that minors undergo genetic testing until they can understand the implications of genetic testing and provide informed consent [66].

**Table 2.2** UK national testing familial pulmonary fibrosis genetic testing criteria [71]

| **Pulmonary Fibrosis Familial Testing Criteria—ILD and ONE of the following** |
|---|
| ILD, no identifiable cause or association, and age < 50 years |
| Family history of ILD regardless of identifiable cause or association |
| For suspected telomerase complex mutations, testing to be considered in the absence of 1 and 2. Above if one or more of the following are present in addition to ILD: |
| Unexplained hematological abnormalities including macrocytosis, anemia, thrombocytopenia, leukopenia, and/or lymphopenia; premature graying |
| Or unexplained liver function abnormalities |
| Consideration of lung transplantation |

## *How to Screen Relatives of FPF Patients*

There is no clear pathway or optimal age for screening relatives of FPF patients [71]. As there is a 1–3-year delay between symptom onset and diagnosis for FPF patients, this represents an opportunity for early diagnosis [72].

The European Respiratory Society statement on familial pulmonary fibrosis recommends that all adult first-degree relatives of FPF patients have a screening chest high-resolution computed tomography (HRCT) scan, especially if they have non-resolving respiratory symptoms such as chronic cough and dyspnea [2]. The prevalence of interstitial lung changes on CT screening of first-degree relatives of FPF patients has been reported as 14–25% [2]. Among first-degree relatives of FPF without overt ILD at screening, 19.4% developed extensive HRCT abnormalities or clinical ILD at 5 years [73]. Also, 63.3% of patients with limited interstitial lung abnormalities (ILA) at enrollment experienced progression compared to only 6.1% of patients with normal HRCT at baseline [73].

Lung function is important for screening and follow-up, but simple spirometry may not identify early cases, since predicted forced vital capacity (FVC) less than 80% in asymptomatic relatives is uncommon [71]. However, relatives with ILA have a lower diffusing capacity of the lung for carbon monoxide (DLCO) than those with normal HRCT [73, 74]. Annual pulmonary function testing may identify trends of decline. The role for home spirometry monitoring has not been explored in this population but may hold promise for the future [71]. Due to the high prevalence of other telomere shortening features, a full blood count (FBC) and liver function testing should also be performed in first-degree relatives [2].

The presence of a disease-causing variant in an affected family member offers potential actionable information for their relatives. In such cases, genetic counseling with targeted gene sequencing for the specific variant should be offered to other interested relatives to aid in susceptibility risk stratification [66]. Those relatives who also harbor the variant should be considered at higher risk for disease development; however, disease penetrance and severity are highly variable, and currently no known pharmacological interventions exist that prevent disease onset [66].

In general, the risk of inheriting an identified variant and of disease developing is gene dependent and may range from 0% to 50%, depending on how the gene is inherited (autosomal dominant, autosomal recessive, or X-linked recessive). Autosomal dominant inheritance is the most common scenario in FPF, resulting in a 50% chance that the parents, children, and siblings of individuals with positive test results will inherit the same mutation. Because pulmonary fibrosis usually manifests in middle to late adulthood, asymptomatic individuals may not suspect that they carry a disease-causing variant until they undergo genetic testing [66]. Genetic anticipation can be observed in relatives harboring rare telomere gene variants resulting from progressive shortening of telomere length across generations. This can result in earlier age of PF onset and higher risk of bone marrow failure developing as the initial manifestation in subsequent generations [7, 40, 75].

To date, there is no consensus on the frequency and duration of clinical, functional, and radiological evaluations of first-degree relatives of FPF patients.

Management could be customized through a risk assessment, considering resources available in each country and national health system.

## Predicting Progression of Familial Pulmonary Fibrosis

Progression of FPF can be measured in different ways. All measurements represent either physiological, architectural, or functional evidence of pulmonary fibrosis disease progression. Within FPF cohort studies, transplant-free survival and change (Δ) in forced vital capacity (FVC) are historically most used [3, 36, 76–78]. Progression data is particularly important in the FPF patient group, as FPF patients are more frequently good transplant candidates, with earlier age at diagnosis and fewer comorbidities than their older sIPF counterparts [2]. Further, unlike in sPF, FPF patients are likely to have lived experience of the disease prior to diagnosis, and additional considerations from genetic testing which may lead to both greater disease knowledge and anxiety over the future [79]. Finally, with expanding antifibrotic medication use, there is a need to identify non-IPF FPF individuals with a progressive phenotype for early antifibrotic therapy [2, 80].

FPF has clinical and radiological heterogeneity [34, 35, 40, 77]. Several studies focusing on the effect of genetic variants associated with IPF risk found similar contributions to disease risk and characteristics in fibrotic hypersensitivity pneumonitis, unclassifiable ILD, and rheumatoid arthritis associated with ILD (RA-ILD) [39, 40, 81–83]. Not only does this heterogeneity exist between unrelated individuals but also within FPF kindreds [40]. One study showed an 80% discordance in clinical and radiological pattern in kindreds with a shared mutation [40]. It has been shown that self-reported specific environmental exposures are associated with distinct HRCT radiological patterns in FPF patients [84]. With this heterogeneity comes increased complexity in defining risk and speed of disease progression in patients with FPF. Further, it underscores the likelihood of intersection between gene and environment effects that necessitate a precision medicine approach to FPF patients. Below, we examine evidence for disease progression of FPF comparative to sPF, as well as evidence within specific groups of FPF and sPF.

### *Familial Pulmonary Fibrosis Disease Progression Compared to Sporadic Pulmonary Fibrosis*

It has been suggested that FPF patients experience a more rapid decline than sPF [35, 77]. In a North American multicenter study of 1262 participants including 224 FPF patients and 1038 sPF patients, there was significantly worse transplant-free survival and mortality which was maintained across different fibrosing ILDs with family aggregation (HR 1.8; CI 1.37–2.37 familial IPF vs. sIPF: HR 2.08; 95% CI, 1.46–2.96 non-IPF FPF vs. sporadic non-IPF PF) [77]. Within the FPF cohort, familial IPF (FIPF) carried a worse prognosis compared to other fibrosing ILDs, mirroring the relative risk of sIPF compared to other fibrosing ILDs. These findings are supported by a European study across two centers that showed greater 6 month decline in FVC in FIPF ($n = 28$) compared to sIPF ($n = 147$) (4.94%, CI 3.16–6.71% vs. 2.48%, CI 1.57–3.38%) [35]. This study also raised concerns regarding genetic anticipation with second-generation FPF patients having earlier onset, although sub-analysis of lung function is not presented [35]. The number of affected relatives was not a significant survival variable [35].

There is, however, conflict between study findings comparing FPF and sPF (Table 2.3). Earlier single-center retrospective studies indicate similar clinical and radiological findings and outcomes between FIPF and sIPF [3, 36, 76]. A prospective Belgian and Luxembourg registry study of sIPF ($n$ = 586) and FIPF ($n$ = 76) showed similar transplant-free survival, time to 10% FVC decline, and time to 15% DLCO decline [78]. Earlier retrospective studies showed no difference in survival

**Table 2.3** Summary of studies comparing spontaneous and familial pulmonary fibrosis progression. Red represents increased speed of progression and blue lower, with circles representing cohort size

| Study design | Measure of progression | Sporadic pulmonary fibrosis | Sporadic idiopathic pulmonary fibrosis | Familial pulmonary fibrosis | Familial idiopathic pulmonary fibrosis |
|---|---|---|---|---|---|
| Cutting et al.(78) Multi-centre retrospective | Survival | N=638 | N=400 | N=90 | N=104 |
| Lee et al.(36) Retrospective case series | Survival | | N=104 | | N=27 |
| Ravaglia et al.(76) Retrospective case series | Survival | | N=127 | | N=30 |
| Krauss et al.(35) Prospective multi-centre | FVC | | N=147 | | N=28 |
| Froidure et al.(79) Multi-centre prospective | FVC | | | | |
| | Survival | | N=542 | N=76 | |
| Klay et al.(101) Multi-centre retrospective | FVC | | N=575 | N=248 | |

despite similar patient profiles (such as younger age of onset and less smoking exposure in familial compared to spontaneous IPF) [3, 36, 76, 78].

Age is a recognized prognostic factor within sIPF [85]. Study recruitment criteria, design, and FPF definition all likely contribute to differences in findings of progression speed compared to sIPF as well. Compared to sPF, FPF study participant numbers have historically been low, due to both the lower prevalence, but also a lack of routine genetic testing in clinical practice [2]. The definition of FPF is variable, from requiring a family member diagnosed with IPF to a broader definition that encompasses other fibrosing ILDs and those with onset younger than 50 years of age without family aggregation [3, 35, 36, 76, 77].

Many studies to date that show increased progression risk in FPF rely upon self-reporting for diagnosis of FPF and do not have genetic testing data available [77, 84]. This supports the role of family history as a tool to assess progression risk and prompt referral to specialist pulmonary fibrosis clinics where available. However, current study size and heterogeneity of findings means there is not yet robust data with which to quantify the magnitude of this risk. Stratifying FPF patients into FIPF and non-IPF FPF is supported by progression and mortality data in some studies [35, 77]. Stratification of outcome in a FPF cohort based on radiological appearance demonstrated that probable usual interstitial pneumonia (UIP) and definite UIP patterns, commonly associated with sIPF, were linked with progressive disease, while inconsistent UIP pattern was less progressive and displayed distinct demographic and BAL features [34].

However, it has also been reported that within a cohort of patients with telomere rare variants that progression and survival are unrelated to clinical and radiological characteristics [40]. This study also showed kindreds with shared genetic background develop differing ILDs, suggesting that while gene-environment interactions are likely important to developing FPF, genetic risk has a large magnitude of effect in progression risk [40].

## *Genomic Markers, Disease Progression, and Prognosis of Familial Pulmonary Fibrosis*

Shorter circulating leukocyte telomere length is associated with worse transplant-free survival across different methodologies of measurement and different fibrosing ILDs [40, 45, 47, 54, 82, 86, 87]. Importantly, this finding has been validated across racial groups [88]. The vast majority of FPF studies are not racially diverse and overrepresent Caucasians (especially North Americans and Europeans) [88]. Telomere shortening is not only associated with genetic mutations, but also other prognostic variables including aging, environmental exposures, and immunosuppressive medications [86, 89–91]. Telomere length also has a dose-dependent inverse relationship with smoking status [92]. Age-adjusted leukocyte telomere length shortening is also seen in sPF, although in a lower proportion than FPF, demonstrating a likely environmental contribution to telomere attrition [47]. In vivo murine studies suggest alveolar type 2 epithelial cell telomere shortening specifically may be a critical driver of pulmonary fibrosis [93]. Thus, circulating leukocyte telomere length measurement may have predictive and prognostic value for disease progression beyond being a surrogate for TRG mutations.

While research has heterogeneity between specific TRG pathogenic variants with regard to clinical characteristics, there are few studies comparing differences in prognosis. Studies comparing outcomes across individual TRG rare variants demonstrate a uniformly progressive disease [39, 40]. It should be noted that while individual pathogenic TRG rare variants have similar trajectory in their lung function decline and transplant-free survival, there are extrapulmonary features may predict worse survival. For example, TRGs with severe hematological or hepatic involvement have worse posttransplant morbidity and survival [2, 94, 95]. Further, TRGs that affect immune cell function such as DKC1 and TERC may predispose patients to pulmonary infections such as pneumocystis, with implications for progression and prognosis [96].

TRGs account for approximately 20% of FPF. Clinical questioning with recognized criteria (Table 2.4) can be used as a tool to identify patients who may not have a recognized TRG pathogenic variant but do have telomere shortening or dysfunction due to other unmeasured factors [71, 97]. Further, it is a useful tool in regions where genetic or leukocyte telomere length testing is not available. These established criteria are based upon family history, pulmonary, and extrapulmonary features of telomere dysfunction [71, 97]. Further studies are required on whether clinical criteria have a role in clinical practice as a screening tool for further genomic testing.

Surfactant proteins have been studied as prognostic biomarkers in sIPF as they are dysregulated during loss of alveolar homeostasis [98]. SRG mutations are rarer in FPF patients than TRGs, and as such, there is a smaller evidence base to ascertain the speed of disease progression [99]. In comparison with other FPF patients, those with SRG mutations tend to be younger and more likely to have indeterminate UIP HRCT patterns, often demonstrating ground glass and have lower FVC and DLCO

**Table 2.4** Clinical criteria for suspecting short telomere syndrome

| ***One or more* of the following should be present with pulmonary fibrosis in patients or first-degree family members** |
|---|
| Early onset (<50 years) |
| Hematological abnormalities (macrocytosis, cytopenias, myelodysplasia, leukemia) |
| Liver abnormalities (cirrhosis, hepatopulmonary syndrome, portal hypertension) |
| Early gray hair (<30 years) |
| Early menopause (<45 years) |
| Frequent malignancy in the family |
| Dyskeratosis congenita or aplastic anemia |

Adapted from ERS statement on familial pulmonary fibrosis, [2] Stanel et al. [71], and Molina Molina et al. [97]

at diagnosis [3, 14, 16, 91, 100]. A single cohort study has compared FPF patients with SRGs ($n = 23$) with FPF patients without SRGs ($n = 248$) and sIPF ($n = 575$) [100]. Transplant-free survival time in patients with an SRG mutation (44 months, SE 11.7) was comparable to other FPF patients (38 months, SE 3.5) and sIPF (36 months, SE 2.0) [100]. ΔFVC in the SRG cohort (mls/year, −84, IQR -35, −382, $n = 21$) was not significantly different to FPF and sIPF cohorts [100]. There was, however, large ΔFVC variability between SRG individuals (range −310, +870 mls/year) with limited numbers preventing comparison of individual SRG mutations [100].

MUC5B polymorphisms are associated with reduced decline in FVC in sIPF and FPF [31, 101–104]. The application of MUC5B variant testing in FPF cohorts is contentious, and thus so is its place as a prognostic biomarker [2]. Some clinicians proposed its use in the absence of monogenic rare variants [2] (Fig. 2.1).

## *Interstitial Lung Abnormalities and Asymptomatic Screening*

Increasingly ILAs are identified on thoracic CT scans which are performed with increasing frequency, especially in the context of cancer investigations [105]. PF and lung cancer screening studies have provided insights into which patients are at increased risk of interstitial lung abnormalities, with family aggregation of pulmonary fibrosis increasing risk of interstitial lung abnormality from 7% (CI 4–10%) to 26% (95% CI 20–32%) [74, 106]. With evidence that antifibrotic therapy is effective in patients with FPF, and a high prevalence of ILAs in kindreds of FPF patients, further FPF CT screening studies of relatives are planned [107].

Data on FPF kindred ILA progression is currently limited, although available data suggests the majority ($n = 13/20$) have progressive disease within 2 years [108]. In a spontaneous ILA cohort, median progression time was 3.2 years (CI 3.0–3.4 years), with 17.2% developing a UIP radiological pattern over 11.2 years (median follow-up time) [109]. This supports increased risk of progressive disease in familial compared to spontaneous ILA cohorts. While polygenic risk scores have shown ability in identifying patients at risk of ILA progression (AUC 0.81; OR 1.16), the clinical applicability has not been assessed, nor any studies conducted specifically in cohorts of FPF kindreds [32]. Individual monogenic rare variant risk data has not yet been generated. Integrating genetic information to ILA progression risk is an important future area for research. For example, it would provide much-needed evidence to inform clinical decisions, and patient counseling, regarding initiating antifibrotic therapy in asymptomatic patients. Arguably, greater knowledge of the natural history of ILA progression to PPF—along with proven efficacy of antifibrotics for preventing progression—is required before Wilson Junger criteria (Table 2.5) would be met for clinical CT scan screening of high-risk populations such as FPF kindreds [110].

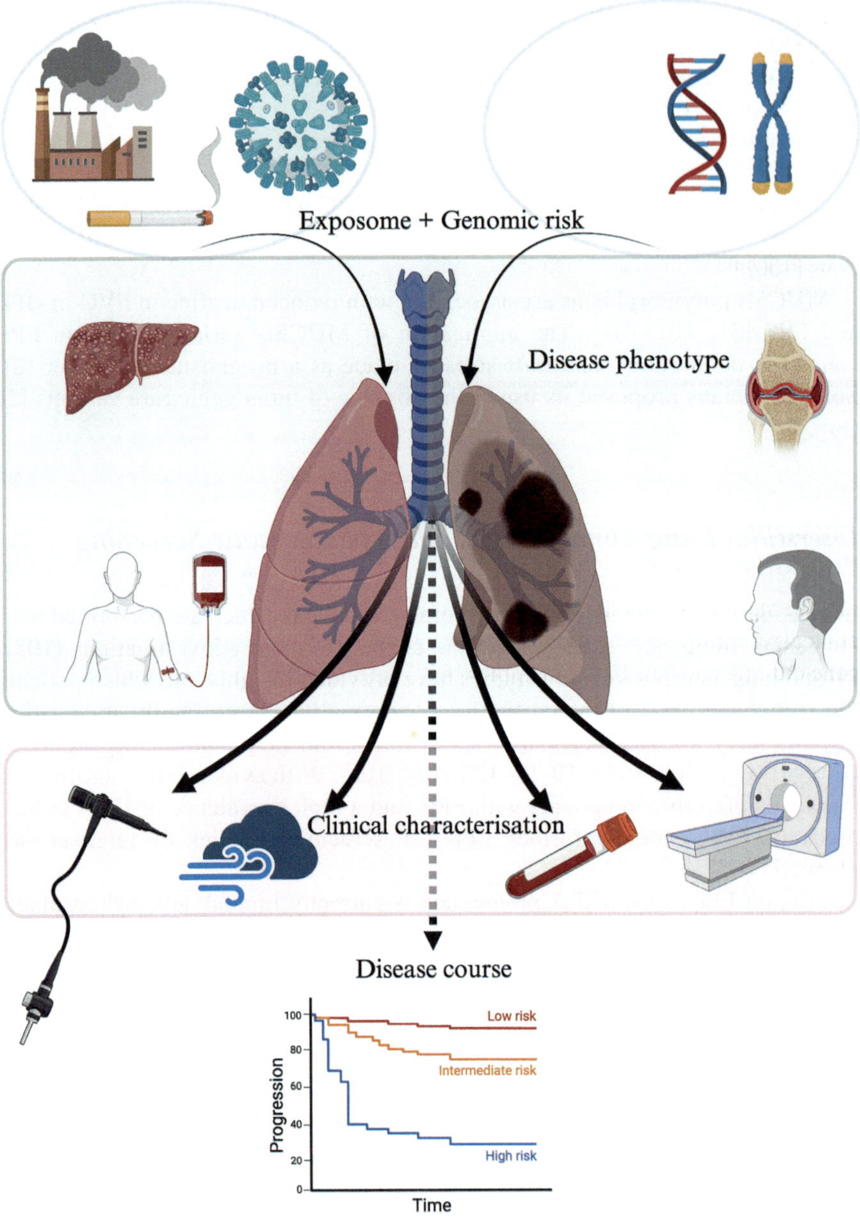


**Fig. 2.1** The interaction between lifetime exposures and genomic risk determines development of pulmonary fibrosis and specific disease phenotypes (e.g., connective tissue disease, anemia, liver fibrosis, early graying of hair), which can be characterized by clinical testing. Familial pulmonary fibrosis clinics can help with the holistic identification and characterisation of the disease phenotype. They are also key to facilitating research on the use of genetics and telomere biology to predict disease outcomes and personalized treatment. (Created with Biorender.com. Pearmain (2025) https://BioRender.com/b49r281)

**Table 2.5** Wilson Junger criteria for a screening program

| **Wilson Junger criteria for a screening program** |
|---|
| The condition sought should be an important health problem |
| There should be an accepted treatment for patients with recognized disease |
| Facilities for diagnosis and treatment should be available |
| There should be a recognizable latent or early symptomatic stage |
| There should be a suitable test or examination |
| The test should be acceptable to the population |
| **The natural history of the condition, including development from latent to declared disease, should be adequately understood** |
| **There should be an agreed policy on whom to treat as patients** |
| The cost of case finding (including diagnosis and treatment of patients diagnosed) should be economically balanced in relation to possible expenditure on medical care as a whole |
| Case finding should be a continuing process and not a "once and for all" project |

Adapted from Wilson and Junger [110]. Bold criteria especially require ongoing research to facilitate screening of high-risk ILD patients, such as those with family aggregation

## Harnessing Precision Medicine to Alter Disease Course Through Personalized Treatment of Familial Pulmonary Fibrosis

Treatment options for FPF are currently similar to sPF and may broadly be characterized as [1] avoidance of triggering exposures (smoking, environmental exposures, drug induced), [2] treatment of an identified cause, [3] antifibrotic medication (nintedanib or pirfenidone), and [4] lung transplantation. Patients may also be referred for therapeutic clinical trials if available in their local area.

Leveraging information on family history, disease-associated pathogenic variants and telomere length measurement provide opportunities for personalized care across all therapeutic modalities.

### *Preventing Disease: Avoiding Environmental Exposures in FPF*

Environmental and occupational exposures increase the risk of developing sIPF [111, 112]. Environmental exposures include mold and birds alongside air pollution and cigarette smoke [113–115]. Cumulative exposure to air pollution progressively increases the hazard ratio of developing sIPF and is additive to genetic predisposition [112]. Similarly, cigarette smoke increases risk of developing sIPF, and there is a dose-response association of cigarette smoking to shorter telomere length [92]. In vitro studies have shown human bronchial epithelial cells exposed to PM2.5 particulates have dose-dependent telomere shortening, altered telomerase activity, and epigenetic modifications [116].

Occupational exposures identified with increased risk of developing sIPF include metal dust, wood dust, silica dust, agricultural dust, and pesticides alongside general exposure to unspecified gas, vapor, dust, and fumes [111, 117]. Therefore, occupations such as farming, carpentry, and stone cutting/polishing are more likely to be extremely hazardous to patients and relatives with a family history or confirmed genetic predisposition to developing FPF.

The existing data therefore emphasizes the importance of discussing both lifestyle and occupational considerations with FPF patients and relatives. Referring or signposting patients to smoking cessation services is a critical intervention that is often underappreciated. Firm data on risk of pulmonary fibrosis from specific exposures is nascent with existing studies often grouping exposures, which makes discussing and advising on changing workplaces or occupations to avoid specific exposures challenging [89, 111, 117]. This is especially true given the significant financial impact on individuals. Genetic testing of FPF patients does, perhaps, offer an opportunity at disease prevention in kindreds through counseling to enable minimization of exposures. This is perhaps one of the most powerful current arguments for genetic screening of kindreds. However, research studies are required on the efficacy of such strategies. Referral to specialist familial ILD services can help facilitate counseling on these complex issues and maximize benefit from genetic testing of kindreds.

## *Personalized Antifibrotic Prescribing for FPF*

Antifibrotic medication is recommended for FPF, regardless of whether the diagnosis is IPF or another form of PPF [2, 41]. The efficacy of antifibrotics in telomere-related gene variant pulmonary fibrosis appears to be comparable to sporadic cases (based on retrospective data) [118]. Pirfenidone was also found to be beneficial regardless of telomere length [119]. Available evidence indicates antifibrotics are effective in SRG variant FPF [100]. Currently, there are no dedicated antifibrotic prescribing criteria for FPF; hence, sIPF and sPPF guidelines are applied.

In FPF, nintedanib is still prescribed for PPF patients according to the INBUILD criteria used in sPF [80]. There should be a low threshold to conduct investigations for progression in non-IPF FPF patients with known genomic predisposition to PF and proactive disease monitoring. This includes serial pulmonary function testing and HRCT to evidence INBUILD criteria [80]. Antifibrotics (pirfenidone or nintedanib) should be considered and initiated at diagnosis of familial IPF, as in sporadic disease.

Non-IPF FPF progression data ($\Delta$FVC and survival) is similar to sIPF (see section “Familial pulmonary fibrosis disease progression compared to sporadic pulmonary fibrosis”). Telomere length diagnostic tests, HRCT radiological patterns, family history, and genetic testing are all available with evidence they can identify patients with poorer prognosis [34, 35, 77]. We would advocate for international guideline committees to consider dedicated antifibrotic prescribing criteria for non-IPF FPF patients, independent of sporadic PPF criteria, and adoption of a more proactive approach to antifibrotic prescribing given evidence the diagnosis has a highly progressive phenotype in those with family history, telomere dysfunction, or TRG/SRG rare variants (Table 2.6) [40, 54, 77, 78, 82, 100].

**Table 2.6** Features that may be present in familial pulmonary fibrosis patients that predict progressive pulmonary fibrosis and support early initiation of antifibrotics

| Features predictive of progressive disease in FPF |
|---|
| Short circulating leukocyte telomere length |
| Telomere related gene mutation |
| Surfactant related gene mutation |
| Definite or probable UIP radiological pattern |

## *Personalized Immunosuppressive Therapy in FPF*

A post hoc analysis of the PANTHER IPF randomized control trial (RCT) demonstrated that patients with leukocyte telomere length < tenth percentile that were administered immunosuppression (azathioprine/prednisolone) had worse outcomes [86]. These findings were replicated in a second independent cohort from the anticoagulant effectiveness in idiopathic pulmonary fibrosis RCT [86]. There have been similar findings of a harmful interaction between immunosuppressive medication and leukocyte telomere length shortening in non-IPF PPF [120, 121]. These studies do not present data on the presence of TRG rare variants or family aggregation in those with leukocyte telomere length below the tenth percentile, although 80% of those with TRG variants have such shortening in other studies [86, 120, 121]. At present, the standard of care for FPF patients with TRG mutations, or clinical features of telomere dysfunction, is the same as their sporadic counterparts. Further prospective studies and biomarker-guided trials are required to alter standard of care or embed these findings in clinical practice. In FPF cases where benefit of immunosuppression is uncertain or ineffective, these findings may support earlier initiation of antifibrotics and referral for transplant assessment.

There is no established standard of care for FPF patients with SRG variants; however, immunosuppressive therapy is often prescribed due to ground-glass opacities on HRCT and interstitial inflammation (often superimposed on background UIP pattern) on histology [13, 100]. Due to the rarity of SRG variants evidence for treatment efficacy is weak. The largest observational study to date comparing SRG to FPF and sIPF outcomes suggested that treatment response to immunosuppression is variable in adult ILD, similar to findings in childhood forms of the disease [13, 100]. However, this study included only 23 SRG variant patients [100]. Antifibrotics had a more consistent stabilizing effect upon lung function [100].

## *Predicting Lung Transplant Outcomes in FPF*

The European Respiratory Society statement on FPF recommends early referral for lung transplant assessment given the potential for rapid progression in FPF cases [2], and it has been recognized that IPF patients have higher mortality while awaiting transplantation compared to other indications [122]. The outcomes of lung transplantation appear to be comparable between sporadic PF cases and those with genomic predisposition or FPF [95, 123, 124]. It is possible that lung transplantation cohorts may actually be enriched with unrecognized FPF patients due to a lack of genomic and telomere testing availability, given that they have a younger age and faster rate of progression [77].

Despite equivocal lung transplant outcomes between FPF and sIPF, posttransplant cytopenias are significantly more common [124]. Standard immunosuppression regimens after lung transplantation were also found to be poorly tolerated in patients harboring pathogenic telomere-related gene variants, particularly owing to hematological toxicity [125–127]. Bone marrow failure and hematological failure are more likely to occur in patients with TRG variants or telomere shortening [95, 127]. There is evidence these patients may also have worse posttransplant outcomes, although transplantation is still beneficial to survival and quality of life [95, 123, 125, 128]. Personalized immunosuppression management of posttransplant FPF patients should be considered, especially those with telomere shortening, and should incorporate closer monitoring.

## *Clinical Trials Using Precision Medicine to Predict Treatment Outcome in FPF*

The clinical development pipeline for improving treatments and diagnostic tests for pulmonary fibrosis has increased significantly in recent years. As of May 2024, there were 183 actively recruiting interventional trials registered on ClinicalTrials.gov, which offer further opportunities for personalized care.

Genomic testing has been recognized as an integral part of PF trial data analysis after post hoc analysis indicated patients with leukocyte telomere length below the tenth percentile are the main driver of unfavorable outcomes in the immunosuppressive arms of PANTHER-IPF study [86]. Additional post hoc analysis of the PANTHER-IPF trial also revealed that TOLLIP TT and TOLLIP CC genotypes were associated with better and worse responses to N-acetylcysteine, respectively [101].

Building on these findings, interventional trials have been designed which aim at targeting specific patient endotypes and genotypes. Current examples of clinical trials include TELO-SCOPE which aims to restore telomere length using danazol (an androgen hormone) as a TERT activator [129] and ANDROTELO (NCT03710356). Further data is awaited to understand if this treatment strategy has clinical applicability, as another trial of danazol in advanced IPF ($n$ = 50 patients) recently reported negative results [130]. The PRECISIONS RCT, assessing efficacy of N-acetylcysteine in TOLLIP TT genotype IPF patients, is also ongoing. There are no variant-specific therapies currently available in clinical trials for FPF; however, successful animal studies involving cytomegalovirus (CMV) or mRNA delivery of TERT in preclinical models have shown promising results [131, 132].

## *Familial Pulmonary Fibrosis Dedicated Clinical Services*

There is wide support among patients and clinicians to implement genomic testing for ILD [133]. Conducting genomic tests as part of dedicated clinics has the advantage of access to trained staff and specialized facilities for managing all aspects of FPF care. FPF clinics are also ideal for implementing ILD screening programs. The experience of healthy relatives of PF patients who undergo screening for early disease and/or genomic testing was found to be mostly positive, though more negative feelings were expressed when ILAs were identified [134]. Having direct access to trained clinicians for counseling and follow-up care can help patients navigate a potentially life-changing diagnosis of FPF.

There is also a pressing need for standardization, with no publications summarizing the core requirements for FPF services. Genomic testing for PF-related pathogenic variants and telomere shortening requires appropriate training and an effective informed consent process, but how this is conducted and the level of detail provided to patients vary around the world. Patients are concerned about the impact of their genetic predisposition on children and other relatives, and how the genomic abnormalities may affect their care, tolerance to treatments for ILD (e.g., immunosuppression), and the risk-benefit discussion of lung transplantation in their case. Early involvement of genetic counselors in FPF care is essential; however, local practice can vary [135].

Multidisciplinary team (MDT) collaboration is essential to provide holistic care and also allows specialists to share experience and learn from each other [136]. ILD MDT for FPF should ideally also include advice from lung transplant and clinical genetics specialists. Due to the sensitive nature of discussions and perceptions around genomic predisposition, staff providing care for FPF should always be tactful and put the desires of their patients at the forefront of decision-making while highlighting the evolving nature of the field [71]. Psychological support is often required and should be available for patients. Clinical psychologists should understand familial pulmonary fibrosis and have experience in managing cases of hereditary conditions. Finally, it is important to note that significant disparities remain in access to genomic testing and counseling around the world, which represents another barrier that needs to be overcome (Fig. 2.2).

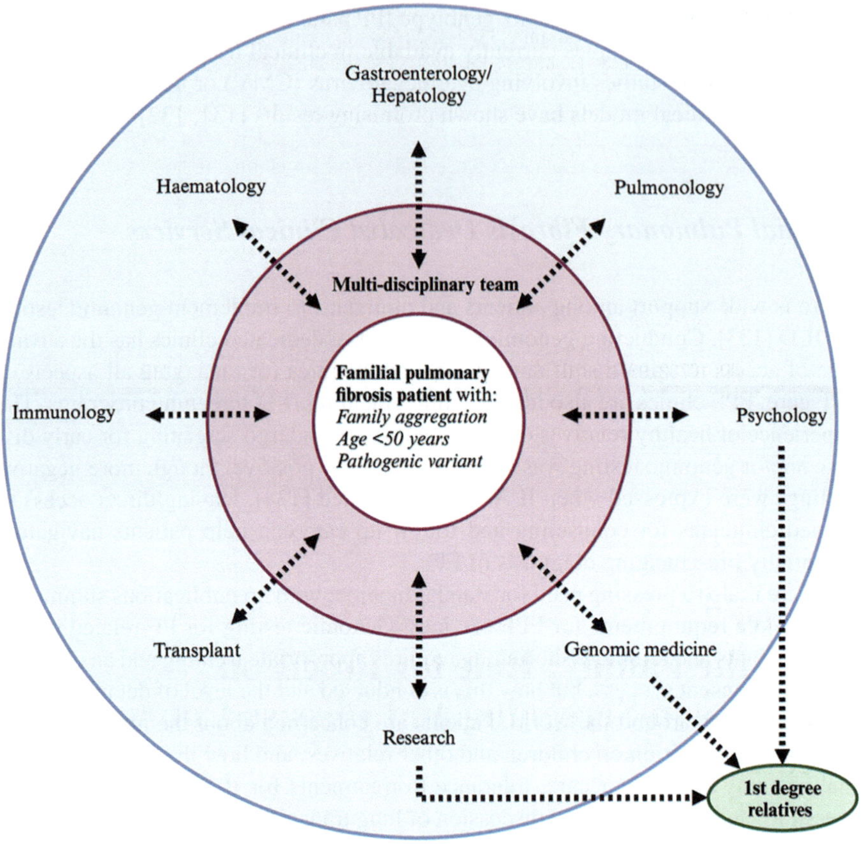


**Fig. 2.2** Composition of familial pulmonary fibrosis services and MDT. (Created with Biorender.com. Pearmain (2025) https://BioRender.com/o48j040)

## Conclusion

The era of genomic and precision medicine is upon us; however, the shape that takes in familial pulmonary fibrosis is still not certain. This is reflected in the current evidence-base, with variation in definitions, testing technologies, and measurement of progression. Additionally, a host of access barriers need to be addressed across society, with protections put in place against discrimination (e.g., health insurance eligibility) and provision of universal access related to genetic testing, not only within countries but globally. The complexity of FPF disease and the sensitive nature of testing mean an MDT approach is needed to deliver FPF services, and our existing workforce need upskilling in genomic medicine. We must overcome these practical challenges to fulfill the promise of early diagnosis and personalized prognosis and treatment, enabled by precision-medicine approaches.

## References

1. Zeng Q, Jiang D. Global trends of interstitial lung diseases from 1990 to 2019: an age-period-cohort study based on the global burden of disease study 2019, and projections until 2030. Front Med (Lausanne). 2023;10:1141372.
2. Borie R, et al. European respiratory society statement on familial pulmonary fibrosis. Eur Respir J. 2023;61
3. van Moorsel CH, et al. Surfactant protein C mutations are the basis of a significant portion of adult familial pulmonary fibrosis in a dutch cohort. Am J Respir Crit Care Med. 2010;182:1419–25.
4. Borie R, et al. Management of suspected monogenic lung fibrosis in a specialised centre. Eur Respir Rev. 2017;26
5. Cottin V, et al. French practical guidelines for the diagnosis and management of idiopathic pulmonary fibrosis. From the National Reference and the Competence centers for rare diseases and the Société de Pneumologie de Langue Française. Rev Mal Respir. 2013;30:879–902.
6. Armanios M, Blackburn EH. The telomere syndromes. Nat Rev Genet. 2012;13:693–704.
7. Armanios M, et al. Haploinsufficiency of te lomerase reverse transcriptase leads to anticipation in autosomal dominant dyskeratosis congenita. Proc Natl Acad Sci. 2005;102:15960–4.
8. Grill S, Nandakumar J. Molecular mechanisms of telomere biology disorders. J Biol Chem. 2021;296
9. Alder JK, et al. Short telomeres are a risk factor for idiopathic pulmonary fibrosis. Proc Natl Acad Sci. 2008;105:13051–6.
10. Alder JK, et al. Ancestral mutation in telomerase causes defects in repeat addition processivity and manifests as familial pulmonary fibrosis. PLoS Genet. 2011;7:e1001352.
11. Whitsett JA, Wert SE, Weaver TE. Alveolar surfactant homeostasis and the pathogenesis of pulmonary disease. Annu Rev Med. 2010;61:105–19.
12. Legendre M, et al. Functional assessment and phenotypic heterogeneity of SFTPA1 and SFTPA2 mutations in interstitial lung diseases and lung cancer. Eur Respir J. 2020;56
13. van Moorsel CH, van der Vis JJ, Grutters JC. Genetic disorders of the surfactant system: focus on adult disease. Eur Respir Rev. 2021;30
14. Wang Y, et al. Genetic defects in surfactant protein A2 are associated with pulmonary fibrosis and lung cancer. Am J Hum Genet. 2009;84:52–9.
15. Nathan N, et al. Germline SFTPA1 mutation in familial idiopathic interstitial pneumonia and lung cancer. Hum Mol Genet. 2016;25:1457–67.
16. van Moorsel CH, et al. SFTPA2 mutations in familial and sporadic idiopathic interstitial pneumonia. Am J Respir Crit Care Med. 2015;192:1249–52.
17. Flamein F, et al. Molecular and cellular characteristics of ABCA3 mutations associated with diffuse parenchymal lung diseases in children. Hum Mol Genet. 2012;21:765–75.
18. Hamdan H, et al. Structure of the human Nkx2. 1 gene. Biochim et Biophys Acta (BBA). 1998;1396:336–48.
19. Nattes E, et al. Heterogeneity of lung disease associated with NK2 homeobox 1 mutations. Respir Med. 2017;129:16–23.
20. Thorwarth A, et al. Comprehensive genotyping and clinical characterisation reveal 27 novel NKX2-1 mutations and expand the phenotypic spectrum. J Med Genet. 2014;51:375–87.
21. Wambach JA, et al. Genotype–phenotype correlations for infants and children with ABCA3 deficiency. Am J Respir Crit Care Med. 2014;189:1538–43.
22. Kröner C, et al. Lung disease caused by ABCA3 mutations. Thorax. 2017;72:213–20.
23. Kröner C, et al. Genotype alone does not predict the clinical course of SFTPC deficiency in paediatric patients. Eur Respir J. 2015;46:197–206.
24. Klay D, Platenburg MG, van Rijswijk RH, Grutters JC, van Moorsel CH. ABCA3 mutations in adult pulmonary fibrosis patients: a case series and review of literature. Curr Opin Pulm Med. 2020;26:293–301.

25. Epaud R, et al. Combined pulmonary fibrosis and emphysema syndrome associated with ABCA3 mutations. Eur Respir J. 2014;43:638–41.
26. Young LR, et al. Usual interstitial pneumonia in an adolescent with ABCA3 mutations. Chest. 2008;134:192–5.
27. Cottin V, Cordier J-F. SFTPC mutations in patients with familial pulmonary fibrosis: combined with emphysema? Am J Respir Crit Care Med. 2011;183:–1113.
28. Nakano Y, et al. MUC5B promoter variant rs35705950 affects MUC5B expression in the distal airways in idiopathic pulmonary fibrosis. Am J Respir Crit Care Med. 2016;193:464–6.
29. Helling BA, Yang IV. Epigenetics in lung fibrosis: from pathobiology to treatment perspective. Curr Opin Pulm Med. 2015;21:454–62.
30. Zhang Y, Noth I, Garcia JG, Kaminski N. A variant in the promoter of MUC5B and idiopathic pulmonary fibrosis. N Engl J Med. 2011;364:1576–7.
31. Seibold MA, et al. A common MUC5B promoter polymorphism and pulmonary fibrosis. N Engl J Med. 2011;364:1503–12.
32. Moll M, et al. A polygenic risk score for idiopathic pulmonary fibrosis and interstitial lung abnormalities. Am J Respir Crit Care Med. 2023;208:791–801.
33. Mars N, et al. Systematic comparison of family history and polygenic risk across 24 common diseases. Am J Hum Genet. 2022;109:2152–62.
34. Bennett D, et al. Familial pulmonary fibrosis: Clinical and radiological characteristics and progression analysis in different high resolution-CT patterns. Respir Med. 2017;126:75–83.
35. Krauss E, et al. Clinical characteristics of patients with familial idiopathic pulmonary fibrosis (f-IPF). BMC Pulm Med. 2019;19:130.
36. Lee HL, et al. Familial idiopathic pulmonary fibrosis: clinical features and outcome. Chest. 2005;127:2034–41.
37. Steele MP, et al. Clinical and pathologic features of familial interstitial pneumonia. Am J Respir Crit Care Med. 2005;172:1146–52.
38. Diaz de Leon A, et al. Telomere lengths, pulmonary fibrosis and telomerase (TERT) mutations. PLoS One. 2010;5:e10680.
39. Borie R, et al. Prevalence and characteristics of TERT and TERC mutations in suspected genetic pulmonary fibrosis. Eur Respir J. 2016;48:1721–31.
40. Chad AN, et al. Telomere-related lung fibrosis is diagnostically heterogeneous but uniformly progressive. Eur Respir J. 2016;48:1710.
41. Raghu G, et al. Idiopathic pulmonary fibrosis (an update) and progressive pulmonary fibrosis in adults: an official ATS/ERS/JRS/ALAT clinical practice guideline. Am J Respir Crit Care Med. 2022;205:e18–47.
42. Papiris SA, et al. Myelodysplastic syndromes and idiopathic pulmonary fibrosis: a dangerous liaison. Respir Res. 2019;20:1–4.
43. Parry EM, Alder JK, Qi X, Chen JJ-L, Armanios M. Syndrome complex of bone marrow failure and pulmonary fibrosis predicts germline defects in telomerase. Blood J Am Soc Hematol. 2011;117:5607–11.
44. Gorgy AI, et al. Hepatopulmonary syndrome is a frequent cause of dyspnea in the short telomere disorders. Chest. 2015;148:1019–26.
45. Newton CA, et al. Telomere length and genetic variant associations with interstitial lung disease progression and survival. Eur Respir J. 2019;53:1801641.
46. Borie R, et al. Regulator of telomere length 1 (RTEL1) mutations are associated with heterogeneous pulmonary and extra-pulmonary phenotypes. Eur Respir J. 2019;53
47. Stuart BD, et al. Effect of telomere length on survival in patients with idiopathic pulmonary fibrosis: an observational cohort study with independent validation. Lancet Respir Med. 2014;2:557–65.
48. Tsakiri KD, et al. Adult-onset pulmonary fibrosis caused by mutations in telomerase. Proc Natl Acad Sci USA. 2007;104:7552–7.
49. van der Vis JJ, van der Smagt JJ, Hennekam FAM, Grutters JC, van Moorsel CHM. Pulmonary fibrosis and a TERT founder mutation with a latency period of 300 years. Chest. 2020;158:612–9.

50. Cogan JD, et al. Rare variants in RTEL1 are associated with familial interstitial pneumonia. Am J Respir Crit Care Med. 2015;191:646–55.
51. Kannengiesser C, et al. Heterozygous RTEL1 mutations are associated with familial pulmonary fibrosis. Eur Respir J. 2015;46:474–85.
52. Philippot Q, et al. Interstitial lung diseases associated with mutations of poly (A)-specific ribonuclease: a multicentre retrospective study. Respirology. 2022;27:226–35.
53. Kropski JA, et al. Rare genetic variants in PARN are associated with pulmonary fibrosis in families. Am J Respir Crit Care Med. 2017;196:1481–4.
54. Planas-Cerezales L, et al. Predictive factors and prognostic effect of telomere shortening in pulmonary fibrosis. Respirology. 2019;24:146–53.
55. Demanelis K, et al. Determinants of telomere length across human tissues. Science. 2020;369:eaaz6876.
56. Stock CJW, Renzoni EA. Telomeres in interstitial lung disease. J Clin Med. 2021;10
57. Mirabello L, et al. The association of telomere length and genetic variation in telomere biology genes. Hum Mutat. 2010;31:1050–8.
58. Stuart BD, et al. Exome sequencing links mutations in PARN and RTEL1 with familial pulmonary fibrosis and telomere shortening. Nat Genet. 2015;47:512–7.
59. Fan Y, et al. Telomerase gene variants and telomere shortening in patients with silicosis or asbestosis. Occup Environ Med. 2020;
60. Alder JK, et al. Diagnostic utility of telomere length testing in a hospital-based setting. Proc Natl Acad Sci USA. 2018;115:E2358–e2365.
61. Snetselaar R, et al. Telomere length in interstitial lung diseases. Chest. 2015;148:1011–8.
62. Mangaonkar AA, et al. Clinical correlates and treatment outcomes for patients with short telomere syndromes. Mayo Clin Proc. 2018;93:834–9.
63. Ley B, et al. Telomere length in patients with unclassifiable interstitial lung disease: a cohort study. Eur Respir J. 2020;56
64. Dodson LM, et al. From incomplete penetrance with normal telomere length to severe disease and telomere shortening in a family with monoallelic and biallelic PARN pathogenic variants. Hum Mutat. 2019;40:2414–29.
65. van der Vis JJ, et al. Pulmonary fibrosis in non-mutation carriers of families with short telomere syndrome gene mutations. Respirology. 2021;26:1160–70.
66. Newton CA, et al. The role of genetic testing in pulmonary fibrosis: a perspective from the pulmonary fibrosis foundation genetic testing work group. Chest. 2022;162:394–405.
67. Richards S, et al. Standards and guidelines for the interpretation of sequence variants: a joint consensus recommendation of the American College of Medical Genetics and Genomics and the Association for Molecular Pathology. Genet Med. 2015;17:405–24.
68. Claustres M, et al. Recommendations for reporting results of diagnostic genetic testing (biochemical, cytogenetic and molecular genetic). Eur J Hum Genet. 2014;22:160–70.
69. MacArthur DG, et al. Guidelines for investigating causality of sequence variants in human disease. Nature. 2014;508:469–76.
70. Resta R, et al. A new definition of genetic counseling: national society of genetic counselors' task force report. J Genet Couns. 2006;15:77–83.
71. Stanel SC, Callum J, Rivera-Ortega P. Genetic and environmental factors in interstitial lung diseases: current and future perspectives on early diagnosis of high-risk cohorts. Front Med (Lausanne). 2023;10
72. Fernandez BA, et al. A Newfoundland cohort of familial and sporadic idiopathic pulmonary fibrosis patients: clinical and genetic features. Respir Res. 2012;13:64.
73. Salisbury ML, et al. Development and progression of radiologic abnormalities in individuals at risk for familial interstitial lung disease. Am J Respir Crit Care Med. 2020;201:1230–9.
74. Hunninghake GM, et al. Interstitial lung disease in relatives of patients with pulmonary fibrosis. Am J Respir Crit Care Med. 2020;201:1240–8.
75. Rojas NR, et al. De novo heme proteins from designed combinatorial libraries. Protein Sci. 1997;6:2512–24.

76. Ravaglia C, et al. Features and outcome of familial idiopathic pulmonary fibrosis. Sarcoidosis Vasc Diffuse Lung Dis. 2014;31:28–36.
77. Cutting CC, et al. Family history of pulmonary fibrosis predicts worse survival in patients with interstitial lung disease. Chest. 2021;159:1913–21.
78. Froidure A, Bondue B, Dahlqvist C, Guiot J, Gusbin N, Wirtz G, Brusselle G, Strens D, Slabbynck H, Wuyts WA. Clinical course of suspected familial and sporadic idiopathic pulmonary fibrosis: data from the PROOF-next registry. Respirology. 2024;29(4):304–11.
79. Grant-Orser A, et al. Perceptions of genetic testing: a mixed-methods study of patients with pulmonary fibrosis and their first-degree relatives. Ann Am Thorac Soc. 2022;19:1305–12.
80. Flaherty KR, et al. Nintedanib in progressive fibrosing interstitial lung diseases. N Engl J Med. 2019;381:1718–27.
81. Juge PA, et al. MUC5B promoter variant and rheumatoid arthritis with interstitial lung disease. N Engl J Med. 2018;379:2209–19.
82. Ley B, et al. The MUC5B promoter polymorphism and telomere length in patients with chronic hypersensitivity pneumonitis: an observational cohort-control study. Lancet Respir Med. 2017;5:639–47.
83. van der Vis JJ, et al. Effect of Muc5b promoter polymorphism on disease predisposition and survival in idiopathic interstitial pneumonias. Respirology. 2016;21:712–7.
84. Copeland CR, et al. The association between exposures and disease characteristics in familial pulmonary fibrosis. Ann Am Thorac Soc. 2022;19:2003–12.
85. Ley B, et al. Unified baseline and longitudinal mortality prediction in idiopathic pulmonary fibrosis. Eur Respir J. 2015;45:1374–81.
86. Newton CA, et al. Telomere Length and Use of Immunosuppressive Medications in Idiopathic Pulmonary Fibrosis. Am J Respir Crit Care Med. 2018;200:336–47.
87. Duckworth A, et al. Telomere length and risk of idiopathic pulmonary fibrosis and chronic obstructive pulmonary disease: a mendelian randomisation study. Lancet Respir Med. 2021;9:285–94.
88. Adegunsoye A, et al. Telomere length associates with chronological age and mortality across racially diverse pulmonary fibrosis cohorts. Nat Commun. 2023;14:1489.
89. Xiao Z, Shao L, William EF, Lifang H. Environmental and occupational exposure to chemicals and telomere length in human studies. Occup Environ Med. 2013;70:743.
90. Cronkhite JT, et al. Telomere shortening in familial and sporadic pulmonary fibrosis. Am J Respir Crit Care Med. 2008;178:729–37.
91. Rossiello F, Jurk D, Passos JF, d'Adda di Fagagna F. Telomere dysfunction in ageing and age-related diseases. Nat Cell Biol. 2022;24:135–47.
92. Astuti Y, Wardhana A, Watkins J, Wulaningsih W. Cigarette smoking and telomere length: a systematic review of 84 studies and meta-analysis. Environ Res. 2017;158:480–9.
93. Piñeiro-Hermida S, et al. Consequences of telomere dysfunction in fibroblasts, club and basal cells for lung fibrosis development. Nat Commun. 2022;13:5656.
94. Phillips-Houlbracq M, et al. Determinants of survival after lung transplantation in telomerase-related gene mutation carriers: a retrospective cohort. Am J Transplant. 2022;22:1236–44.
95. Planas-Cerezales L, et al. Lung transplant improves survival and quality of life regardless of telomere dysfunction. Front Med (Lausanne). 2021;8:695919.
96. Hoffman TW, van Moorsel CHM, Borie R, Crestani B. Pulmonary phenotypes associated with genetic variation in telomere-related genes. Curr Opin Pulm Med. 2018;24:269–80.
97. Molina-Molina M, Borie R. Clinical implications of telomere dysfunction in lung fibrosis. Curr Opin Pulm Med. 2018;24:440–4.
98. Greene KE, et al. Serum surfactant proteins-A and -D as biomarkers in idiopathic pulmonary fibrosis. Eur Respir J. 2002;19:439–46.
99. Sutton RM, et al. Rare surfactant-related variants in familial and sporadic pulmonary fibrosis. Hum Mutat. 2022;43:2091–101.
100. Klay D, Grutters JC, van der Vis JJ, Platenburg MG, Kelder JC, Tromp E, van Moorsel CH. Progressive disease with low survival in adult patients with pulmonary fibrosis carrying surfactant-related gene mutations: an observational study. Chest. 2023;163(4):870–80.

101. Oldham JM, et al. TOLLIP, MUC5B, and the response to N-acetylcysteine among individuals with idiopathic pulmonary fibrosis. Am J Respir Crit Care Med. 2015;192:1475–82.
102. Fingerlin TE, et al. Genome-wide association study identifies multiple susceptibility loci for pulmonary fibrosis. Nat Genet. 2013;45:613–20.
103. Cai S, Allen RJ, Wain LV, Dudbridge F. Reassessing the association of MUC5B with survival in idiopathic pulmonary fibrosis. Ann Hum Genet. 2023;87:248–53.
104. Peljto AL, et al. Association between the MUC5B promoter polymorphism and survival in patients with idiopathic pulmonary fibrosis. JAMA. 2013;309:2232–9.
105. Hatabu H, et al. Interstitial lung abnormalities detected incidentally on CT: a position paper from the fleischner society. Lancet Respir Med. 2020;8:726–37.
106. Grant-Orser A, Min B, Elmrayed S, Podolanczuk AJ, Johannson KA. Prevalence, risk factors, and outcomes of adult interstitial lung abnormalities: a systematic review and meta-analysis. Am J Respir Crit Care Med. 2023;208:695–708.
107. Maus MTK, Groen K, van der Vis JJ, Grutters JC, van Moorsel CHM. Optimizing screening for early disease detection in familial pulmonary fibrosis (FLORIS): a prospective cohort study design. J Clin Med. 2023;12
108. Rose JA, et al. Progressive interstitial lung disease in relatives of patients with pulmonary fibrosis. Am J Respir Crit Care Med. 2023;207:211–4.
109. Park S, et al. Long-term follow-up of interstitial lung abnormality: implication in follow-up strategy and risk thresholds. Am J Respir Crit Care Med. 2023;208:858–67.
110. Wilson, J., & Jungner, G. (1968). Principles and practice of screening. WHO: Geneva, 69(5), 1085.
111. Park Y, Ahn C, Kim TH. Occupational and environmental risk factors of idiopathic pulmonary fibrosis: a systematic review and meta-analyses. Sci Rep. 2021;11:4318.
112. Cui F, et al. Air pollutants, genetic susceptibility and risk of incident idiopathic pulmonary fibrosis. Eur Respir J. 2023;61
113. De Sadeleer LJ, et al. Clinical behaviour of patients exposed to organic dust and diagnosed with idiopathic pulmonary fibrosis. Respirology. 2018;23:1160–5.
114. Yoon HY, Kim SY, Kim OJ, Song JW. Nitrogen dioxide increases the risk of mortality in idiopathic pulmonary fibrosis. Eur Respir J. 2021;57
115. Sesé L, et al. Role of atmospheric pollution on the natural history of idiopathic pulmonary fibrosis. Thorax. 2018;73:145–50.
116. Leclercq B, et al. Genetic and epigenetic alterations in normal and sensitive COPD-diseased human bronchial epithelial cells repeatedly exposed to air pollution-derived PM(2.5). Environ Pollut. 2017;230:163–77.
117. Gandhi SA, et al. The impact of occupational exposures on the risk of idiopathic pulmonary fibrosis: a systematic review and meta-analysis. Ann Am Thorac Soc. 2024;21:486–98.
118. Justet A, et al. Safety and efficacy of pirfenidone and nintedanib in patients with idiopathic pulmonary fibrosis and carrying a telomere-related gene mutation. Eur Respir J. 2021;57
119. Dressen A, et al. Analysis of protein-altering variants in telomerase genes and their association with MUC5B common variant status in patients with idiopathic pulmonary fibrosis: a candidate gene sequencing study. Lancet Respir Med. 2018;6:603–14.
120. Zhang D, et al. Telomere length and immunosuppression in non-idiopathic pulmonary fibrosis interstitial lung disease. Eur Respir J. 2023;62
121. Adegunsoye A, et al. Leukocyte telomere length and mycophenolate therapy in chronic hypersensitivity pneumonitis. Eur Respir J. 2021;57
122. Kistler KD, Nalysnyk L, Rotella P, Esser D. Lung transplantation in idiopathic pulmonary fibrosis: a systematic review of the literature. BMC Pulm Med. 2014;14:139.
123. Bennett D, et al. Lung transplant in patients with familial pulmonary fibrosis. J Bras Pneumol. 2020;46:e20200032.
124. Lari SM, et al. Lung transplantation for familial pulmonary fibrosis. J Heart Lung Transplant. 2019;38:S325–6.

125. Borie R, et al. Severe hematologic complications after lung transplantation in patients with telomerase complex mutations. J Heart Lung Transplant. 2015;34:538–46.
126. Tokman S, et al. Clinical outcomes of lung transplant recipients with telomerase mutations. J Heart Lung Transplant. 2015;34:1318–24.
127. Silhan LL, et al. Lung transplantation in telomerase mutation carriers with pulmonary fibrosis. Eur Respir J. 2014;44:178.
128. Courtwright AM, et al. Shorter telomere length following lung transplantation is associated with clinically significant leukopenia and decreased chronic lung allograft dysfunction-free survival. ERJ Open Res. 2020;6
129. Mackintosh JA, et al. TELO-SCOPE study: a randomised, double-blind, placebo-controlled, phase 2 trial of danazol for short telomere related pulmonary fibrosis. BMJ Open Respir Res. 2021;8
130. Hoffman TW, van Moorsel CHM, van der Vis JJ, Biesma DH, Grutters JC. No effect of danazol treatment in patients with advanced idiopathic pulmonary fibrosis. ERJ Open Res. 2023;9
131. Jaijyan DK, et al. New intranasal and injectable gene therapy for healthy life extension. Proc Natl Acad Sci USA. 2022;119:e2121499119.
132. Ramunas J, et al. Transient delivery of modified mRNA encoding TERT rapidly extends telomeres in human cells. FASEB J. 2015;29:1930–9.
133. Terwiel M, et al. Genetic testing in interstitial lung disease: an international survey. Respirology. 2022;27:747–57.
134. Carmichael N, et al. Psychological impact of genetic and clinical screening for pulmonary fibrosis on asymptomatic first-degree relatives of affected individuals. Thorax. 2021;76:621–3.
135. Abacan M, et al. The global state of the genetic counseling profession. Eur J Hum Genet. 2019;27:183–97.
136. Glenn LM, Troy LK, Corte TJ. Diagnosing interstitial lung disease by multidisciplinary discussion: a review. Front Med (Lausanne). 2022;9:1017501.

# Chapter 3
# Genetic Biomarkers for Interstitial Lung Disease

**David Zhang and Chad A. Newton**

## Introduction

The Human Genome Project brought forward the idea that an individual's genetic variation could be leveraged to personalize clinical care [1]. Since then, major technologic and analytic advancements along with drastically reduced costs have ushered genomics into clinical practice. In fact, it is now standard practice to utilize genetic information for routine management of patients with cancer and cystic fibrosis [2] or to personalize medication strategies and dosage for a wide range of diseases [3]. Our understanding of the genetic underpinnings of interstitial lung diseases has greatly improved with a plethora of studies highlighting complex genetic contributions to disease susceptibility. In addition, recent studies have demonstrated that genomic features also contribute to disease progression and influence the response to ILD-directed therapies. These seminal findings have not only improved understanding of the pathobiology of the ILDs but also provided a framework for the potential utility of genetics-based biomarkers that could advance disease categorization and management. The ILD field is on the verge of embracing genetic evaluations for subsets of ILD patients, which has the potential to usher in a new era of ILD personalized management for subsets of patients who meet specific criteria. In this chapter, we will review research and clinical requirements of genetic biomarkers and discuss their potential impact on patient care. We will also review the current understanding of the genetic contributors to ILD and highlight key

D. Zhang
Department of Medicine, Columbia University Irving Medical Center, New York, NY, USA
e-mail: dz2409@cumc.columbia.edu

C. A. Newton (✉)
Department of Internal Medicine, University of Texas Southwestern Medical Center, Dallas, TX, USA
e-mail: Chad.Newton@UTSouthwestern.edu



B. F. Collins, S. B. Montesi (eds.), *Precision Medicine in Interstitial Lung Disease*, Respiratory Medicine, https://doi.org/10.1007/978-3-031-87183-2_3

findings that suggest genetic information could be leveraged in the current ILD management schema. Lastly, we will extrapolate recent findings to frame how genetic biomarkers could be used to improve management of interstitial lung diseases.

## Genetic Biomarkers

Biomarkers have become an increasingly utilized tool to inform care for patients who suffer from disease. In general, biomarkers allow for objectively defining disease states, refining risk and natural history expectations, and informing management decisions [4]. Because of this, there have been massive efforts to leverage molecular information to identify, validate, and implement the use of biomarkers to improve the delivery of care in hopes of improving patient health.

Genomic biomarkers are unique in that they can, at birth, inform the likelihood to which an individual person is to develop a disease or a specific manifestation. Genetic biomarkers alone can be diagnostic for specific genetic syndromes that cluster within families. Unlike transcriptomic- or proteomic-based biomarkers, the germline genomic sequence is immutable and allows researchers to study the ontologically earliest consequences of genetic variation on disease manifestations. Therefore, genomic markers not only inform pathobiology of Mendelian disorders but offer insights into complex disorders driven by both genetic and nongenetic etiologies.

Although there is significant potential for genomic biomarkers to impact patient care, their translation to from discovery to clinical implementation must follow systematic evaluations that demonstrate increasingly stringent evidence of the utility and validity of the biomarker (Fig. 3.1) [5]. As with any biomarker, genomic biomarkers must have established characteristics that allow its clinical use. First, biomarkers must be plausibly linked with the biologic processes that are known or suspected to cause disease. Second, biomarkers must be easily measured without causing substantial risk, inexpensive, and produce timely results. The costs and lag

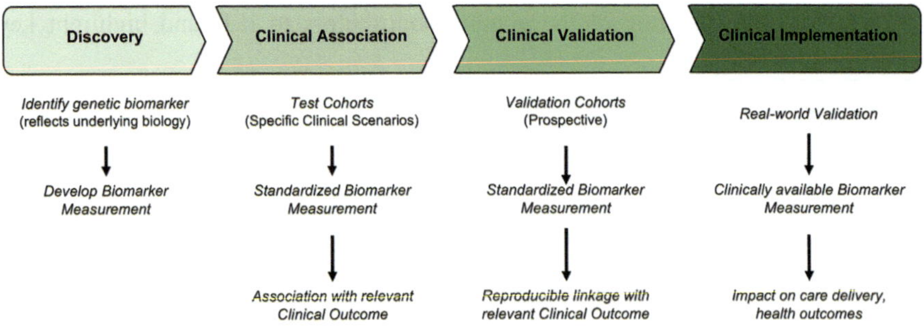


**Fig. 3.1** Discovery to implementation pipeline for genetic biomarkers

time of genetic evaluations are improving, and the bodily risk is not a significant limitation for germline genetic markers which can easily be assessed from peripheral blood or buccal mucosa cells. However, assessing somatic genetic variation in diseased lung tissue of ILD patients may carry substantial risk [6]. Third, genetic biomarkers should be precisely measured and objectively defined. For genetic variants, clinicians and researchers can reference curated variant databases like ClinGen [7] to determine variant pathogenicity. The interpretation algorithm is well established by the American College of Medical Genetics Guidelines (ACMG) which recommends categorizing variants into five categories to denote evidence of pathogenicity [8]. At times, genetic variants are unable to be confidently categorized as either pathogenic or benign so are labeled variants of undetermined significance (VUS). Although the ACMG outlines steps to take for patients with VUS, the presence of yet to be classified variants highlights challenges with interpretation of genetic sequencing. Interpretation of other genomic biomarkers such as telomere length and polygenic risk scores is also challenging given the continuous nature of these variables is dependent on the context in which they are evaluated. Lastly, genetic biomarkers must be rigorously linked with clinically meaningful endpoints. These translational studies should calculate test performance characteristics to demonstrate the biomarker's ability to improve decision-making or care delivery over standard practices. Larger studies are then needed to assess the clinical implementation of the biomarker with respect to decision-making, patient outcomes, and costs in the real-world setting. Collectively, these arduous steps serve as gatekeepers to ensure that validated and helpful biomarkers survive the journey from discovery to clinical use.

## Genetic ILD Biomarker Domains

The domain in which a biomarker offers clinically actionable information should be context specific (Table 3.1). In the ILD realm, genetic biomarkers may offer insight into disease susceptibility, diagnosis, prognosis, or response to therapy. Although the general steps from discovery to validation to implementation are similar, the study design and analyses differ across domains.

### *Susceptibility Genetic Biomarkers in ILD*

The logical application of genomic biomarkers is in assessing the ILD development risk in a healthy individual. Examples of genomic susceptibility markers include the *BRCA1/2* mutations linked to breast and ovarian cancer predisposition [9, 10]. Case-control study designs with both healthy and diseased individuals are typically used to identify and validate susceptibility biomarkers which include genome-wide association studies (for common variants) and candidate gene studies (for rare

**Table 3.1** Genomic biomarker domains, definitions, and potential ILD applications

| Biomarker domain | Definition | Potential population | Potential ILD application |
|---|---|---|---|
| Susceptibility | Informs risk of unaffected individual developing disease | Unaffected relatives within FPF kindred, high-risk occupations | Targeted ILD screening, surveillance programs |
| Diagnostic | Identify disease presence, differentiate between disease subtypes | Newly established ILD patients | Group into current subtypes and/or identify novel subtypes |
| Prognostic | Informs risk of clinically relevant future event | All ILD patients | Estimate prognosis, set monitoring frequency, timing of treatment and/or lung transplant referral |
| Predictive | Informs response to treatment or intervention | ILD patients requiring therapy | Medication selection and sequence |

variants). These approaches often employ regression-based methods to demonstrate that a variant, or group of variants, is enriched in either the cases (disease-associated) or controls (protective). However, statistical enrichment alone is insufficient to classify a variant as a susceptibility biomarker. Functional analyses are required to confirm that the variant impacts biologic pathways to produce disease.

Susceptibility biomarkers are generally used to guide entry into screening programs or to institute effective preventative strategies for high-risk but unaffected individuals. The presence of *BRCA1/2* mutations provides information that informs timing and frequency of screening breast imaging mammography or even preventative surgeries. Unfortunately, there are no validated preventative options that reduce the risk of ILD development. Therefore, studies evaluating genetic ILD susceptibility markers have focused on screening and surveillance to identify early disease which may be more amenable to disease-modifying therapies.

## *Diagnostic Genetic ILD Biomarkers*

Diagnostic biomarkers are utilized to detect or confirm the presence of a disease or to separate individuals into subcategories of disease. Genetic biomarkers are not needed to establish the presence of ILD itself, which is easily detected by chest radiology. For patients with clinical history or exam findings concerning for ILD, high-resolution computed tomography is widely utilized and sufficient to determine if ILD is present. Therefore, it is unlikely that biomarkers, genetic or otherwise, will supplant the use of radiology to establish ILD diagnosis. However, diagnostic biomarkers could potentially be useful for identifying disease states that precede gross radiographic findings. In addition, diagnostic biomarkers could also aid in ILD subclassification akin to the *EGFR* mutations and *ALK* rearrangements used to subclassify lung adenocarcinomas. The current classification schema utilizes clinical, radiologic, and pathologic features to group patients into seemingly discrete diagnostic groups according to phenotype and suspected underlying disease etiology [11–14]. Recently, disease course has also been incorporated into the ILD diagnostic classification with the advent of the progressive pulmonary fibrosis designation [12]. Novel biomarkers also offer the potential to refine diagnostic categorization according to underlying biology, which may offer additional insights into disease behavior and therapeutic targets.

Regardless of the categorization schema, the analytic process of defining and validating diagnostic biomarkers is similar. Cohort and case-control studies are used to determine if a genetic biomarker is statistically enriched in patients with disease or disease subcategory. Further analyses to calculate performance characteristics (sensitivity, specificity), diagnostic accuracy (positive and negative predictive value), and discriminative ability (area under the receiver operating characteristic curve) to inform diagnosis and/or diagnostic subgrouping are required to grade the ability of the biomarker to inform categorization beyond standard practices. Although reasonable performance of a diagnostic genetic ILD biomarker is necessary, the diagnosis or disease subcategory must also be clinically relevant. In the lung cancer example, *EGFR* mutations are associated with poor prognosis and differential response to specific therapeutic agents which justifies *EGFR* status assessment. Therefore, incorporating potential genetic biomarkers into the ILD diagnostic process could not only improve disease subcategorization but also improve understanding of the underlying disease processes.

## Prognostic Genetic ILD Biomarkers

A prognostic biomarker reliably indicates the differential risk of a clinical event occurring at some point in the future. The "event" is dependent on the disease and the potential clinical utility of the marker. Time to death is the ultimate outcome for fatal conditions like many ILDs; however, more proximal events such as symptomatic worsening, lung function decline, radiographic progression, or the need for lung transplantation can be utilized depending on the clinical context and the aim of the biomarker usage. Composite endpoints can also be used to increase the event rate and retain statistical power using smaller datasets. Typically, potential prognostic biomarkers are first evaluated in longitudinal cohort studies where the biomarker is assessed at a predetermined baseline and then patients are followed over time to collect event occurrence data. The potential biomarker is linked to future events using time-to-event analyses that often account for other factors that could influence the biomarker and time to the event (i.e., confounders). These analyses not only quantify key associations between the biomarker and the outcome event but also quantify the relative impact of other factors that may affect event risk.

Although typical prognostic markers forecast the risk for a binary event during follow-up, linking a biomarker with differential disease course also falls under the prognostic biomarker domain. For ILD, most studies focus on change in lung function over time using a repeated measures framework. Given that progressive decline in serial lung function is a poor prognostic indicator alone, biomarkers that are linked to both progression and survival offer a distinct advantage to clinicians whose main focus is to mitigate progression. Although the clinical relevance of prognostic biomarkers is clear, they also could be leveraged in the design of clinical trials through enrichment strategies that preferentially enroll high-risk patients that are more likely to experience the primary outcome to reduce sample size and duration of the study.

### Predictive Genetic ILD Biomarkers

Predictive genetic biomarkers are used to identify individuals that differentially respond to a particular intervention or treatment. For ILD studies, "response" could indicate differential change in lung function or time-to-event, depending on the clinical context and potential application of the biomarker. In general, predictive biomarkers are often assessed using interaction testing within statistical models to determine if the presence of a genetic marker modifies the effect of treatment on an outcome. Because of this framework, predictive biomarkers should be measured at or before treatment and then linked to future response to the intervention. Initial discovery of predictive genetic biomarkers may be borne out of observational cohort studies, although care to account for systematic bias related to treatment exposure and effect is needed. Another avenue to explore predictive biomarkers is through post hoc analyses of randomized controlled trials which take advantage of the random treatment allocation to overcome some potential biases intrinsic to observational studies. Ideally, these analyses would generate information needed to conduct prospective stratified or enriched prospective clinical trials in which the biomarker is used to select or group study participants. These trials not only validate the ability of the predictive biomarker but also quantify the effect of the intervention across biomarker stratified groups which ultimately informs clinical care.

## Genetic Architecture of ILD

The initial description of familial pulmonary fibrosis came in 1907 by Sandoz et al., detailing twin sisters who were found to have stiff lungs and increased interstitial tissue on necropsy [15]. This observation was extended in the 1950s through a series of reports describing relatives with fibrotic lung disease, further solidifying the idea that heritable traits may contribute to familial transmission of ILD [16–18]. This entity is now called familial pulmonary fibrosis (FPF) which is defined by the presence of fibrotic ILD occurring in at least two blood relatives [19]. The prevalence of FPF among more common diagnoses of ILD ranges from 5% of patients with connective tissue disease-related ILD (CTD-ILD) to upward of 25% of patients with idiopathic pulmonary fibrosis (IPF). Relatives within FPF kindred are enriched for heritable genetic factors that predispose ILD; however, individuals with sporadic forms of ILD may also harbor similar genetic architecture to their FPF counterparts. While patients are often separated into either familial or sporadic subsets based on family history, the underlying biology likely represents a spectrum of genetic variations that contribute to disease development. This suggests that studying FPF kindreds can provide insight into pathobiology that also underlies the broader population of ILD and allows clinicians to leverage genetic discoveries in both FPF and sporadic ILD patients. These observations have led to in-depth investigations into genetic explanations for the heritable risk underlying various forms of ILD.

The current known genetic landscape of ILD is best understood through discoveries made in its prototypic form, IPF. Over the past two decades, genetic studies have implicated numerous genetic factors in the risk of developing IPF. These include common variants identified through genome-wide association studies (GWAS) [20–23], rare variants discovered through whole exome sequencing studies (WES) [24–28] or familial aggregation studies [29–36], and structural elements including telomere length [37–42]. To date, these genetic discoveries have led to recognition of highly penetrant rare mutations in telomere maintenance genes or surfactant metabolism genes in large kindreds of familial pulmonary fibrosis. Despite the advancements in genetic analyses, inclusion of larger number of individuals and families, and the improvement in genetic sequencing interpretation, a sizable portion of familial cases remain without a genetic diagnosis [26–28, 43]. This missing heritability is likely due to several factors including single small effect and rare mutations, additive multigenic variation, and the complex interplay between underlying genetic variation and specific environmental exposure that contributes to lung fibrosis.

## Overview of Individual ILD Genetic Biomarkers

### *Rare Genetic Variants*

The advent of next-generation sequencing technology, including whole exome and whole genome sequencing, has led to increasing efforts to catalog rare genetic mutations in ILD. While initial studies focused on these mutations as risk factors for developing idiopathic pulmonary fibrosis (IPF) or familial pulmonary fibrosis (FPF), it has become increasingly recognized that carrying such mutations can impact prognosis and management. In contrast to common single-nucleotide polymorphisms (SNPs), a rare mutation is present in far less than 1% of the alleles in the general population and causes a disruption or full loss of function of the gene's protein product. Because of this, rare and pathogenic variants are sufficient to cause ILD.

One of the first rare mutations described in ILD is in genes that govern surfactant metabolism including *SFTPC* [44, 45]. These mutations were initially found in families of patients with ILD but subsequently identified in sporadic cases as well. Importantly, initial reports described both adult and pediatric patients linking these cases to already described reports of neonatal lung disease in infants with autosomal recessive *SFTPB* mutations. Subsequently, mutations in *SFTPA1* and *SFTPA2* were also linked with ILD as well as lung cancer [46, 47]. These surfactant gene mutations are rare even among adult FPF patients, accounting for 1–2% of such cases. A recent large report cataloging surfactant gene mutation carriers also identified an increased prevalence of lung cancer which may be driven by a few highly penetrant families with such mutations [48].

Rare damaging mutations in telomere-related genes, such as *TERT*, *TERC*, *PARN*, and *RTEL1*, are the most well-characterized rare variants in IPF and FPF and increase the odds of developing disease by 8- to 40-fold [24, 26–28]. These genes serve primarily to maintain the telomere length of cells to prevent critical shortening that triggers cellular consequences such as DNA damage and senescence. Rare variants in these four genes alone can be identified in 20% of FPF patients [26–28, 43] and 10% of IPF patients undergoing transplant regardless of family history [24]. Additional genes that impact telomere biology have been identified in case series or large families with pulmonary fibrosis or syndromic cases of dyskeratosis congenita including *DKC1*, *TINF2*, *NAF1*, *NHP2*, *NOP10*, *WRAP53*, *CTC1*, *ZCCHC8*, and *ACD* [29, 31, 33, 35, 49, 50]. In general, carriers of these mutations have pathologically short age-adjusted telomere lengths, often below the first percentile [51], as well as a uniformly poor prognosis regardless of the clinical subtype of ILD diagnosed [52].

Recent reports have highlighted rare mutations in *KIF15* [26–28] and *SPDL1* [53] enriched in patients with pulmonary fibrosis. These genes encode proteins that play key roles in mitotic spindle formation and cell division. Rare damaging variants in *KIF15* were identified in about 1% of patients with IPF or FPF and collectively conferred fourfold increased odds of developing disease in both patients of European and non-European ancestry [26–28]. One *KIF15* variant (rs138043992) that encodes for a rare missense mutation was associated with earlier onset of IPF as well as earlier time to death or transplant [54]. In a separate study, a rare missense mutation in *SPDL1* (rs116483731) was also noted to be associated with risk of developing IPF. This missense mutation was noted to be present in about 2% of sporadic IPF cases and conferred a twofold increased odds of disease [53]. Notably, both the *KIF15* missense (rs138043992) and the *SPDL1* missense (rs116483731) mutation were significantly more enriched in the general Finnish population compared to non-Finnish Europeans, suggesting additional ancestry-specific risk. However, in contrast to common variants which are heavily influenced by genetic ancestry, rare variants in *TERT*, *PARN*, *RTEL1*, and *KIF15* generally confer similar risk regardless of European vs. non-European ancestry [26–28].

Rare germline mutations are strong ILD susceptibility biomarkers given their large effect size on not only the patient but also family members who inherit the mutation. In one study of asymptomatic family members who carry rare *TERT* mutations associated with IPF demonstrated that 80% of them had quantifiable interstitial abnormalities on chest CT [55]. Therefore, clinicians can couple the family history with rare variant testing to inform susceptibility risk for unaffected relatives. In this scenario, genetic sequencing is first performed in an affected FPF patient. If a pathogenic or likely pathogenic variant is found, then unaffected relatives can then undergo testing for the same variant to personalize their susceptibility risk. For unaffected relatives who harbor disease-causing rare variants, active surveillance using symptoms assessments, physical exams, pulmonary function tests, and/or HRCT should allow clinicians to identify the earliest manifestation ILD to institute management plans. Although ongoing longitudinal studies are examining optimal screening and surveillance strategies, rare variants in FPF-causing genes represent clear genetic susceptibility markers that can be utilized to identify at-risk unaffected relatives within FPF kindred.

Rare variants can also serve as diagnostic genetic biomarkers for patients with syndromic presentations. Hermansky-Pudlak Syndrome (HPS) is typified by oculocutaneous albinism, bleeding diathesis due to platelet dysfunction, colitis, and pulmonary fibrosis [56, 57]. In total, there are ten genetic subtypes of HPS, of which the HPS-1 (*HPS1* gene), HPS-2 (*AP3B1* gene), and HSP-4 (*HPS4* gene) subtypes confer higher prevalence of pulmonary fibrosis [58–61]. These genetic disorders arise from pathogenic mutations in genes that contribute to lysosomal organelle formation and intracellular vesicle trafficking, although the exact mechanism by which this leads to pulmonary fibrosis remains unclear. For kindred with FPF and extrapulmonary manifestations suggestive of HPS, rare variants in the HPS genes are diagnostic.

Individuals who harbor rare variants in known genes can exhibit a wide variety of ILD phenotypes. Although IPF tends to be the most common subtype attributed to patients who harbor rare variants in telomere and surfactant gene variants, individuals can develop other idiopathic interstitial pneumonias and ILD of known causes such as hypersensitivity pneumonitis and connective tissue disease ILD. In fact, relatives within FPF kindred who harbor the same disease-causing rare variant can manifest discordant ILD diagnoses suggesting poor genotype-phenotype correlation [52]. This means that rare variants poorly discriminate across the current diagnostic subtypes. Despite this, rare variants in telomere genes still offer prognostic information. Multiple observational studies have demonstrated that variants in *TERT*, *TERC*, *PARN*, and *RTEL1* are associated with rapid loss of lung function and worse survival compared to non-carriers [52, 62, 63]. Although prospective validation is required, these data may allow clinicians to use these prognostic genomic markers to inform monitoring for individual patients.

## *Telomere Length*

The prevalence of rare telomere gene mutations in FPF and sporadic ILD has led to the recognition of telomere length, which is maintained by telomere genes, as an independent genomic contributor to ILD development. Telomeres are the caps of six nucleotide repeats on the ends of chromosomes that protect the exome from progressive loss during cellular replication. The length of the telomere is maintained by telomerase, a ribonucleoprotein composed of a reverse transcriptase (*TERT*) and an RNA template (*TERC*) [64, 65]. Telomeres normally shorten with cellular replication and advancing age; therefore, older individuals have, on average, shorter telomeres than younger individuals [66]. However, pathologic telomere shortening occurs when telomeres are unexpectedly short based on the age of the individual. Therefore, the assessment of excessive telomere shortening requires age adjustment using nomograms generated from healthy control subjects.

Although rare variants in telomere maintenance genes cause pathologic telomere shortening, other factors such as chronic infection [67], inflammation [68, 69], smoking [70], and socioeconomic stressors [71–76] can also contribute to telomere attrition. It is estimated that while rare damaging telomere gene mutations are present in upward of 10% of IPF patients [26–28], short telomere length below the tenth percentile adjusted for age can be found in 30–50% IPF patients regardless of mutation status [77, 78]. Cases of "unexplained" short telomeres without rare variants may be attributable to common variant polygenic risk [26–28] or to rare variants in yet-to-be identified telomere genes. A recent Mendelian randomization study suggested that genetic liability to short telomere length may be causal for IPF [79].

Dyskeratosis congenita is a pediatric genetic disorder resulting from extreme telomere shortening that classically manifests as oral leukoplakia, lacy reticular skin pigmentation, and dystrophic nails. The life-limiting manifestation for most DC patients is bone marrow failure; however, pulmonary fibrosis often develops in later adolescence or early adulthood. Up to 70% of patients with DC have rare variants in telomere genes, which largely overlap with adult-onset FPF genes but are transmitted through various inheritance patterns (X-linked, autosomal recessive, autosomal dominant) [80]. Although genetic sequencing can identify rare variants in telomere genes, extremely short age-adjusted telomere length < first percentile is diagnostic of DC in the correct clinical context [81, 82]. Therefore, telomere length is a diagnostic biomarker for short telomere syndromes such as DC. In patients with pulmonary fibrosis with or without extrapulmonary manifestations such as premature hair greying, cryptogenic cirrhosis, or cytopenias, telomere length below the first percentile can increase the pretest probability for identifying a pathogenic telomere-gene mutation [51]. These mutations can also provide supporting evidence for the pathogenicity of variants of uncertain significance (VUS) in telomere-related genes.

As a parallel to telomere gene rare variants, short telomere length can be found in patients with a variety of ILD subtypes. In non-IPF ILDs, telomere length below tenth percentile is prevalent and found in ~30% of patients with hypersensitivity pneumonitis, rheumatoid arthritis ILD, and unclassifiable ILD and 10% of patients with other forms of connective tissue disease ILD [42, 77, 78, 83]. While telomere length does not discriminate between clinical ILD diagnoses, telomere shortening represents a common genetic and biologic vulnerability to progressive pulmonary fibrosis. Studies have demonstrated shorter telomere length as a reliable prognostic biomarker as it is associated with increased mortality and progressive lung function decline in multiple subtypes of ILD including IPF, unclassifiable ILD, fibrotic hypersensitivity pneumonitis, and connective tissue disease ILD. Therefore, recognition of this prognostic factor could prompt increased vigilance for progressive pulmonary fibrosis in non-IPF patients, so that appropriate therapies and/or transplant referral can be instituted in a timely fashion.

Recent studies have also postulated that telomere length may serve as a predictive ILD biomarker. In a post hoc analysis of the PANTHER study, combination treatment with prednisone, azathioprine, and N-acetylcysteine (NAC) was associated with worse composite endpoint-free survival for IPF patients who harbored age-adjusted telomere length < tenth percentile and was replicated in two additional IPF cohorts [77, 78]. The predictive ability of telomere length has also been extended to non-IPF forms of ILD through multicenter studies which demonstrated that mycophenolate or azathioprine exposure was associated with reduced transplant-free survival for patients with age-adjusted telomere length < tenth percentile [83]. Together, these data suggest that telomere length may represent a predictive biomarker that crosses ILD diagnostic categories and could inform medication selection pending prospective validation of the harmful pharmacogenomic interaction. However, in cases where empiric immunosuppressive therapy is being considered, identifying a telomere length below the tenth percentile may confer additional risk of harm and help inform the risks and benefits of treatment for ILDs without approved therapies.

## *Common Genetic Variants*

Increasingly larger GWAS studies have now identified over 20 independent genetic loci associated with IPF in clinical cohorts and multi-ancestry biobanks. These loci harbor common SNPs that are often located within intronic gene regulatory elements that influence gene transcription. Importantly, common variants are prevalent in at least 5% of alleles within the general population but are statistically enriched in individuals with disease. While many identified common variants confer small but significant susceptibility risk of IPF, a few well-characterized polymorphisms have been additionally identified as prognostic, predictive, or susceptibility biomarkers for non-IPF ILDs as well.

A polymorphism in *MUC5B* (rs35705950) was initially found to be enriched in a cohort of sporadic and familial pulmonary fibrosis [84] and subsequently validated as the single highest effect size common variant for IPF risk [20]. It is estimated that the rs35705950 polymorphism is present in nearly three quarters of patients with IPF compared to roughly 20% of healthy controls of European ancestry, conferring nearly fourfold increased odds of IPF. This SNP lies in the promoter region of *MUC5B* and is linked to increased expression of MUC5B, a mucin with key roles in lung mucociliary clearance. Studies carried out in mice suggest that overexpression of *Muc5b* exaggerates fibrosis induced by bleomycin [85]. Further investigation of this polymorphism identified its role in conferring disease risk for several other forms of ILD including chronic hypersensitivity pneumonitis [42], rheumatoid arthritis-associated ILD [86], and certain forms of unclassifiable ILD such as interstitial pneumonitis with autoimmune features [77, 78]. Recent large-scale analyses of healthy adults have also demonstrated a link between the *MUC5B* polymorphism and increased risk of developing interstitial lung abnormalities [87], which can be a precursor to clinically significant pulmonary fibrosis. Common polymorphisms in *FAM13A* (rs2013701) and *DSP* (rs2076295) have also been identified as risk alleles for IPF [20]. Interestingly, both SNPs have also been associated with genetic risk of COPD, but with opposite directions of effect [88, 89]. Additionally, the rs2076295 *DSP* SNP may also be associated with longitudinal change in quantitative emphysema [90] but was not found to be associated with longitudinal lung function in IPF [91].

Initial studies suggested an intriguing effect of increased survival among IPF carriers of the *MUC5B* variant. This paradoxical effect was initially attributed to index-case bias [92], but more recent reports debunk this in favor of a more neutral effect on survival [93]. Indeed, a recent large GWAS on IPF survival did not identify *MUC5B* as associated with increased or decreased survival [91, 94]. However, in non-IPF forms of ILD, the *MUC5B* SNP may predispose to an "IPF-like" phenotype and differential survival. In patients with hypersensitivity pneumonitis, connective tissue disease ILD, and interstitial pneumonia with autoimmune features, the presence of the *MUC5B* polymorphism was associated with around twofold higher mortality risk [77, 78]. Recent GWAS studies focusing on outcomes in IPF have implicated additional SNPs in *PKN2* (rs115982800, associated with longitudinal lung function) [91] and *PCSK6* (rs35647788, associated with mortality) [91, 94]. Interestingly, previous SNPs associated with IPF disease risk were not associated with either lung function trajectory or mortality, including the *MUC5B* promoter SNP. However, both of these prognostic SNPs are relatively rare in IPF patients, present in 1–6% of alleles and account for a small minority of outcomes overall.

The genetic region surrounding *MUC5B* also contains SNPs in the region of the *TOLLIP* gene (rs111521887, rs5743894, rs5743890) initially identified as risk alleles for developing disease [23]. However, follow-up studies confirmed that this risk was tied to its proximity to the *MUC5B* SNP (rs35705950) [20]. These *TOLLIP* SNPs are thought to mediate the pulmonary innate immune system through toll-like receptor signaling. Another *TOLLIP* SNP has been postulated to represent a predictive genomic biomarker. The rs3750920 was associated with differential survival for IPF patients exposed to NAC therapy with the TT genotype showing protection, whereas the GG genotype conferred harm in a post hoc analysis of the PANTHER trial data [95]. Based on the function of *TOLLIP*, it is postulated that this effect may be related to host defense and dysbiosis in the lung microbiome [96]. Importantly, the first genomic-driven randomized controlled trial in the ILD field is currently underway to validate the TOLLIP-NAC relationship which will undoubtedly pave the way for future molecularly enriched clinical trials of ILD patients [97].

While common variants may have utility as predictive ILD biomarkers as evidenced by the pharmacogenetic interactions with *TOLLIP* and NAC, they generally provide limited utility as susceptibility biomarkers given their high prevalence among the general populace. Aside from the unusually high effect size of the highly prevalent *MUC5B* polymorphism, most common variants related to ILD are identified in GWAS studies and confer less than twofold odds of disease [20]. When factoring in the rarity of ILD and the high prevalence of common variants, the attributable risk of each common variant individually explains less than 1% of the genetic liability in the general population [98]. Even among a preselected population with increased risk of ILD, such as first-degree relatives of patients with ILD, the *MUC5B* polymorphism was present in about 40% of relatives without interstitial lung abnormalities [99, 100], considered to be a preclinical precursor to ILD.

## *Polygenic Risk Scores*

A combination of common genetic variation comprises a polygenic risk score that encapsulates additive genetic risk of ILD that goes beyond the effect of individual SNPs. These scores may include just a few dozen common variants with the highest significance in GWAS studies or thousands of SNPs with fine-tuned effect sizes calculated via regression methods. These polygenic scores improved clinical prediction of IPF diagnosis beyond baseline clinical attributes. Even with exclusion of the high effect *MUC5B* rs35705950 polymorphism, polygenic scores remained highly associated with disease risk with those in the highest quintile of polygenic score having sevenfold odds of disease compared to those in the lowest quintile [101]. Therefore, polygenic scores may represent an avenue to combine multiple genetic contributors into an objective marker with defined thresholds to serve as a susceptibility genomic marker. Although further studies are needed, recent construction and evaluation of the IPF polygenic score also predicted both the prevalence and progression of interstitial lung abnormalities (ILA), thus furthering the potential utility of these scores in the future.

Polygenic risk scores of other phenotypes may also interact with IPF polygenic risk. A polygenic score associated with a healthy lifestyle score was additive to an IPF polygenic risk score when predicting incident risk of IPF [102]. A telomere length polygenic score was associated with "unexplained" short telomere length in IPF and FPF patients without rare telomere gene variants [26–28]. Of note, all existing polygenic scores are derived from GWAS studies that excluded patients of non-European ancestry and do not predict genetic risk of IPF in these ethnic and ancestry groups.

As a biomarker for ILD, polygenic risk scores can serve as a more robust susceptibility biomarker than individual common variants. In contrast to individual common variants which explain ~1% of IPF genetic risk, a polygenic risk score explained 4–14% of IPF genetic liability [101]. Predictive models that include this polygenic score improved discrimination of IPF when compared to a model that only included clinical characteristics in a selected cohort enriched for lung disease. Similarly, this IPF polygenic score improved discrimination of detecting subclinical ILA in a population-based cohort but with less discriminating power [101]. Further studies will be needed to understand the performance of such a test in a broader testing population.

## *Multi-Omic Markers in ILD*

In contrast to relatively static genetic markers, markers obtained from transcriptomic, epigenomic, and proteomic analyses can reflect a combination of host factors and lifetime exposures that influence disease activity. As such, these dynamic -omics markers may vary depending on the time of collection, whereas genetic germline markers are immutable since birth. Furthermore, due to ease and availability, -omics markers for ILD are commonly measured in peripheral blood samples which serve as surrogates for biologic processes occurring in the lung. Germline genetic markers on the other hand generally reflect inherited DNA changes present in every cell in the body. Nevertheless, transcriptomic, epigenomic, and proteomic markers can play a role in prognostication of IPF and non-IPF ILD.

Peripheral blood gene expression profiles correlate with several aspects of IPF including disease severity, transplant-free survival, and progressive lung function decline implicating both T lymphocytes [103, 104] and natural killer cells [105] in the disease process. Epigenetic DNA methylation profiles of fibrotic lung tissue in IPF differ when compared to healthy lung tissue and correspond to changes in gene expression [106]. Aptamer-based proteomic studies have uncovered proteomic signatures that correspond to transplant-free survival in IPF [94, 107] as well as progressive fibrosis in non-IPF ILD [108].

Studies that utilize multi-omics analyses incorporating two or more -omics layers have begun to refine the clinical relevance of these biomarkers. Integration of multi-omic features can help strengthen the biologic basis of identified biomarkers as being truly relevant to the pathobiology of disease. These early efforts have yielded hypothesis-generating data describing unique endotypes or novel disease pathways of disease. Larger -omics datasets paired with clinical data may be able to yield additional multi-omic markers that can be helpful for clinical care of ILD patients.

## Precision Diagnosis and Management Informed by Genetics

In-depth genetic evaluations in larger and deeply phenotyped cohorts are needed to further refine the validity of genomic biomarkers within specific clinical scenarios which could aid in decision-making and improve patient health (Table 3.2). However, studies to date have demonstrated the clear utility of genetics to inform susceptibility risk for relatives of FPF kindred. These monogenic forms of FPF serve as a testing ground to understand the risks and benefits of incorporating

**Table 3.2** Interstitial lung disease genomic biomarkers and domain

| | Susceptibility | Diagnostic | | Prognostic | | Predictive |
|---|---|---|---|---|---|---|
| | At risk for ILD | Define diagnosis | Define ILD subtype | Survival | progression | Interaction effects |
| *Rare variants* | | | | | | |
| Telomere genes (*TERT, TERC, PARN, RTEL1, TINF2, DKC1, NAF1, NHP2, NOP10, WRAP53, CTC1, ZCCHC8, ACD*) | ++ | – | – | + | + | – |
| Surfactant genes (*SFTPC, SFTPA1/2, ABCA3*) | ++ | – | – | – | – | – |
| HPS genes (*HPS1, HSP4, AP3B1*) | ++ | ++ HPS | – | – | – | – |
| KIF15, SPDL1 | ++ | – | | – | – | – |
| *Common variants* | | | | | | |
| *MUC5B* | + | – | – | ± | – | – |
| *TOLLIP* | ± | – | – | ± | – | + NAC |
| *PCSK6* | – | – | – | + | – | – |
| *PKN2* | – | – | – | – | + | – |
| Age-adjusted telomere length | – | ++ DC | – | + | + | + IS |
| Polygenic risk scores | + | – | – | – | + ILA | – |

Abbreviations: *ILD* interstitial lung disease, *HPS* Hermansky-Pudlak syndrome, *DC* Dyskeratosis congenita, *NAC-N*-acetylcysteine, *IS* immunosuppression, *ILA* interstitial lung abnormalities

genetic testing into clinical practice and to identify potential implementation barriers that must be overcome prior to widespread use. In addition, the evolution of the diagnostic categorization process has opened the door to incorporate molecular signatures, including genomic biomarkers, in the diagnostic process. Patients with specific genomic characteristics appear to experience differential progression and survival, which may serve as a substrate to further refine subclasses of ILD. The foundation has also been laid for how to discover and validate predictive genomic biomarkers. The list of potential genomic predictors of treatment response is only expected to grow as more therapeutics are being tested in larger and diverse ILD cohorts. Although these advances will undoubtedly impact the care and health of ILD patients, efforts must also be undertaken to reduce costs, streamline molecular testing, and educate clinicians and patients on the use and misuse of these technologies. The last 20 years have seen an explosion of genetics research, and the ILD field is now on the precipice of being able to leverage these discoveries to inform management.

## References


1. International Human Genome Sequencing, Consortium. Finishing the euchromatic sequence of the human genome. Nature. 2004;431:931–45.
2. Farrell PM, White TB, Ren CL, Hempstead SE, Accurso F, Derichs N, Howenstine M, McColley SA, Rock M, Rosenfeld M, Sermet-Gaudelus I, Southern KW, Marshall BC, Sosnay PR. Diagnosis of cystic fibrosis: consensus guidelines from the cystic fibrosis foundation. J Pediatr. 2017;181:S4-S15.
3. Relling MV, Klein TE. CPIC: clinical pharmacogenetics implementation consortium of the pharmacogenomics research network. Clin Pharmacol Ther. 2011;89:464–7.
4. Group, FDA-NIH Biomarker Working. *BEST (Biomarkers, EndpointS, and other Tools) Resource* (Food and Drug Administration (US); National Institutes of Health (US): Silver Spring (MD) Bethesda (MD)); 2016.
5. Pepe MS, Etzioni R, Feng Z, Potter JD, Thompson ML, Thornquist M, Winget M, Yasui Y. Phases of biomarker development for early detection of cancer. J Natl Cancer Inst. 2001;93:1054–61.
6. Hutchinson JP, Fogarty AW, McKeever TM, Hubbard RB. In-hospital mortality after surgical lung biopsy for interstitial lung disease in the United States. 2000 to 2011. Am J Respir Crit Care Med. 2016;193:1161–7.
7. Rehm HL, Berg JS, Brooks LD, Bustamante CD, Evans JP, Landrum MJ, Ledbetter DH, Maglott DR, Martin CL, Nussbaum RL, Plon SE, Ramos EM, Sherry ST, Watson MS. ClinGen – the clinical genome resource. N Engl J Med. 2015;372:2235–42.
8. Richards S, Aziz N, Bale S, Bick D, Das S, Gastier-Foster J, Grody WW, Hegde M, Lyon E, Spector E, Voelkerding K, Rehm HL. Standards and guidelines for the interpretation of sequence variants: a joint consensus recommendation of the American College of Medical Genetics and Genomics and the Association for Molecular Pathology. Genet Med. 2015;17:405–24.
9. Hall JM, Friedman L, Guenther C, Lee MK, Weber JL, Black DM, King MC. Closing in on a breast cancer gene on chromosome 17q. Am J Hum Genet. 1992;50:1235–42.
10. Wooster R, Neuhausen SL, Mangion J, Quirk Y, Ford D, Collins N, Nguyen K, Seal S, Tran T, Averill D, et al. Localization of a breast cancer susceptibility gene, BRCA2, to chromosome 13q12-13. Science. 1994;265:2088–90.
11. Fernández Pérez ER, Travis WD, Lynch DA, Brown KK, Johannson KA, Selman M, Ryu JH, Wells AU, Tony Huang YC, Pereira CAC, Scholand MB, Villar A, Inase N, Evans RB, Mette SA, Frazer-Green L. Executive summary: diagnosis and evaluation of hypersensitivity pneumonitis: chest guideline and expert panel report. Chest. 2021;160:595–615.
12. Raghu G, Remy-Jardin M, Richeldi L, Thomson CC, Inoue Y, Johkoh T, Kreuter M, Lynch DA, Maher TM, Martinez FJ, Molina-Molina M, Myers JL, Nicholson AG, Ryerson CJ, Strek ME, Troy LK, Wijsenbeek M, Mammen MJ, Hossain T, Bissell BD, Herman DD, Hon SM, Kheir F, Khor YH, Macrea M, Antoniou KM, Bouros D, Buendia-Roldan I, Caro F, Crestani B, Ho L, Morisset J, Olson AL, Podolanczuk A, Poletti V, Selman M, Ewing T, Jones S, Knight SL, Ghazipura M, Wilson KC. Idiopathic pulmonary fibrosis (an update) and progressive pulmonary fibrosis in adults: an official ATS/ERS/JRS/ALAT clinical practice guideline. Am J Respir Crit Care Med. 2022;205:e18–47.
13. Raghu G, Remy-Jardin M, Ryerson CJ, Myers JL, Kreuter M, Vasakova M, Bargagli E, Chung JH, Collins BF, Bendstrup E, Chami HA, Chua AT, Corte TJ, Dalphin JC, Danoff SK, Diaz-Mendoza J, Duggal A, Egashira R, Ewing T, Gulati M, Inoue Y, Jenkins AR, Johannson KA, Johkoh T, Tamae-Kakazu M, Kitaichi M, Knight SL, Koschel D, Lederer DJ, Mageto Y, Maier LA, Matiz C, Morell F, Nicholson AG, Patolia S, Pereira CA, Renzoni EA, Salisbury ML, Selman M, Walsh SLF, Wuyts WA, Wilson KC. Diagnosis of hypersensitivity pneumonitis in adults. An official ATS/JRS/ALAT clinical practice guideline. Am J Respir Crit Care Med. 2020;202:e36–69.

14. Travis WD, Costabel U, Hansell DM, King TE Jr, Lynch DA, Nicholson AG, Ryerson CJ, Ryu JH, Selman M, Wells AU, Behr J, Bouros D, Brown KK, Colby TV, Collard HR, Cordeiro CR, Cottin V, Crestani B, Drent M, Dudden RF, Egan J, Flaherty K, Hogaboam C, Inoue Y, Johkoh T, Kim DS, Kitaichi M, Loyd J, Martinez FJ, Myers J, Protzko S, Raghu G, Richeldi L, Sverzellati N, Swigris J, Valeyre D. An official American Thoracic Society/European respiratory society statement: update of the international multidisciplinary classification of the idiopathic interstitial pneumonias. Am J Respir Crit Care Med. 2013;188:733–48.
15. Sandoz E. Uber zwei Falle von fötaler Bronchektasie. Beitr Pathol Anat. 1907;41:495.
16. Donohue WL, Laski B, Uchida I, Munn JD. Familial fibrocystic pulmonary dysplasia and its relation to Hamman-Rich syndrome. Pediatrics. 1959;24:786–813.
17. Mac MJ. Familial pulmonary fibrosis. Dis Chest. 1951;20:426–36.
18. Peabody JW, Peabody JW Jr, Hayes EW, Hayes EW Jr. Idiopathic pulmonary fibrosis; its occurrence in identical twin sisters. Dis Chest. 1950;18:330–44.
19. Newton CA, Oldham JM, Applegate C, Carmichael N, Powell K, Dilling D, Schmidt SL, Scholand MB, Armanios M, Garcia CK, Kropski J, Talbert J. The role of genetic testing in pulmonary fibrosis: a perspective from the pulmonary fibrosis foundation genetic testing work group. Chest. 2022;
20. Allen RJ, Guillen-Guio B, Oldham JM, Ma SF, Dressen A, Paynton ML, Kraven LM, Obeidat M, Li X, Ng M, Braybrooke R, Molina-Molina M, Hobbs BD, Putman RK, Sakornsakolpat P, Booth HL, Fahy WA, Hart SP, Hill MR, Hirani N, Hubbard RB, McAnulty RJ, Millar AB, Navaratnam V, Oballa E, Parfrey H, Saini G, Whyte MKB, Zhang Y, Kaminski N, Adegunsoye A, Strek ME, Neighbors M, Sheng XR, Gudmundsson G, Gudnason V, Hatabu H, Lederer DJ, Manichaikul A, Newell JD Jr, O'Connor GT, Ortega VE, Xu H, Fingerlin TE, Bosse Y, Hao K, Joubert P, Nickle DC, Sin DD, Timens W, Furniss D, Morris AP, Zondervan KT, Hall IP, Sayers I, Tobin MD, Maher TM, Cho MH, Hunninghake GM, Schwartz DA, Yaspan BL, Molyneaux PL, Flores C, Noth I, Jenkins RG, Wain LV. Genome-wide association study of susceptibility to idiopathic pulmonary fibrosis. Am J Respir Crit Care Med. 2020;201:564–74.
21. Allen RJ, Porte J, Braybrooke R, Flores C, Fingerlin TE, Oldham JM, Guillen-Guio B, Ma SF, Okamoto T, John AE, Obeidat M, Yang IV, Henry A, Hubbard RB, Navaratnam V, Saini G, Thompson N, Booth HL, Hart SP, Hill MR, Hirani N, Maher TM, McAnulty RJ, Millar AB, Molyneaux PL, Parfrey H, Rassl DM, Whyte MKB, Fahy WA, Marshall RP, Oballa E, Bosse Y, Nickle DC, Sin DD, Timens W, Shrine N, Sayers I, Hall IP, Noth I, Schwartz DA, Tobin MD, Wain LV, Jenkins RG. Genetic variants associated with susceptibility to idiopathic pulmonary fibrosis in people of European ancestry: a genome-wide association study. Lancet Respir Med. 2017;5:869–80.
22. Fingerlin TE, Murphy E, Zhang W, Peljto AL, Brown KK, Steele MP, Loyd JE, Cosgrove GP, Lynch D, Groshong S, Collard HR, Wolters PJ, Bradford WZ, Kossen K, Seiwert SD, du Bois RM, Garcia CK, Devine MS, Gudmundsson G, Isaksson HJ, Kaminski N, Zhang Y, Gibson KF, Lancaster LH, Cogan JD, Mason WR, Maher TM, Molyneaux PL, Wells AU, Moffatt MF, Selman M, Pardo A, Kim DS, Crapo JD, Make BJ, Regan EA, Walek DS, Daniel JJ, Kamatani Y, Zelenika D, Smith K, McKean D, Pedersen BS, Talbert J, Kidd RN, Markin CR, Beckman KB, Lathrop M, Schwarz MI, Schwartz DA. Genome-wide association study identifies multiple susceptibility loci for pulmonary fibrosis. Nat Genet. 2013;45:613–20.
23. Noth I, Zhang Y, Ma SF, Flores C, Barber M, Huang Y, Broderick SM, Wade MS, Hysi P, Scuirba J, Richards TJ, Juan-Guardela BM, Vij R, Han MK, Martinez FJ, Kossen K, Seiwert SD, Christie JD, Nicolae D, Kaminski N, Garcia JGN. Genetic variants associated with idiopathic pulmonary fibrosis susceptibility and mortality: a genome-wide association study. Lancet Respir Med. 2013;1:309–17.
24. Petrovski S, Todd JL, Durheim MT, Wang Q, Chien JW, Kelly FL, Frankel C, Mebane CM, Ren Z, Bridgers J, Urban TJ, Malone CD, Finlen Copeland A, Brinkley C, Allen AS, O'Riordan T, McHutchison JG, Palmer SM, Goldstein DB. An exome sequencing study to

assess the role of rare genetic variation in pulmonary fibrosis. Am J Respir Crit Care Med. 2017;196:82–93.
25. Stuart BD, Choi J, Zaidi S, Xing C, Holohan B, Chen R, Choi M, Dharwadkar P, Torres F, Girod CE, Weissler J, Fitzgerald J, Kershaw C, Klesney-Tait J, Mageto Y, Shay JW, Ji W, Bilguvar K, Mane S, Lifton RP, Garcia CK. Exome sequencing links mutations in PARN and RTEL1 with familial pulmonary fibrosis and telomere shortening. Nat Genet. 2015;47:512–7.
26. Zhang D, Newton CA, Wang B, Povysil G, Noth I, Martinez FJ, Raghu G, Goldstein D, Kim Garcia C. Utility of whole genome sequencing in assessing risk and clinically-relevant outcomes for pulmonary fibrosis. Eur Respir J. 2022a;
27. Zhang D, Povysil G, Kobeissy PH, Li Q, Wang B, Amelotte M, Jaouadi H, Newton CA, Maher TM, Molyneaux PL, Noth I, Martinez FJ, Raghu G, Todd JL, Palmer SM, Haefliger C, Platt A, Petrovski S, Garcia JA, Goldstein DB, Garcia CK. Rare and common variants in KIF15 contribute to genetic risk of idiopathic pulmonary fibrosis. Am J Respir Crit Care Med. 2022b;206:56–69.
28. Zhang D, Povysil G, Newton CA, Maher TM, Molyneaux PL, Noth I, Martinez FJ, Raghu G, Todd JL, Palmer SM, Platt A, Petrovski S, Goldstein DB, Garcia CK. Genome-wide enrichment of TERT rare variants in idiopathic pulmonary fibrosis patients of Latino ancestry. Am J Respir Crit Care Med. 2022c;206:903–5.
29. Alder JK, Stanley SE, Wagner CL, Hamilton M, Hanumanthu VS, Armanios M. Exome sequencing identifies mutant TINF2 in a family with pulmonary fibrosis. Chest. 2015;147:1361–8.
30. Armanios MY, Chen JJ, Cogan JD, Alder JK, Ingersoll RG, Markin C, Lawson WE, Xie M, Vulto I, Phillips JA 3rd, Lansdorp PM, Greider CW, Loyd JE. Telomerase mutations in families with idiopathic pulmonary fibrosis. N Engl J Med. 2007;356:1317–26.
31. Benyelles M, O'Donohue MF, Kermasson L, Lainey E, Borie R, Lagresle-Peyrou C, Nunes H, Cazelles C, Fourrage C, Ollivier E, Marcais A, Gamez AS, Morice-Picard F, Caillaud D, Pottier N, Menard C, Ba I, Fernandes A, Crestani B, de Villartay JP, Gleizes PE, Callebaut I, Kannengiesser C, Revy P. NHP2 deficiency impairs rRNA biogenesis and causes pulmonary fibrosis and Hoyeraal-Hreidarsson syndrome. Hum Mol Genet. 2020;29:907–22.
32. Cogan JD, Kropski JA, Zhao M, Mitchell DB, Rives L, Markin C, Garnett ET, Montgomery KH, Mason WR, McKean DF, Powers J, Murphy E, Olson LM, Choi L, Cheng DS, Blue EM, Young LR, Lancaster LH, Steele MP, Brown KK, Schwarz MI, Fingerlin TE, Schwartz DA, Lawson WE, Loyd JE, Zhao Z, Phillips JA 3rd, Blackwell TS. Rare variants in RTEL1 are associated with familial interstitial pneumonia. Am J Respir Crit Care Med. 2015;191:646–55.
33. Gable DL, Gaysinskaya V, Atik CC, Talbot CC Jr, Kang B, Stanley SE, Pugh EW, Amat-Codina N, Schenk KM, Arcasoy MO, Brayton C, Florea L, Armanios M. ZCCHC8, the nuclear exosome targeting component, is mutated in familial pulmonary fibrosis and is required for telomerase RNA maturation. Genes Dev. 2019;33:1381–96.
34. Kropski JA, Reiss S, Markin C, Brown KK, Schwartz DA, Schwarz MI, Loyd JE, Phillips JA 3rd, Blackwell TS, Cogan JD. Rare genetic variants in PARN are associated with pulmonary fibrosis in families. Am J Respir Crit Care Med. 2017;196:1481–4.
35. Stanley SE, Gable DL, Wagner CL, Carlile TM, Hanumanthu VS, Podlevsky JD, Khalil SE, DeZern AE, Rojas-Duran MF, Applegate CD, Alder JK, Parry EM, Gilbert WV, Armanios M. Loss-of-function mutations in the RNA biogenesis factor NAF1 predispose to pulmonary fibrosis-emphysema. Sci Transl Med. 2016;8:351ra107.
36. Tsakiri KD, Cronkhite JT, Kuan PJ, Xing C, Raghu G, Weissler JC, Rosenblatt RL, Shay JW, Garcia CK. Adult-onset pulmonary fibrosis caused by mutations in telomerase. Proc Natl Acad Sci USA. 2007;104:7552–7.
37. Adegunsoye A, Newton CA, Oldham JM, Ley B, Lee CT, Linderholm AL, Chung JH, Garcia N, Zhang D, Vij R, Guzy R, Jablonski R, Bag R, Voogt RS, Ma SF, Sperling AI, Raghu G, Martinez FJ, Strek ME, Wolters PJ, Garcia CK, Pierce BL, Noth I. Telomere length associates with chronological age and mortality across racially diverse pulmonary fibrosis cohorts. Nat Commun. 2023;14:1489.

38. Alder JK, Chen JJ, Lancaster L, Danoff S, Su SC, Cogan JD, Vulto I, Xie M, Qi X, Tuder RM, Phillips JA 3rd, Lansdorp PM, Loyd JE, Armanios MY. Short telomeres are a risk factor for idiopathic pulmonary fibrosis. Proc Natl Acad Sci USA. 2008;105:13051–6.
39. Cronkhite JT, Xing C, Raghu G, Chin KM, Torres F, Rosenblatt RL, Garcia CK. Telomere shortening in familial and sporadic pulmonary fibrosis. Am J Respir Crit Care Med. 2008;178:729–37.
40. Doyle TJ, Juge PA, Peljto AL, Lee S, Walts AD, Esposito AJ, Poli S, Gill R, Hatabu H, Nishino M, Dellaripa PF, Weinblatt ME, Shadick NA, Demoruelle MK, Sparks JA, Rosas IO, Granger B, Deane KD, Crestani B, Wolters PJ, Dieude P, Lee JS. Short peripheral blood leukocyte telomere length in rheumatoid arthritis-interstitial lung disease. Thorax. 2024;79:182–5.
41. Ley B, Liu S, Elicker BM, Henry TS, Vittinghoff E, Golden JA, Jones KD, Wolters PJ. Telomere length in patients with unclassifiable interstitial lung disease: a cohort study. Eur Respir J. 2020;56
42. Ley B, Newton CA, Arnould I, Elicker BM, Henry TS, Vittinghoff E, Golden JA, Jones KD, Batra K, Torrealba J, Garcia CK, Wolters PJ. The MUC5B promoter polymorphism and telomere length in patients with chronic hypersensitivity pneumonitis: an observational cohort-control study. Lancet Respir Med. 2017;5:639–47.
43. Liu Q, Zhou Y, Cogan JD, Mitchell DB, Sheng Q, Zhao S, Bai Y, Ciombor KK, Sabusap CM, Malabanan MM, Markin CR, Douglas K, Ding G, Banovich NE, Nickerson DA, Blue EE, Bamshad MJ, Brown KK, Schwartz DA, Phillips JA 3rd, Martinez-Barricarte R, Salisbury ML, Shyr Y, Loyd JE, Kropski JA, Blackwell TS. The genetic landscape of familial pulmonary fibrosis. Am J Respir Crit Care Med. 2023;207:1345–57.
44. Nogee LM, Dunbar AE 3rd, Wert SE, Askin F, Hamvas A, Whitsett JA. A mutation in the surfactant protein C gene associated with familial interstitial lung disease. N Engl J Med. 2001;344:573–9.
45. Thomas AQ, Lane K, Phillips J 3rd, Prince M, Markin C, Speer M, Schwartz DA, Gaddipati R, Marney A, Johnson J, Roberts R, Haines J, Stahlman M, Loyd JE. Heterozygosity for a surfactant protein C gene mutation associated with usual interstitial pneumonitis and cellular nonspecific interstitial pneumonitis in one kindred. Am J Respir Crit Care Med. 2002;165:1322–8.
46. Nathan N, Giraud V, Picard C, Nunes H, Dastot-Le Moal F, Copin B, Galeron L, De Ligniville A, Kuziner N, Reynaud-Gaubert M, Valeyre D, Couderc LJ, Chinet T, Borie R, Crestani B, Simansour M, Nau V, Tissier S, Duquesnoy P, Mansour-Hendili L, Legendre M, Kannengiesser C, Coulomb-L'Hermine A, Gouya L, Amselem S, Clement A. Germline SFTPA1 mutation in familial idiopathic interstitial pneumonia and lung cancer. Hum Mol Genet. 2016;25:1457–67.
47. Wang Y, Kuan PJ, Xing C, Cronkhite JT, Torres F, Rosenblatt RL, DiMaio JM, Kinch LN, Grishin NV, Garcia CK. Genetic defects in surfactant protein A2 are associated with pulmonary fibrosis and lung cancer. Am J Hum Genet. 2009;84:52–9.
48. Brudon A, Legendre M, Mageau A, Bermudez J, Bonniaud P, Bouvry D, Cadranel J, Cazes A, Crestani B, Degot T, Delestrain C. High risk of lung cancer in surfactant-related gene variant carriers. Eur Respir J. 2024;63(5)
49. Kropski JA, Mitchell DB, Markin C, Polosukhin VV, Choi L, Johnson JE, Lawson WE, Phillips JA 3rd, Cogan JD, Blackwell TS, Loyd JE. A novel dyskerin (DKC1) mutation is associated with familial interstitial pneumonia. Chest. 2014;146:e1–7.
50. Savage SA, Niewisch MR. Dyskeratosis Congenita and related telomere biology disorders. In: Adam MP, Feldman J, Mirzaa GM, Pagon RA, Wallace SE, Bean LJH, Gripp KW, Amemiya A, editors. GeneReviews((R)). Seattle; 1993.
51. Alder JK, Hanumanthu VS, Strong MA, DeZern AE, Stanley SE, Takemoto CM, Danilova L, Applegate CD, Bolton SG, Mohr DW, Brodsky RA, Casella JF, Greider CW, Jackson JB, Armanios M. Diagnostic utility of telomere length testing in a hospital-based setting. Proc Natl Acad Sci USA. 2018;115:E2358–E65.

52. Newton CA, Batra K, Torrealba J, Kozlitina J, Glazer CS, Aravena C, Meyer K, Raghu G, Collard HR, Garcia CK. Telomere-related lung fibrosis is diagnostically heterogeneous but uniformly progressive. Eur Respir J. 2016;48:1710–20.
53. Dhindsa RS, Mattsson J, Nag A, Wang Q, Wain LV, Allen R, Wigmore EM, Ibanez K, Vitsios D, Deevi SVV, Wasilewski S, Karlsson M, Lassi G, Olsson H, Muthas D, Monkley S, Mackay A, Murray L, Young S, Haefliger C, FinnGen C, Maher TM, Belvisi MG, Jenkins G, Molyneaux PL, Platt A, Petrovski S. Identification of a missense variant in SPDL1 associated with idiopathic pulmonary fibrosis. Commun Biol. 2021;4:392.
54. Hollmen M, Laaka A, Partanen JJ, Koskela J, Sutinen E, Kaarteenaho R, Ainola M, Myllarniemi M. KIF15 missense variant is associated with the early onset of idiopathic pulmonary fibrosis. Respir Res. 2023;24:240.
55. Diaz de Leon A, Cronkhite JT, Yilmaz C, Brewington C, Wang R, Xing C, Hsia CCW, Garcia CK. Subclinical lung disease, macrocytosis, and premature graying in kindreds with telomerase (TERT) mutations. Chest. 2011;140:753–63.
56. Hermansky F, Pudlak P. Albinism associated with hemorrhagic diathesis and unusual pigmented reticular cells in the bone marrow: report of two cases with histochemical studies. Blood. 1959;14:162–9.
57. Yokoyama T, Gochuico BR. Hermansky-Pudlak syndrome pulmonary fibrosis: a rare inherited interstitial lung disease. Eur Respir Rev. 2021;30
58. Dell'Angelica EC, Shotelersuk V, Aguilar RC, Gahl WA, Bonifacino JS. Altered trafficking of lysosomal proteins in Hermansky-Pudlak syndrome due to mutations in the beta 3A subunit of the AP-3 adaptor. Mol Cell. 1999;3:11–21.
59. Hermos CR, Huizing M, Kaiser-Kupfer MI, Gahl WA. Hermansky-Pudlak syndrome type 1: gene organization, novel mutations, and clinical-molecular review of non-Puerto Rican cases. Hum Mutat. 2002;20:482.
60. Huizing M, Malicdan MCV, Wang JA, Pri-Chen H, Hess RA, Fischer R, O'Brien KJ, Merideth MA, Gahl WA, Gochuico BR. Hermansky-Pudlak syndrome: mutation update. Hum Mutat. 2020;41:543–80.
61. Martina JA, Moriyama K, Bonifacino JS. BLOC-3, a protein complex containing the Hermansky-Pudlak syndrome gene products HPS1 and HPS4. J Biol Chem. 2003;278:29376–84.
62. Borie R, Tabeze L, Thabut G, Nunes H, Cottin V, Marchand-Adam S, Prevot G, Tazi A, Cadranel J, Mal H, Wemeau-Stervinou L, Bergeron Lafaurie A, Israel-Biet D, Picard C, Reynaud Gaubert M, Jouneau S, Naccache JM, Mankikian J, Menard C, Cordier JF, Valeyre D, Reocreux M, Grandchamp B, Revy P, Kannengiesser C, Crestani B. Prevalence and characteristics of TERT and TERC mutations in suspected genetic pulmonary fibrosis. Eur Respir J. 2016;48:1721–31.
63. Dressen A, Abbas AR, Cabanski C, Reeder J, Ramalingam TR, Neighbors M, Bhangale TR, Brauer MJ, Hunkapiller J, Reeder J, Mukhyala K, Cuenco K, Tom J, Cowgill A, Vogel J, Forrest WF, Collard HR, Wolters PJ, Kropski JA, Lancaster LH, Blackwell TS, Arron JR, Yaspan BL. Analysis of protein-altering variants in telomerase genes and their association with MUC5B common variant status in patients with idiopathic pulmonary fibrosis: a candidate gene sequencing study. Lancet Respir Med. 2018;6:603–14.
64. Feng J, Funk WD, Wang SS, Weinrich SL, Avilion AA, Chiu CP, Adams RR, Chang E, Allsopp RC, Yu J, et al. The RNA component of human telomerase. Science. 1995;269:1236–41.
65. Greider CW, Blackburn EH. Identification of a specific telomere terminal transferase activity in Tetrahymena extracts. Cell. 1985;43:405–13.
66. Kim NW, Piatyszek MA, Prowse KR, Harley CB, West MD, Ho PL, Coviello GM, Wright WE, Weinrich SL, Shay JW. Specific association of human telomerase activity with immortal cells and cancer. Science. 1994;266:2011–5.
67. Wolthers KC, Bea G, Wisman A, Otto SA, de Roda Husman AM, Schaft N, de Wolf F, Goudsmit J, Coutinho RA, van der Zee AG, Meyaard L, Miedema F. T cell telomere length in HIV-1 infection: no evidence for increased CD4+ T cell turnover. Science. 1996;274:1543–7.

68. Jurk D, Wilson C, Passos JF, Oakley F, Correia-Melo C, Greaves L, Saretzki G, Fox C, Lawless C, Anderson R, Hewitt G, Pender SL, Fullard N, Nelson G, Mann J, van de Sluis B, Mann DA, von Zglinicki T. Chronic inflammation induces telomere dysfunction and accelerates ageing in mice. Nat Commun. 2014;2:4172.
69. Shin D, Shin J, Lee KW. Effects of inflammation and depression on telomere length in young adults in the United States. J Clin Med. 2019;8
70. Astuti Y, Wardhana A, Watkins J, Wulaningsih W, Pilar Research Network. Cigarette smoking and telomere length: a systematic review of 84 studies and meta-analysis. Environ Res. 2017;158:480–9.
71. Adler N, Pantell MS, O'Donovan A, Blackburn E, Cawthon R, Koster A, Opresko P, Newman A, Harris TB, Epel E. Educational attainment and late life telomere length in the health, aging and body composition study. Brain Behav Immun. 2013;27:15–21.
72. Fujishiro K, Diez-Roux AV, Landsbergis PA, Jenny NS, Seeman T. Current employment status, occupational category, occupational hazard exposure and job stress in relation to telomere length: the multiethnic study of atherosclerosis (MESA). Occup Environ Med. 2013;70:552–60.
73. Hamad R, Tuljapurkar S, Rehkopf DH. Racial and socioeconomic variation in genetic markers of telomere length: a cross-sectional study of U.S. older adults. EBioMedicine. 2016;11:296–301.
74. Huang Y, Yim OS, Lai PS, Yu R, Chew SH, Gwee X, Nyunt MSZ, Gao Q, Ng TP, Ebstein RP, Gouin JP. Successful aging, cognitive function, socioeconomic status, and leukocyte telomere length. Psychoneuroendocrinology. 2019;103:180–7.
75. Martens DS, Janssen BG, Bijnens EM, Clemente DBP, Vineis P, Plusquin M, Nawrot TS. Association of parental socioeconomic status and newborn telomere length. JAMA Netw Open. 2020;3:e204057.
76. Needham BL, Adler N, Gregorich S, Rehkopf D, Lin J, Blackburn EH, Epel ES. Socioeconomic status, health behavior, and leukocyte telomere length in the national health and nutrition examination survey, 1999-2002. Soc Sci Med. 2013;85:1–8.
77. Newton CA, Oldham JM, Ley B, Anand V, Adegunsoye A, Liu G, Batra K, Torrealba J, Kozlitina J, Glazer C, Strek ME, Wolters PJ, Noth I, Garcia CK. Telomere length and genetic variant associations with interstitial lung disease progression and survival. Eur Respir J. 2019a;53
78. Newton CA, Zhang D, Oldham JM, Kozlitina J, Ma SF, Martinez FJ, Raghu G, Noth I, Garcia CK. Telomere length and use of immunosuppressive medications in idiopathic pulmonary fibrosis. Am J Respir Crit Care Med. 2019b;200:336–47.
79. Duckworth A, Gibbons MA, Allen RJ, Almond H, Beaumont RN, Wood AR, Lunnon K, Lindsay MA, Wain LV, Tyrrell J, Scotton CJ. Telomere length and risk of idiopathic pulmonary fibrosis and chronic obstructive pulmonary disease: a mendelian randomisation study. Lancet Respir Med. 2021;9:285–94.
80. Alter BP, Giri N, Savage SA, Rosenberg PS. Cancer in the National Cancer Institute inherited bone marrow failure syndrome cohort after fifteen years of follow-up. Haematologica. 2018;103:30–9.
81. Alter BP, Baerlocher GM, Savage SA, Chanock SJ, Weksler BB, Willner JP, Peters JA, Giri N, Lansdorp PM. Very short telomere length by flow fluorescence in situ hybridization identifies patients with dyskeratosis congenita. Blood. 2007;110:1439–47.
82. Alter BP, Rosenberg PS, Giri N, Baerlocher GM, Lansdorp PM, Savage SA. Telomere length is associated with disease severity and declines with age in dyskeratosis congenita. Haematologica. 2012;97:353–9.
83. Zhang D, Adegunsoye A, Oldham JM, Kozlitina J, Garcia N, Poonawalla M, Strykowski R, Linderholm AL, Ley B, Ma SF, Noth I, Strek ME, Wolters PJ, Garcia CK, Newton CA. Telomere length and immunosuppression in non-idiopathic pulmonary fibrosis interstitial lung disease. Eur Respir J. 2023;

84. Seibold MA, Wise AL, Speer MC, Steele MP, Brown KK, Loyd JE, Fingerlin TE, Zhang W, Gudmundsson G, Groshong SD, Evans CM, Garantziotis S, Adler KB, Dickey BF, du Bois RM, Yang IV, Herron A, Kervitsky D, Talbert JL, Markin C, Park J, Crews AL, Slifer SH, Auerbach S, Roy MG, Lin J, Hennessy CE, Schwarz MI, Schwartz DA. A common MUC5B promoter polymorphism and pulmonary fibrosis. N Engl J Med. 2011;364:1503–12.
85. Hancock LA, Hennessy CE, Solomon GM, Dobrinskikh E, Estrella A, Hara N, Hill DB, Kissner WJ, Markovetz MR, Grove Villalon DE, Voss ME, Tearney GJ, Carroll KS, Shi Y, Schwarz MI, Thelin WR, Rowe SM, Yang IV, Evans CM, Schwartz DA. Muc5b overexpression causes mucociliary dysfunction and enhances lung fibrosis in mice. Nat Commun. 2018;9:5363.
86. Juge PA, Lee JS, Ebstein E, Furukawa H, Dobrinskikh E, Gazal S, Kannengiesser C, Ottaviani S, Oka S, Tohma S, Tsuchiya N, Rojas-Serrano J, Gonzalez-Perez MI, Mejia M, Buendia-Roldan I, Falfan-Valencia R, Ambrocio-Ortiz E, Manali E, Papiris SA, Karageorgas T, Boumpas D, Antoniou K, van Moorsel CHM, van der Vis J, de Man YA, Grutters JC, Wang Y, Borie R, Wemeau-Stervinou L, Wallaert B, Flipo RM, Nunes H, Valeyre D, Saidenberg-Kermanac'h N, Boissier MC, Marchand-Adam S, Frazier A, Richette P, Allanore Y, Sibilia J, Dromer C, Richez C, Schaeverbeke T, Liote H, Thabut G, Nathan N, Amselem S, Soubrier M, Cottin V, Clement A, Deane K, Walts AD, Fingerlin T, Fischer A, Ryu JH, Matteson EL, Niewold TB, Assayag D, Gross A, Wolters P, Schwarz MI, Holers M, Solomon JJ, Doyle T, Rosas IO, Blauwendraat C, Nalls MA, Debray MP, Boileau C, Crestani B, Schwartz DA, Dieude P. MUC5B promoter variant and rheumatoid arthritis with interstitial lung disease. N Engl J Med. 2018;379:2209–19.
87. Hunninghake GM, Hatabu H, Okajima Y, Gao W, Dupuis J, Latourelle JC, Nishino M, Araki T, Zazueta OE, Kurugol S, Ross JC, et al. MUC5B promoter polymorphism and interstitial lung abnormalities. N Engl J Med. 2013;368:2192–200.
88. Cho MH, Boutaoui N, Klanderman BJ, Sylvia JS, Ziniti JP, Hersh CP, DeMeo DL, Hunninghake GM, Litonjua AA, Sparrow D, Lange C, Won S, Murphy JR, Beaty TH, Regan EA, Make BJ, Hokanson JE, Crapo JD, Kong X, Anderson WH, Tal-Singer R, Lomas DA, Bakke P, Gulsvik A, Pillai SG, Silverman EK. Variants in FAM13A are associated with chronic obstructive pulmonary disease. Nat Genet. 2010;42:200–2.
89. Hobbs BD, de Jong K, Lamontagne M, Bosse Y, Shrine N, Artigas MS, Wain LV, Hall IP, Jackson VE, Wyss AB, London SJ, North KE, Franceschini N, Strachan DP, et al. Genetic loci associated with chronic obstructive pulmonary disease overlap with loci for lung function and pulmonary fibrosis. Nat Genet. 2017;49:426–32.
90. Kim W, Cho MH, Sakornsakolpat P, Lynch DA, Coxson HO, Tal-Singer R, Silverman EK, Beaty TH. DSP variants may be associated with longitudinal change in quantitative emphysema. Respir Res. 2019;20:160.
91. Allen RJ, Oldham JM, Jenkins DA, Leavy OC, Guillen-Guio B, Melbourne CA, Ma SF, Jou J, Kim JS, U. P. I. P. F. Investigators of the Pulmonary Trials Cooperative Clean, Fahy WA, Oballa E, Hubbard RB, Navaratnam V, Braybrooke R, Saini G, Roach KM, Tobin MD, Hirani N, Whyte MKB, Kaminski N, Zhang Y, Martinez FJ, Linderholm AL, Adegunsoye A, Strek ME, Maher TM, Molyneaux PL, Flores C, Noth I, Jenkins RG, Wain LV. Longitudinal lung function and gas transfer in individuals with idiopathic pulmonary fibrosis: a genome-wide association study. Lancet Respir Med. 2023;11:65–73.
92. Dudbridge F, Allen RJ, Sheehan NA, Schmidt AF, Lee JC, Jenkins RG, Wain LV, Hingorani AD, Patel RS. Adjustment for index event bias in genome-wide association studies of subsequent events. Nat Commun. 2019;10:1561.
93. Cai S, Allen RJ, Wain LV, Dudbridge F. Reassessing the association of MUC5B with survival in idiopathic pulmonary fibrosis. Ann Hum Genet. 2023;87:248–53.
94. Oldham JM, Allen RJ, Lorenzo-Salazar JM, Molyneaux PL, Ma SF, Joseph C, Kim JS, Guillen-Guio B, Hernandez-Beeftink T, Kropski JA, Huang Y, Lee CT, Adegunsoye A, Pugashetti JV, Linderholm AL, Vo V, Strek ME, Jou J, Munoz-Barrera A, Rubio-Rodriguez

LA, Hubbard R, Hirani N, Whyte MKB, Hart S, Nicholson AG, Lancaster L, Parfrey H, Rassl D, Wallace W, Valenzi E, Zhang Y, Mychaleckyj J, Stockwell A, Kaminski N, Wolters PJ, Molina-Molina M, Banovich NE, Fahy WA, Martinez FJ, Hall IP, Tobin MD, Maher TM, Blackwell TS, Yaspan BL, Jenkins RG, Flores C, Wain LV, Noth I. PCSK6 and survival in idiopathic pulmonary fibrosis. Am J Respir Crit Care Med. 2023a;207:1515–24.

95. Oldham JM, Ma SF, Martinez FJ, Anstrom KJ, Raghu G, Schwartz DA, Valenzi E, Witt L, Lee C, et al. TOLLIP, MUC5B, and the response to N-Acetylcysteine among individuals with idiopathic pulmonary fibrosis. Am J Respir Crit Care Med. 2015;192:1475–82.
96. Lipinski JH, Erb-Downward JR, Huffnagle GB, Flaherty KR, Martinez FJ, Moore BB, Dickson RP, Noth I, O'Dwyer DN. Toll-interacting protein and altered lung microbiota in idiopathic pulmonary fibrosis. Am J Respir Crit Care Med. 2022;206:224–7.
97. Podolanczuk AJ, Kim JS, Cooper CB, Lasky JA, Murray S, Oldham JM, Raghu G, Flaherty KR, Spino C, Noth I, Martinez FJ, Precisions Study Team. Design and rationale for the prospective treatment efficacy in IPF using genotype for NAC selection (PRECISIONS) clinical trial. BMC Pulm Med. 2022;22:475.
98. Leavy OC, Ma SF, Molyneaux PL, Maher TM, Oldham JM, Flores C, Noth I, Jenkins RG, Dudbridge F, Wain LV, Allen RJ. Proportion of idiopathic pulmonary fibrosis risk explained by known common genetic loci in European populations. Am J Respir Crit Care Med. 2021;203:775–8.
99. Hunninghake GM, Quesada-Arias LD, Carmichael NE, Martinez Manzano JM, Poli De Frias S, Baumgartner MA, DiGianni L, Gampala-Sagar SN, Leone DA, Gulati S, El-Chemaly S, Goldberg HJ, Putman RK, Hatabu H, Raby BA, Rosas IO. Interstitial lung disease in relatives of patients with pulmonary fibrosis. Am J Respir Crit Care Med. 2020;201:1240–8.
100. Rose JA, Planchart Ferretto MA, Maeda AH, Perez Garcia MF, Carmichael NE, Gulati S, Rice MB, Goldberg HJ, Putman RK, Hatabu H, Raby BA, Rosas IO, Hunninghake GM. Progressive interstitial lung disease in relatives of patients with pulmonary fibrosis. Am J Respir Crit Care Med. 2023;207:211–4.
101. Moll M, Peljto AL, Kim JS, Xu HF, Debban CL, Chen XF, Menon A, Putman RK, Ghosh AJ, Saferali A, Nishino M, Hatabu H, Hobbs BD, Hecker J, McDermott G, Sparks JA, Wain LV, Allen RJ, Tobin MD, Raby BA, Chun S, Silverman EK, Zamora AC, Ortega VE, Garcia CK, Barr RG, Bleecker ER, Meyers DA, Kaner RJ, Rich SS, Manichaikul A, Rotter JI, Dupuis J, O'Connor GT, Fingerlin TE, Hunninghake GM, Schwartz DA, Cho MH. A polygenic risk score for idiopathic pulmonary fibrosis and interstitial lung abnormalities. Am J Respir Crit Care Med. 2023;208:791–801.
102. Ma Y, Cui F, Li D, Wang J, Tang L, Xie J, Hu Y, Tian Y. Lifestyle, genetic susceptibility, and the risk of idiopathic pulmonary fibrosis: a large prospective cohort study. Chest. 2023;164:929–38.
103. Herazo-Maya JD, Noth I, Duncan SR, Kim S, Ma SF, Tseng GC, Feingold E, Juan-Guardela BM, Richards TJ, Lussier Y, Huang Y, Vij R, Lindell KO, Xue J, Gibson KF, Shapiro SD, Garcia JG, Kaminski N. Peripheral blood mononuclear cell gene expression profiles predict poor outcome in idiopathic pulmonary fibrosis. Sci Transl Med. 2013;5:205ra136.
104. Herazo-Maya JD, Sun J, Molyneaux PL, Li Q, Villalba JA, Tzouvelekis A, Lynn H, Juan-Guardela BM, Risquez C, Osorio JC, Yan X, Michel G, Aurelien N, Lindell KO, Klesen MJ, Moffatt MF, Cookson WO, Zhang Y, Garcia JGN, Noth I, Prasse A, Bar-Joseph Z, Gibson KF, Zhao H, Herzog EL, Rosas IO, Maher TM, Kaminski N. Validation of a 52-gene risk profile for outcome prediction in patients with idiopathic pulmonary fibrosis: an international, multicentre, cohort study. Lancet Respir Med. 2017;5:857–68.
105. Huang Y, Oldham JM, Ma SF, Unterman A, Liao SY, Barros AJ, Bonham CA, Kim JS, Vij R, Adegunsoye A, Strek ME, Molyneaux PL, Maher TM, Herazo-Maya JD, Kaminski N, Moore BB, Martinez FJ, Noth I. Blood transcriptomics predicts progression of pulmonary fibrosis and associated natural killer cells. Am J Respir Crit Care Med. 2021;204:197–208.

106. Sanders YY, Ambalavanan N, Halloran B, Zhang X, Liu H, Crossman DK, Bray M, Zhang K, Thannickal VJ, Hagood JS. Altered DNA methylation profile in idiopathic pulmonary fibrosis. Am J Respir Crit Care Med. 2012;186:525–35.
107. Oldham JM, Huang Y, Bose S, Ma SF, Kim JS, Schwab A, Ting C, Mou K, Lee CT, Adegunsoye A, Ghodrati S, Pugashetti JV, Nazemi N, Strek ME, Linderholm AL, Chen CH, Murray S, Zemans RL, Flaherty KR, Martinez FJ, Noth I. Proteomic biomarkers of survival in idiopathic pulmonary fibrosis. Am J Respir Crit Care Med. 2023b;
108. Bowman WS, Newton CA, Linderholm AL, Neely ML, Pugashetti JV, Kaul B, Vo V, Echt GA, Leon W, Shah RJ, Huang Y, Garcia CK, Wolters PJ, Oldham JM. Proteomic biomarkers of progressive fibrosing interstitial lung disease: a multicentre cohort analysis. Lancet Respir Med. 2022;10:593–602.

# Chapter 4
# Molecular Biomarkers in Interstitial Lung Diseases

**Umberto Zanini, Paola Faverio, and Fabrizio Luppi**

Interstitial lung diseases (ILDs), or interstitial pneumonias, encompass a diverse set of conditions that impact the tissue and space surrounding the air sacs in our lungs, known as the interstitium [1–3]. ILDs are a heterogeneous disease, including more than 200 different types of ILDs. These conditions are characterized by inflammation and scarring of the interstitium, which can lead to impaired lung function and adversely impact survival [4]. Various factors can contribute to the development of ILDs, including exposure to environmental and occupational toxins, autoimmune disorders, infections, and unknown causes [4]. The diagnosis of ILD can be challenging due to its intricate and overlapping patterns. A multidisciplinary team is often necessary to accurately diagnose the condition [5]. In certain instances, open surgical lung biopsy may be required, but it should be noted that this procedure carries a high risk of mortality [6]. The correct diagnosis of ILD is crucial for effective treatment and evaluation of disease prognosis. In fact, the natural history of some ILDs can be very poor (e.g., idiopathic pulmonary fibrosis (IPF) survival is 2–5 years) [7, 8]. Early and accurate diagnosis, personalized treatment strategies, and ongoing medical management are essential for optimizing patient outcomes [9]. Identifying molecular fingerprints and biomarkers can also improve ILD diagnosis and follow-up.

Since most ILD patients are elderly with multiple comorbidities, within the context of ILD serum biomarkers have been explored more than biomarkers in bronchoalveolar lavage (BAL) or lung tissue, since they are more accessible and less invasive [10]. Biomarkers can be used to distinguish between individuals with a particular disease and those without it as well as predict the severity or outcome of the disease. Ideal biomarkers should complement established clinical or functional disease criteria or replace invasive diagnostic or prognostic procedures [9]. The

U. Zanini · P. Faverio · F. Luppi (✉)
University of Milano-Bicocca, Fondazione IRCCS "San Gerardo dei Tintori", Monza, Italy
e-mail: u.zanini@campus.unimib.it; paola.faverio@unimib.it; fabrizio.luppi@unimib.it



B. F. Collins, S. B. Montesi (eds.), *Precision Medicine in Interstitial Lung Disease*, Respiratory Medicine, https://doi.org/10.1007/978-3-031-87183-2_4

diagnosis of ILDs can be intricate, necessitating the use of highly accurate diagnostic tools. The use of molecular biomarkers might help to overcome current diagnostic limitations and to advance personalized medicine for patients with ILD.

## Serum Biomarkers, Where Are We Now?

Currently, no molecular biomarkers are commonly used to diagnose ILDs. Despite investigations into multiple potential candidate biomarkers, none have been implemented in clinical practice [11, 12]. Available biomarkers can be divided into three categories according to the pathogenic pathway involved (Fig. 4.1): epithelial

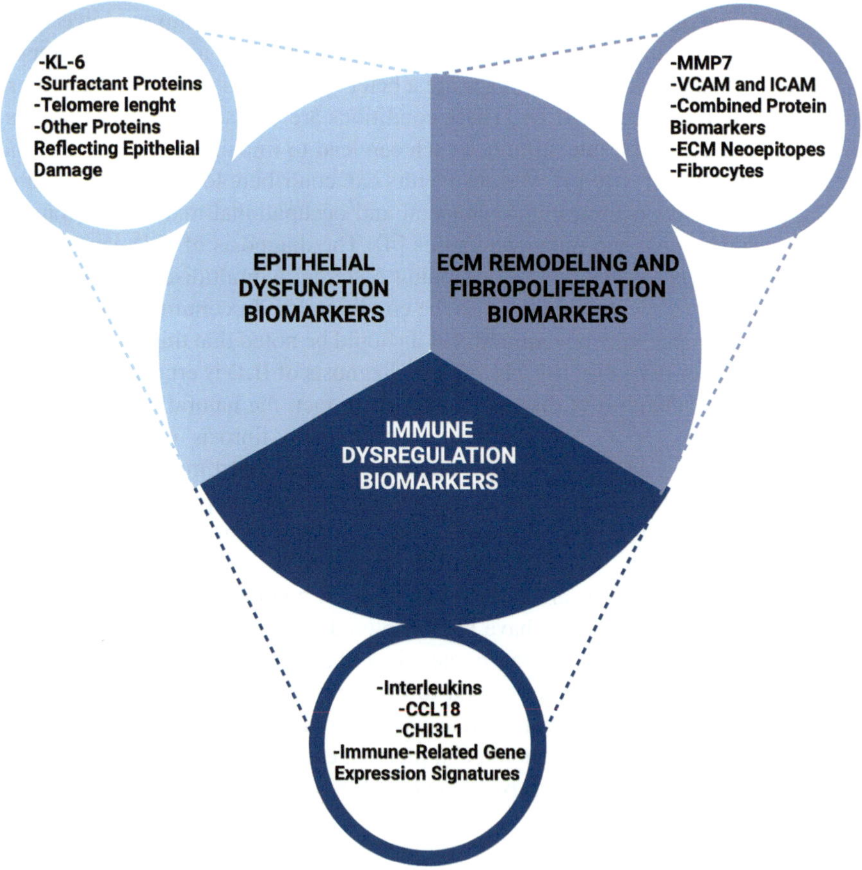


**Fig. 4.1** Serum biomarkers in patients with interstitial lung disease divided according to the pathogenic pathways involved. *CCL-18* CC-chemokine ligand 18, *ECM* extracellular matrix, *ICAM* intercellular cell adhesion molecule, *KL*-6 Krebs Von Den Lungen 6, *MMP* matrix metalloproteinase, *VCAM* vascular cell adhesion molecule

dysfunction, extracellular matrix (ECM) remodeling and fibroproliferation, and immune dysregulation [11].

ILDs are characterized by epithelial dysfunction, which can be evaluated by specific biomarkers such as Krebs von den Lungen-6 (KL-6) and surfactant protein (SP). These two biomarkers have potential to aid in the diagnosis and prognosis of ILDs.

Other biomarkers, such as matrix metalloproteinase-7 (MMP-7) and chitinase 3-like-1 (CHI3L1), offer insights into the progression and severity of ILDs by indicating, respectively, proteolytic activity in extracellular matrix remodeling and fibroproliferative responses. These biomarkers have also the potential to help in the development of targeted treatment approaches.

Immune dysregulation also plays a crucial role in ILDs. Cytokines like IL-6 and TNF-α are indicators of immune system activation and inflammation, while CD4+ T lymphocytes can help to characterize the immune terrain of ILDs. These biomarkers could assist in diagnosis and offer potential avenues for regulating aberrant immune responses. Continuous research is critical for efficacious clinical management.

We categorized the most available biomarkers based on the systems in Table 4.1 and described some of the biomarkers below.

**Table 4.1** Serum biomarker in patients with interstitial lung disease

| | Prognostic | Diagnosis of lung fibrosis | Diagnosis of specific ILD |
|---|---|---|---|
| KL-6 | +++++ | ++++ | +/− |
| CCL-18 | ++++ | +++ | + |
| SPA and SPD | ++++ | +++ | + |
| MMP7 | ++++ | +++ | + |
| IL-6 | ++++ | ++ | − |
| VCAM and ICAM-1 | +++ | + | +/− |
| CCL-2 | ++ | ++ | +/− |
| YKL-40 | + | + | −/+ |
| IL-10 | +/− | +/− | − |
| CA 15-3, CA19-9 | + | ++ | − |
| IL-8 | ++ | + | +/− |
| CXCL13 | ++ | + | + |
| CD28 | ++ | − | − |
| S100A12 | ++ | + | − |

Modified from De Lauretis et al. [11]. "−" no association, "+/−" uncertain association, "+" mild association, "++" moderate association, "+++" strong association, "++++" very strong association, "+++++" extremely strong association. *CA* carbohydrate antigen, *CD* cluster of differentiation, *CCL* chemokine (C-C motif) ligand, *CCL*-18 CC-chemokine ligand 18, *CXCL* C-X-C motif chemokine, *ICAM* intercellular cell adhesion molecule, *IL* interleukin, *KL*-6 Krebs Von Den Lungen 6, *MMP* matrix metalloproteinase, *SP* surfactant protein, S100A12 S100 calcium-binding protein A12, *VCAM* vascular cell adhesion molecule, *YKL*-40 also called human cartilage glycoprotein 39, and chitinase 3-like 1

## Epithelial Dysfunction Biomarkers

### *Surfactant Proteins*

Surfactant proteins (SPs) are a group of water-soluble proteins that belong to the C-type lectin superfamily [13]. The genes for lung collectins, such as SP-A, SP-D, and MBL, are located on human chromosome 10 [14, 15]. These SPs are secreted by alveolar epithelial type II cells, playing a vital role in transporting and utilizing surfactant lipids to reduce alveolar surface tension and prevent lung collapse [16]. Moreover, these proteins also serve as host defense against infectious agents in the terminal airways [17, 18]. Patients with IPF and other ILDs have shown increased levels of surfactant proteins A (SP-A) and D (SP-D) in their serum and BAL [19, 20]. Research has found that elevated levels of serum SP-A and SP-D can predict mortality in IPF patients, while SP-D levels have been linked to deteriorating lung function values and acute exacerbations (AE) [21]. A meta-analysis investigating SP-A and SP-D as biomarkers for the diagnosis and prognosis of IPF found that patients with IPF had higher SP-A levels than patients with other ILDs and that SP-D was associated with the frequency of acute exacerbations and prognosis [22]. *Song and colleagues* evaluated blood biomarkers from 118 patients with IPF. The results showed that matrix metalloproteinase-7 (MMP-7) and SP-A were noteworthy indicators of survival, combined with age, FVC, and extent of honeycombing. Patients with elevated levels of MMP-7 and SP-A had a greater likelihood of experiencing a shorter lifespan and more frequent decline in lung function [23]. In a study by Kinder et al., the prognostic significance of serum SP-A and D was examined in 82 patients diagnosed with biopsy-proven IPF [24]. Results showed that elevated levels of baseline SP-A were associated with a 3.3-fold increase in mortality risk within the first year. Furthermore, combining SP-A and SP-D with clinical predictors, such as age, gender, smoking status, pulmonary function test, and blood sample, enhanced the accuracy of mortality prediction [24]. Ishii et al. found significantly elevated SP-A, SP-D, and KL-6 serum levels in 57 ILD patients compared to healthy control groups [25]. Importantly, SP-A levels in UIP patients were significantly higher than in NSIP patients. The findings suggest that serum SP-A levels could be a clinically valuable biomarker for differentiating UIP and NSIP in ILD patients [25]. Moreover, genetic variations of the surfactant protein A2 (SFTPA2) and surfactant protein C (SFTPC) genes have been linked to the development of lung fibrosis, while variants of the gene encoding SP-A1 (SFTPA1) and SFTPA2 have been associated with a disease phenotype of IPF that coexists with lung cancer [26, 27]. Surfactant proteins may serve as biomarkers of abnormal function, injury, apoptosis, or proliferation of alveolar epithelial cells (AECs), but further research is necessary to determine their ability to reflect disease activity over time and their clinical usefulness.

## *Krebs von den Lungen-6*

Krebs von den Lungen-6 (KL-6) is a mucinous high-molecular-weight (200 kDa) glycoprotein expressed on type 2 pneumonocytes. When these cells are damaged or are growing back after being damaged, they release KL-6 into the bloodstream [28]. KL-6 can be measured in the patient's blood or BAL, helping to identify ILD patients. In fact, KL-6 protein is reported to be elevated in the serum and bronchoalveolar lavage fluid of patients with interstitial pneumonia [29]. Serum concentrations of this glycoprotein have been proposed as a diagnostic helpful biomarker to distinguish IPF from fibrotic hypersensitivity pneumonitis and other ILDs [30, 31]. Previous studies demonstrated the superiority of KL-6 as a diagnostic marker for ILDs compared to SP-A, SP-D, and MCP-1 [32]. In fact, KL-6 demonstrated the highest diagnostic accuracy, sensitivity, specificity, and odds ratio [32]. Notably, KL-6 levels remained normal in bacterial pneumonia cases, distinguishing it from SP-A and SP-D. A recent study found that serum KL-6 concentration, alone or combined with gender, effectively stratifies ILD patients for risk of disease progression [33]. In the same way, another study investigated serum KL-6 levels in IPF patients and found that levels below 1000 U/mL at diagnosis correlate with a more favorable 3-year survival rate [34]. A retrospective study explored KL-6 as a potential biomarker for connective tissue disease-associated interstitial lung disease (CTD-ILD) [35]. Serum KL-6 levels were significantly higher in CTD-ILD patients, correlating with ILD severity on chest HRCT. Also, serial KL-6 measurements could aid in monitoring ILD exacerbation, with a cutoff value below 275.1 U/mL indicating no AE-ILD [35].

Kohno et al. conducted a study to examine levels of KL-6 in bronchoalveolar lavage fluid (BALF) of healthy individuals and those with interstitial pneumonitis [36]. The study found that abnormally high levels of KL-6 were present in patients with IPF (70%), sarcoidosis (64%), and hypersensitivity pneumonitis (100%) [36]. These high levels correlated significantly with total cell count, lymphocytes, neutrophils, albumin, total protein in BALF, and serum KL-6 levels [36]. These findings suggest elevated serum KL-6 in pneumonitis patients reflects production from damaged or regenerating type 2 pneumocytes in the lower respiratory tract.

Another study conducted on patients with polymyositis (PM) or dermatomyositis (DM) and ILD found that those with ILD had significantly higher levels of KL-6 in their serum as compared to those without ILD [37]. The study also found a significant inverse correlation between KL-6 levels and lung function parameters [37]. In a retrospective longitudinal study of 39 patients with systemic sclerosis, Yanaba et al. revealed that elevated initial KL-6 levels, especially in those with PF, correlated with disease progression [38]. Rapid KL-6 increases were observed in patients with anti-topo I Abs, indicating PF progression, while those with inactive PF maintained elevated but stable KL-6 levels [38]. Similarly, in the fibrotic nonspecific interstitial pneumonia (f-NSIP) investigation involving 26 patients, elevated KL-6 levels correlated with the extent of fibrotic abnormalities on high-resolution computed tomography (HRCT) [39]. Traction bronchiectasis on HRCT showed a significant association with serum KL-6 in multivariate analysis, suggesting its potential as a marker for fibrosis [39]. Hisata et al. conducted a study to assess the individual effects and clinical outcomes of SP-D and KL-6/MUC1 in patients with interstitial pneumonia. The study revealed that KL-6 levels were higher in symptomatic IPF patients, indicating its potential as a prognostic marker [40]. Another study focused on serum KL-6 levels as a prognostic marker for diffuse alveolar haemorrhage (DAH) and suggested that a peak level of ≥700 U/mL could be a clinically useful marker for predicting poor prognosis in DAH patients [41]. Furthermore, a study was conducted on sarcoidosis patients to evaluate the discriminative value of serum CC16, KL-6, and SP-D as markers for [42]ILD. The study found that KL-6 was the best discriminative marker reflecting disease severity and outcome [42].

## *Telomeres*

Telomeres are repeating sequences that cap chromosomes, preventing shortening during replication [43]. Their maintenance involves the shelterin, telomerase, and CST complexes, and various genes [43]. Mutations in these genes cause shortened telomeres, leading to cell death [44]. Organs with high replicative demands are especially vulnerable. Among the ILDs, IPF is a well-known condition linked to telomere-related mutations, with up to 30% of familial IPF cases showing such mutations [45, 46]. Telomere-related mutations also occur in other ILDs, including pleuroparenchymal fibroelastosis (PPFE) and rheumatoid arthritis ILD [47]. Studies suggest that the onset of ILD is connected to the degree of telomere shortening, with radiologic abnormalities preceding clinically significant ILD. While IPF is a common manifestation, other ILDs like unclassifiable pulmonary fibrosis and chronic hypersensitivity pneumonitis are also observed in people with telomere-related mutations [47, 48]. Environmental factors, such as smoking or exposure to pulmonary toxicants, may contribute to ILD development in individuals with telomere-related mutations, which exhibit incomplete penetrance [49]. Those with short telomeres and/or telomere-related mutations experience more rapid disease progression and decreased transplant-free survival [48, 50].

## *Other Proteins Reflecting Epithelial Damage*

Several different proteins reflecting epithelial damage have been studied. Different studies have evaluated the level of specific tumor markers in ILD patients. In rheumatoid arthritis-associated interstitial lung disease (RA-ILD), a recent study revealed elevated levels of serum CEA, CA19-9, and CA125, indicating potential correlations with ILD development [51]. Tumor markers CA125, CA19-9, and CEA, reflecting epithelial injury, were implicated as potential diagnostic indicators [52].

## ECM Remodeling and Fibroproliferation Biomarkers

### *Matrix Metallopeptidase 7*

Matrix metalloproteinases (MMPs) are zinc-dependent endoproteases crucial for extracellular matrix remodeling [53]. The activity of MMPs is regulated by tissue inhibitors of metalloproteinase (TIMPs) [54]. Microarray studies revealed upregulation of several MMP family members (MMP-1, 2, 3, 7, 8, 9) in IPF lungs, and elevated protein expression is detected in bronchoalveolar lavage fluid and blood of IPF patients [55–58].

Rosas et al. reported that elevated MMP1 and MMP7 levels in plasma correlated with IPF lung changes, distinguishing it from other lung diseases [56]. The study suggested MMPs as potential biomarkers for IPF, with MMP7 correlating with disease severity.

Bauer and colleagues investigated the prognostic potential of MMP-7 in IPF using serum samples from the BUILD-3 clinical trial [55]. MMP-7 showed consistently elevated levels, with progressive increases longitudinally. High baseline MMP-7 levels predicted worsening over time and correlated with decreased FVC. Despite differences in treatment, MMP-7 levels consistently correlated with prognosis. Baseline MMP-7 assessment could help predict disease progression and tailor treatment strategies in IPF patients.

Studies also highlight their potential utility as biomarkers for IPF, aiding the disease's differential diagnosis [55, 56, 59]. High expression of MMP-1 and MMP-7 has been observed in IPF compared to other ILDs, such as sarcoidosis and hypersensitivity pneumonitis [56].

In the Multi-Ethnic Study of Atherosclerosis (MESA), baseline levels of MMP7 were associated with decreased lung function, the future development of interstitial lung abnormalities, and an increased risk of all-cause mortality [60]. MMP7 measurements have shown promise in aiding the early detection of ILD. However, the clinical use of MMP7 as a potential biomarker in IPF has faced challenges due to varying cutoff points used in different studies and inconsistent protocols for measuring its levels, including using different collection matrices such as serum, EDTA, and heparin plasma.

### *Intercellular Adhesion Molecule and Vascular Cell Adhesion Molecule*

Intercellular Adhesion Molecule-1 (ICAM-1) and Vascular Cell Adhesion Molecule-1 (VCAM-1) are cell adhesion molecules that play crucial roles in immune responses and inflammatory processes, facilitating the interaction between endothelial cells and immune cells [61, 62].

Ihn and colleagues investigated serum levels of intercellular adhesion molecule-1 (ICAM-1) in systemic sclerosis (SSc) patients and healthy controls [63]. Results showed significantly higher ICAM-1 levels in SSc patients, especially those with diffuse cutaneous SSc. Elevated ICAM-1 correlated with clinical features like phalangeal contracture, pulmonary fibrosis, joint involvement, and increased erythrocyte sedimentation rate.

In another study, serum levels of soluble vascular cell adhesion molecule-1 (sVCAM-1) and soluble E-selectin (sE-selectin) were evaluated in patients with systemic sclerosis (SSc) [64]. The findings revealed significantly elevated sVCAM-1 and sE-selectin levels in SSc patients compared to healthy controls. Moreover, associations were observed between sVCAM-1 level and pulmonary fibrosis, joint involvement, and elevated erythrocyte sedimentation rate, while sE-selectin levels were correlated with pulmonary fibrosis.

## *Combined Protein Biomarkers*

Using combined biomarker approaches along with multiple variable scoring systems has shown great potential. A study involving 241 IPF patients analyzed 95 different cytokines, chemokines, MMPs, and other markers [58]. Only five of them (MMP-7, VCAM-1, S100A12, ICAM-1, and IL-8) were found to predict outcomes independently of age, sex, or baseline pulmonary function tests. Validation in an independent cohort confirmed their predictive value for reduced and progression-free survival. The Personal Clinical and Molecular Mortality Prediction Index (PCMI), combining physiological, clinical, and biomarker variables, accurately predicted mortality. This panel of proteins offers insights into IPF progression, paving the way for improved classification, management, and potential therapeutic monitoring in IPF patients [58]. In another study involving 97 IPF patients, the prognostic accuracy of plasma MMP-7, SP-D, and osteopontin concentrations was validated [57]. Plasma levels of SP-D (>31 ng/ml), MMP-7 (>1.75 ng/ml), and osteopontin (>6 ng/ml) significantly distinguished patients with IPF from patients with other forms of ILD, both individually and in a combined index.

## *Extracellular Matrix Neoepitopes*

Extracellular matrix (ECM)-associated biomarkers are vital for assessing fibrosis [65, 66]. Collagens, the primary ECM proteins, undergo dynamic balance through fibroblast synthesis and matrix metalloproteinase-mediated degradation [67]. Proteolytic cleavage of the ECM produces neoepitopes, measurable biomarkers indicating ECM synthesis and degradation. Due to a simple blood sample, these neo-epitopes are valuable for serological quantification of fibrotic processes [67].

A recent study explored the use of collagen neoepitopes as biomarkers to predict extracellular matrix remodeling in those with systemic sclerosis [67]. The findings indicated that type III and IV collagen neo-epitopes were present in higher concentrations in patients with the disease, with a significant association observed. Furthermore, degradation neo-epitopes showed a distinction between progressors and non-progressors. Specifically, higher serum concentrations of certain neo-epitopes in skin progressors suggested their potential for predicting fibrosis progression.

The PROFILE study, the largest prospective cohort study on incident idiopathic fibrotic lung disease, revealed that the changes in circulating protein concentrations over time can predict IPF disease progression and outcomes [52]. The study particularly examined six neoepitopes that hold promise as theragnostic biomarkers, facilitating clinical decision-making and potentially reducing future clinical trials [52].

### *Fibrocytes*

Fibrocytes, derived from bone marrow, are circulating progenitor cells involved in scar formation at injury sites [68]. In mouse fibrotic lung disease models, these cells swiftly leave the bone marrow post-injury, enter the bloodstream, and migrate to the lungs [69, 70]. Elevated circulating fibrocyte levels in human ILD, particularly in IPF and in fibrotic lung diseases linked to rheumatoid arthritis and scleroderma, correlate with poor outcomes [71–73]. Odackal et al. revealed that circulating fibrocytes in patients with autoimmune ILD showed elevated concentrations, especially in activated subsets and those with specific signaling pathways [74]. Initiating immunosuppressive therapy led to a decline in fibrocyte concentration. Higher peak fibrocyte levels correlated with a 5% increased risk of death or lung function decline [73].

## Immune Dysregulation Biomarkers

### *Chitinase 1 and Chitinase 3 Like 1*

Recent studies have highlighted the significant involvement of chitinase 1 (CHIT1) and chitinase 3-like-1 (CHI3L1), members of the 18-Glycosyl hydrolase (18-GH) family, in the pathogenesis of inflammatory and remodeling-related human diseases [75–77]. Dysregulated expression of CHIT1 and CHI3L1 has been observed in patients with pulmonary fibrosis, and their levels correlate inversely with clinical outcomes [78, 79]. Macrophages, mainly, play a significant role in expressing these chitinases, influencing profibrotic macrophage activation, fibroblast proliferation, myofibroblast transformation, and TGF-β signaling [78–81]. Preclinical studies using animal models further suggest the necessity of CHIT1 and CHI3L1 for fibroproliferative responses, opening up the possibility of reprogramming profibrotic cells to reverse established pulmonary fibrosis by intervening with these chitinases [82].

In pulmonary fibrosis, CHIT1 is elevated, correlating with disease severity [79, 80]. It is mainly expressed in profibrotic macrophages, influencing their differentiation. CHIT1 also enhances fibroblast activity and TGF-β signaling, which is crucial in fibrosis development [80]. Studies in mice suggest CHIT1 is necessary for TGF-β-induced pulmonary fibrosis, interacting with Tgfbrap1 and FoxO3 [80]. This interaction negatively regulates FoxO3, potentially amplifying TGF-β signaling. CHIT1 emerges as a key player in pulmonary fibrosis pathogenesis [82].

On the other hand, CHI3L1, known also like YKL-40, is a protein linked to inflammation and remodeling-related diseases, especially pulmonary fibrosis [82, 83]. It interacts with IL-13Rα2 and CRTH2 receptors, which can have protective effects and promote fibrosis [84]. Gal-3 is a β-galactoside-binding lectin with profibrotic effects, who interferes with CHI3L1 signaling and impacts epithelial cells and macrophages [85, 86]. CHI3L1 dysregulation has been identified in Hermansky-Pudlak syndrome-associated lung fibrosis and in potential therapeutic targets [81]. High levels of CHI3L1 are associated with poor survival in cases of IPF [87]. For instance, a study on 85 patients with IPF and 126 controls found that IPF patients with high CHI3L1 levels in serum or BALF had significantly shorter survival than those with low CHI3L1 levels [88]. In contrast, patients with low serum and BALF CHI3L1 levels did not experience IPF-related mortality, suggesting that serum CHI3L1 could be a useful prognostic marker. Similarly, another study found that elevated levels of CHI3L1 were associated with severe disease progression in 64 IPF patients with IPF [78]. Furthermore, other studies have also reported that patients with other types of ILD, such as connective tissue-related ILD, sarcoidosis, cryptogenic organizing pneumonia, asbestosis-ILD, and idiopathic nonspecific interstitial pneumonia, have increased levels of serum CHI3L1 [89–95].

## *Interleukins*

Interleukins are small proteins known as cytokines. They play a vital role in regulating immune responses and inflammation in the body. IL-6 promotes immune responses and inflammation, while IL-10 counteracts these effects by suppressing inflammation and preventing an excessive immune reaction. IL-8 works as a chemoattractant for immune system cells, especially neutrophils, thereby contributing to inflammation and the body's defense against pathogens.

De Lauretis et al. conducted a study to examine the role of serum cytokines in patients with SSc and IPF [96]. The study found that only interleukin 6 (IL-6) was an independent predictor of DLCO decline. Serum IL-6 levels greater than 7.67 pg/ml predicted a decline in forced vital capacity (FVC) and DLCO within the first year and death within the first 30 months. Notably, for patients with milder disease, elevated levels of IL-6 predicted functional decline or death within the first year [96].

Another study investigated cytokine levels in patients with IPF compared to healthy controls [97]. The serum levels of interleukins (IL-2, IL-4, IL-8, IL-10), interferon-γ (IFN-γ), and IL-12 (p40) were measured in 20 IPF patients and 40 healthy controls. The IPF group showed higher levels of IL-2, IL-8, IL-10, and IL-12 (p40) and lower levels of IFN-γ compared to controls.

On the other hand, a more recent study examined the relationship between genetic polymorphisms in cytokine genes (IL-6, IL-10, IFN-γ, TNF-α, and TGF-β1), serum levels of these cytokines, and the clinical characteristics of patients with IPF [98]. No significant differences emerged in the genotype and allele distributions between IPF patients and healthy controls for the studied cytokines. However, certain genotypes were significantly associated with HRCT (high-resolution computed tomography) scores and physiological parameters.

## *C-C Motif Chemokine Ligand 18*

C-C Motif Chemokine Ligand 18 (CCL18) is a unique CC-chemokine produced by human myeloid cells, distinguishing it from rodents. It is a marker for the alternative activation of macrophages associated with tissue repair and fibrosis [99, 100]. Elevated CCL18 levels are observed in various diseases, including atopic dermatitis, Gaucher disease, and childhood acute lymphoblastic leukemia [101, 102]. Like TGF-β, CCL18 promotes collagen production by lung fibroblasts, and there is a feedback loop where collagen type 1 stimulation increases CCL18 production by alveolar macrophages [103, 104]. In patients with IPF, alveolar macrophages abundantly produce CCL18, and its serum concentrations correlate with spontaneous macrophage production [103, 105]. Prasse et al. investigated the correlation between baseline serum CCL18 concentrations and survival in patients with IPF [106]. Elevated serum CCL18 levels above 150 ng/ml at baseline strongly predicted mortality in IPF patients, with an 8.0 hazard of death after adjusting for various factors [106]. A post hoc analysis based on cohorts from CAPACITY and ASCEND trials evaluated plasma protein biomarkers in patients with IPF receiving pirfenidone or placebo [107]. Among several baseline biomarkers, CCL18 consistently predicted disease progression, showing prognostic significance for forced vital capacity (FVC%pred) decline in both test and replication cohorts [107].

## *Immune-Related Gene Expression Signatures*

A recent study developed a molecular genomic signature to predict the prognosis of patients with IPF [108]. The study analyzed the immune system's role in IPF and identified immune-related genes (IRGs) to create a five-IRG-based prognostic signature (CXCL14, SLC40A1, RNASE3, CCR3, and RORA) [108]. This signature demonstrated a strong predictive effect and was associated with the progression of IPF. The genes involved in the signature were linked to fibrogenesis and remodeling of lung structure. The study validated the performance of the signature, suggesting its potential use in real-world applications [108].

A study analyzed gene expression profiles of 130 IPF patients to identify peripheral blood biomarkers for early disease progression detection and assessment [109]. 1428 genes were found in mild IPF and 2790 in severe IPF compared to controls immune-related genes (IRGs)). Thirteen transcripts distinguished between mild and severe IPF based on the percent predicted DLCO but not on percent predicted FVC. Findings suggest peripheral blood biomarkers could be utilized for early IPF detection and severity assessment [109].

Sivakumar et al. conducted a study of simultaneous comprehensive analysis of the plasma proteome and lung transcriptome in advanced IPF patients, comparing them with healthy donors [110]. Patients with IPF showed notable irregularities in pathways associated with T-cell activation, chemokine signaling, mast cell maturation, Wnt signaling, and extracellular matrix (ECM) homeostasis in both lung tissue and peripheral blood [110]. The study highlights a chemokine signaling pattern within the IPF group, which may suggest immune-related genes (IRGs)) involvement in inflammation and tissue remodeling [110]. Additionally, chemokines related to mast cells and components of Wnt signaling were upregulated in both lung tissue and plasma of IPF patients. Furthermore, ECM remodeling and proteolysis pathways were significantly dysregulated in the IPF cohort [110].

## Conclusion

Identifying serum markers has indeed constituted a significant stride in pursuing diagnostic precision for ILD. Among the notable serum markers, such as surfactant proteins, monocyte chemoattractant protein-1, and Kerbs von Lungren, other serum biomarkers have emerged as promising candidates.

Despite these promising findings, the clinical role of serum markers in diagnosing ILD remains unclear, and challenges persist. The tests, including those for SP-A, SP-B, MCP-1, and KL-6, are generally not commercially available, limiting their routine clinical application. Furthermore, the complexity of ILD, characterized by a spectrum of subtypes and varying disease trajectories, necessitates a nuanced understanding of the context in which these serum markers may offer optimal diagnostic value.

The analysis of genomic, proteomic, and omics data is expected to yield significant advancements in our understanding of IPF and ILD pathogenesis. This understanding will lead to the discovery of ILD subtypes, which will allow for more tailored therapeutic approaches. Routine biomarker testing will be implemented for patient stratification and personalized treatment. Promising biomarker-therapy candidates will be identified based on pivotal fibrosis pathways.

As the field progresses, addressing these challenges and further elucidating the clinical significance of serum markers in ILD diagnosis is imperative. Continued research endeavors hold the potential to bridge existing diagnostic gaps and contribute to the development of more accessible and reliable diagnostic tools for ILD in clinical practice.

**Acknowledgments** We acknowledge that this research was partially supported by the Grant: Italian MUR Dipartimenti di Eccellenza 2023-2027 (l. 232/2016, art. 1, commi 314-337).

## References

1. Bradley B, Branley HM, Egan JJ, Greaves MS, Hansell DM, Harrison NK, Hirani N, Hubbard R, Lake F, Millar AB, Wallace WAH. Interstitial lung disease guideline: the British Thoracic Society in collaboration with the Thoracic Society of Australia and New Zealand and the Irish thoracic society. Thorax. 2008;63(11):1029.
2. Travis WD, King TE, Bateman ED, Lynch DA, Capron F, Center D, et al. American Thoracic Society/European Respiratory Society international multidisciplinary consensus classification of the idiopathic interstitial pneumonias. This joint statement of the American Thoracic Society (ATS), and the European Respiratory Society (ERS) was adopted by the ATS board of directors, June 2001 and by the ERS executive committee, June 2001. Am J Respir Crit Care Med. 2002;165(2):277–304.
3. Travis WD, Costabel U, Hansell DM, King TE Jr, Lynch DA, Nicholson AG, Ryerson CJ, Ryu JH, Selman M, Wells AU, Behr J. An official American Thoracic Society/European Respiratory Society statement: update of the international multidisciplinary classification of the idiopathic interstitial pneumonias. Am J Respir Crit Care Med. 2013;188(6):733–48.
4. Antoniou KM, Margaritopoulos GA, Tomassetti S, Bonella F, Costabel U, Poletti V. Interstitial lung disease. Eur Respir Rev. 2014;23(131):40–54.
5. Cottin V, Martinez FJ, Smith V, Walsh SL. Multidisciplinary teams in the clinical care of fibrotic interstitial lung disease: current perspectives. Eur Respir Rev. 2022;31(165).
6. Hutchinson JP, Fogarty AW, McKeever TM, Hubbard RB. In-hospital mortality after surgical lung biopsy for interstitial lung disease in the United States. 2000 to 2011. Am J Respir Crit Care Med. 2016;193(10):1161–7.
7. Nathan SD, Shlobin OA, Weir N, Ahmad S, Kaldjob JM, Battle E, et al. Long-term course and prognosis of idiopathic pulmonary fibrosis in the new millennium. Chest. 2011;140(1):221–9.
8. Ley B, Ryerson CJ, Vittinghoff E, Ryu JH, Tomassetti S, Lee JS, et al. A multidimensional index and staging system for idiopathic pulmonary fibrosis. Ann Intern Med. 2012;156(10):684–95.
9. Greiffo FR, Eickelberg O, Fernandez IE. Systems medicine advances in interstitial lung disease. Eur Respir Rev. 2017;26(145):170021.
10. Ley B, Brown KK, Collard HR. Molecular biomarkers in idiopathic pulmonary fibrosis. Am J Physiol Lung Cell Mol Physiol. 2014;307:681–91.
11. De Lauretis A, Renzoni EA. Molecular biomarkers in interstitial lung diseases. Mol Diagn Ther. 2014;18(5):505–22.
12. Nathan N, Corvol H, Amselem S, Clement A. Biomarkers in Interstitial lung diseases. Paediatr Respir Rev. 2015;16(4):219–24.
13. Day AJ. The C-type carbohydrate recognition domain (CRD) superfamily. Biochem Soc Trans. 1994;22(1):83–8.
14. Kölble K, Reid KB. The genomics of soluble proteins with collagenous domains: C1q, MBL, SP-A, SP-D, conglutinin, and CL-43. Behring Inst Mitt. 1993;93:81–6.

15. Kölble K, Lu J, Mole SE, Kaluz S, Reid KB. Assignment of the human pulmonary surfactant protein D gene (SFTP4) to 10q22-q23 close to the surfactant protein a gene cluster. Genomics. 1993;17(2):294–8.
16. Mulugeta S, Nureki SI, Beers MF. Lost after translation: insights from pulmonary surfactant for understanding the role of alveolar epithelial dysfunction and cellular quality control in fibrotic lung disease. Am J Physiol Lung Cell Mol Physiol. 2015;309(6):L507.
17. Honda Y, Kuroki Y, Matsuura E, Nagae H, Takahashi H, Akino T, Abe S. Pulmonary surfactant protein D in sera and bronchoalveolar lavage fluids. Am J Respir Crit Care Med. 1995;152(6):1860–6.
18. Greene KE, Wright JR, Steinberg KP, Ruzinski JT, Caldwell E, Wong WB, et al. Serial changes in surfactant-associated proteins in lung and serum before and after onset of ARDS. Am J Respir Crit Care Med. 2012;160(6):1843–50.
19. Greene KE, King JE, Kuroki Y, Bucher-Bartelson B, Hunninghake GW, Newman LS, et al. Serum surfactant proteins-A and -D as biomarkers in idiopathic pulmonary fibrosis. Eur Respir J. 2002;19(3):439–46.
20. Günther A, Schmidt R, Nix F, Yabut-Perez M, Guth C, Rosseau S, et al. Surfactant abnormalities in idiopathic pulmonary fibrosis, hypersensitivity pneumonitis and sarcoidosis. Eur Respir J. 1999;14(3):565–73.
21. McCormac FX, King TE, Bucher BL, Nielsen L, Mason RJ. Surfactant protein a predicts survival in idiopathic pulmonary fibrosis. Am J Respir Crit Care Med. 2012;152(2):751–9.
22. Wang K, Ju Q, Cao J, Tang W, Zhang J. Impact of serum SP-A and SP-D levels on comparison and prognosis of idiopathic pulmonary fibrosis a systematic review and meta-analysis systematic review and meta-analysis medicine ® OPEN 1. Medicine. 2017;96(23):e7083.
23. Song JW, Do KH, Jang SJ, Colby TV, Han S, Kim DS. Blood biomarkers MMP-7 and SP-A: predictors of outcome in idiopathic pulmonary fibrosis. Chest. 2013;143(5):1422–9.
24. Kinder BW, Brown KK, Mccormack FX, Ix JH, Kervitsky A, Schwarz MI, et al. Serum surfactant protein-a is a strong predictor of early mortality in idiopathic pulmonary fibrosis. Chest. 2009;135(6):1557–63.
25. Ishii H, Mukae H, Kadota J, Kaida H, Nagata T, Abe K, et al. High serum concentrations of surfactant protein a in usual interstitial pneumonia compared with non-specific interstitial pneumonia. Thorax. 2003;58(1):52–7.
26. Van Moorsel CHM, Ten Klooster L, Van Oosterhout MFM, De Jong PA, Adams H, Van Es HW, et al. SFTPA2 mutations in familial and sporadic idiopathic interstitial pneumonia. Am J Respir Crit Care Med. 2015;192(10):1249–52.
27. Nathan N, Giraud V, Picard C, Nunes H, Le MFD, Copin B, et al. Germline SFTPA1 mutation in familial idiopathic interstitial pneumonia and lung cancer. Hum Mol Genet. 2016;25(8):1457–67.
28. Ishizaka A, Matsuda T, Albertine KH, Koh H, Tasaka S, Hasegawa N, et al. Elevation of KL-6, a lung epithelial cell marker, in plasma and epithelial lining fluid in acute respiratory distress syndrome. Am J Physiol Lung Cell Mol Physiol. 2004;286(6).
29. Kobayashi J, Kitamura S. KL-6: a serum marker for interstitial pneumonia. Chest. 1995;108(2):311–5.
30. He J, Zhang J, Ren X. Krebs von den lungen-6 as a clinical marker for hypersensitivity pneumonitis: a meta-analysis and bioinformatics analysis. Front Immunol. 2022;13:1041098.
31. Yokoyama A, Kohno N, Hamada H, Sakatani M, Ueda E, Kondo K, et al. Circulating KL-6 predicts the outcome of rapidly progressive idiopathic pulmonary fibrosis. Am J Respir Crit Care Med. 2012;158(5 PART I):1680–4.
32. Ohnishi H, Yokoyama A, Kondo K, Hamada H, Abe M, Nishimura K, et al. Comparative study of KL-6, surfactant protein-a, surfactant protein-D, and monocyte chemoattractant Protein-1 as serum markers for interstitial lung diseases. Am J Respir Crit Care Med. 2012;165(3):378–81.
33. Jehn LB, Costabel U, Boerner E, Wälscher J, Theegarten D, Taube C, et al. Serum KL-6 as a biomarker of progression at any time in fibrotic interstitial lung disease. J Clin Med. 2023;12(3).

34. Yokoyama A, Kondo K, Nakajima M, Matsushima T, Takahashi T, Nishimura M, et al. Prognostic value of circulating KL-6 in idiopathic pulmonary fibrosis. Respirology. 2006;11(2):164–8.
35. Lee JS, Lee EY, Ha YJ, Kang EH, Lee YJ, Song YW. Serum kl-6 levels reflect the severity of interstitial lung disease associated with connective tissue disease. Arthritis Res Ther. 2019;21(1):1–8.
36. Kohno N, Awaya Y, Oyama T, Yamakido M, Akiyama M, Inoue Y, et al. KL-6, a mucin-like glycoprotein, in bronchoalveolar lavage fluid from patients with interstitial lung disease. Am Rev Respir Dis. 1993;148(3):637–42.
37. Fathi M, Barbasso Helmers S, Lundberg IE. KL-6: a serological biomarker for interstitial lung disease in patients with polymyositis and dermatomyositis. J Intern Med. 2012;271(6):589–97.
38. Yanaba K, Hasegawa M, Hamaguchi Y, Fujimoto M, Takehara K, Sato S. Longitudinal analysis of serum KL-6 levels in patients with systemic sclerosis: association with the activity of pulmonary fibrosis. Clin Exp Rheumatol. 2003.
39. Sakamoto K, Taniguchi H, Kondoh Y, Johkoh T, Sumikawa H, Kimura T, et al. Serum KL-6 in fibrotic NSIP: correlations with physiologic and radiologic parameters. Respir Med. 2010;104(1):127–33.
40. Hisata S, Kimura Y, Shibata N, Ono S, Kobayashi T, Chiba S, et al. A normal range of KL-6/MUC1 independent of elevated SP-D indicates a better prognosis in the patients with honeycombing on high-resolution computed tomography. Pulm Med. 2011.
41. Kida Y, Ohshimo S, Ota K, Tamura T, Otani T, Une K, et al. KL-6, a human MUC1 mucin, as a prognostic marker for diffuse alveolar hemorrhage syndrome. Orphanet J Rare Dis. 2012;7(1):1–8.
42. Janssen R, Sato H, Grutters JC, Bernard A, Van Velzen-Blad H, Du Bois RM, et al. Study of Clara cell 16, KL-6, and surfactant protein-D in serum as disease markers in pulmonary sarcoidosis. Chest. 2003;124(6):2119–25.
43. Wu RA, Upton HE, Vogan JM, Collins K. Telomerase mechanism of telomere synthesis. Annu Rev Biochem. 2017;86:439.
44. MacNeil DE, Bensoussan HJ, Autexier C. Telomerase regulation from beginning to the end. Genes. 2016;7:64.
45. Cronkhite JT, Xing C, Raghu G, Chin KM, Torres F, Rosenblatt RL, et al. Telomere shortening in familial and sporadic pulmonary fibrosis. Am J Respir Crit Care Med. 2012;178(7):729–37.
46. Tsakiri KD, Cronkhite JT, Kuan PJ, Xing C, Raghu G, Weissler JC, et al. Adult-onset pulmonary fibrosis caused by mutations in telomerase. Proc Natl Acad Sci USA. 2007;104(18):7552.
47. Snetselaar R, Van Moorsel CHM, Kazemier KM, Van Der Vis JJ, Zanen P, Van Oosterhout MFM, et al. Telomere length in interstitial lung diseases. Chest. 2015;148(4):1011–8.
48. Newton CA, Batra K, Torrealba J, Kozlitina J, Glazer CS, Aravena C, et al. Telomere-related lung fibrosis is diagnostically heterogeneous but uniformly progressive. Eur Respir J. 2016;48(6):1710–20.
49. Alder JK, Guo N, Kembou F, Parry EM, Anderson CJ, Gorgy AI, et al. Telomere length is a determinant of emphysema susceptibility. Am J Respir Crit Care Med. 2011;198:904.
50. Borie R, Tabèze L, Thabut G, Nunes H, Cottin V, Marchand-Adam S, et al. Prevalence and characteristics of TERT and TERC mutations in suspected genetic pulmonary fibrosis. Eur Respir J. 2016;48(6):1721–31.
51. Zheng M, Lou A, Zhang H, Zhu S, Yang M, Lai W. Serum KL-6, CA19-9, CA125 and CEA are diagnostic biomarkers for rheumatoid arthritis-associated interstitial lung disease in the Chinese population. Rheumatol Ther. 2021;8(1):517.
52. Jenkins RG, Simpson JK, Saini G, Bentley JH, Russell AM, Braybrooke R, et al. Longitudinal change in collagen degradation biomarkers in idiopathic pulmonary fibrosis: an analysis from the prospective, multicentre PROFILE study. Lancet Respir Med. 2015;3(6):462–72.
53. Cui N, Hu M, Khalil RA. Biochemical and biological attributes of matrix metalloproteinases. Prog Mol Biol Transl Sci. 2017;147:1–73.

54. Cabral-Pacheco GA, Garza-Veloz I, La RCCD, Ramirez-Acuña JM, Perez-Romero BA, Guerrero-Rodriguez JF, et al. The roles of matrix metalloproteinases and their inhibitors in human diseases. Int J Mol Sci. 2020;21(24):1–53.
55. Bauer Y, White ES, de Bernard S, Cornelisse P, Leconte I, Morganti A, et al. MMP-7 is a predictive biomarker of disease progression in patients with idiopathic pulmonary fibrosis. ERJ Open Res. 2017;3(1).
56. Rosas IO, Richards TJ, Konishi K, Zhang Y, Gibson K, Lokshin AE, et al. MMP1 and MMP7 as potential peripheral blood biomarkers in idiopathic pulmonary fibrosis. PLoS Med. 2008;5(4):0623–33.
57. Tzouvelekis A, Herazo-Maya JD, Slade M, Chu J-H, Deiuliis G, Ryu C, et al. Validation of the prognostic value of MMP-7 in idiopathic pulmonary fibrosis. Respirology. 2017;22(3):486–93.
58. Richards TJ, Kaminski N, Baribaud F, Flavin S, Brodmerkel C, Horowitz D, et al. Peripheral blood proteins predict mortality in idiopathic pulmonary fibrosis. Am J Respir Crit Care Med. 2012;185(1):67–76.
59. Morais A, Beltrão M, Sokhatska O, Costa D, Melo N, Mota P, et al. Serum metalloproteinases 1 and 7 in the diagnosis of idiopathic pulmonary fibrosis and other interstitial pneumonias. Respir Med. 2015;109(8):1063–8.
60. Armstrong HF, Podolanczuk AJ, Barr RG, Oelsner EC, Kawut SM, Hoffman EA, et al. Serum matrix Metalloproteinase-7, respiratory symptoms, and mortality in community-dwelling adults. MESA (multi-ethnic study of atherosclerosis). Am J Respir Crit Care Med. 2017;196(10):1311–7.
61. Altmann DM, Hogg N, Trowsdale J, Wilkinson D. Cotransfection of ICAM-1 and HLA-DR reconstitutes human antigen-presenting cell function in mouse L cells. Nature. 1989;338:6215.
62. Springer TA. Adhesion receptors of the immune system. Nature. 1990;346:6283.
63. Ihn H, Sato S, Fujimoto M, Kikuchi K, Kadono T, Tamaki K, et al. Circulating intercellular adhesion molecule-1 in the sera of patients with systemic sclerosis: enhancement by inflammatory cytokines. Rheumatology. 1997;36(12):1270–5.
64. Ihn H, Sato S, Fujimoto M, Takehara K, Tamaki K. Increased serum levels of soluble vascular cell adhesion molecule-1 and E-selectin in patients with systemic sclerosis. Br J Rheumatol. 1998;37:1188–92.
65. Karsdal M. Biochemistry of collagens, laminins and elastin: structure, function and biomarkers. Elsevier; 2023.
66. Tatler AL. Recent advances in the non-invasive assessment of fibrosis using biomarkers. Curr Opin Pharmacol. 2019;49:110–5.
67. Dobrota R, Jordan S, Juhl P, Maurer B, Wildi L, Bay-Jensen AC, et al. Circulating collagen neo-epitopes and their role in the prediction of fibrosis in patients with systemic sclerosis: a multicentre cohort study. Lancet Rheumatol. 2021;3(3):e175–84.
68. Mehrad B, Strieter RM. Fibrocytes and the pathogenesis of diffuse parenchymal lung disease. Fibrogenesis Tissue Repair. 2012;5(Suppl 1).
69. Mehrad B, Burdick MD, Strieter RM. Fibrocyte CXCR4 regulation as a therapeutic target in pulmonary fibrosis. Int J Biochem Cell Biol. 2009;41(8–9):1708–18.
70. Moore BB, Murray L, Das A, Wilke CA, Herrygers AB, Toews GB. The role of CCL12 in the recruitment of fibrocytes and lung fibrosis. Am J Respir Cell Mol Biol. 2006;35(2):175–81.
71. Just SA, Lindegaard H, Hejbøl EK, Davidsen JR, Bjerring N, Hansen SWK, et al. Fibrocyte measurement in peripheral blood correlates with number of cultured mature fibrocytes in vitro and is a potential biomarker for interstitial lung disease in rheumatoid arthritis. Respir Res. 2017;18(1).
72. Trimble A, Gochuico BR, Markello TC, Fischer R, Gahl WA, Lee JK, et al. Circulating fibrocytes as biomarker of prognosis in Hermansky-Pudlak syndrome. Am J Respir Crit Care Med. 2014;190(12):1395–401.
73. Moeller A, Gilpin SE, Ask K, Cox G, Cook D, Gauldie J, et al. Circulating fibrocytes are an indicator of poor prognosis in idiopathic pulmonary fibrosis. Am J Respir Crit Care Med. 2009;179(7):588–94.

74. Odackal J, Yu V, Gomez-Manjerres D, Field JJ, Burdick MD, Mehrad B. Circulating fibrocytes as prognostic biomarkers of autoimmune interstitial lung disease. ERJ Open Res. 2020;6(4):1–9.
75. Zhao T, Su Z, Li Y, Zhang X, You Q. Chitinase-3 like-protein-1 function and its role in diseases. Signal Transduct Target Ther. 2020;5(1):201.
76. Hong JY, Kim M, Sol IS, Kim KW, Lee CM, Elias JA, Sohn MH, Lee CG. Chitotriosidase inhibits allergic asthmatic airways via regulation of TGF-β expression and Foxp3+ Treg cells. Allergy. 2018;73(8):1686–99.
77. Kanneganti M, Kamba A, Mizoguchi E. Role of chitotriosidase (chitinase 1) under normal and disease conditions. J Epithel Biol Pharmacol. 2012;5:1–9.
78. Zhou Y, Peng H, Sun H, Peng X, Tang C, Gan Y, et al. Chitinase 3-like 1 suppresses injury and promotes fibroproliferative responses in mammalian lung fibrosis. Sci Transl Med. 2014;6(240).
79. Lee CG, Herzog EL, Ahangari F, Zhou Y, Gulati M, Lee C-M, et al. Chitinase 1 is a biomarker for and therapeutic target in scleroderma-associated interstitial lung disease that augments TGF-β1 signaling. J Immunol. 2012;189(5):2635–44.
80. Lee CM, He CH, Park JW, Lee JH, Kamle S, Ma B, et al. Chitinase 1 regulates pulmonary fibrosis by modulating TGF-β/SMAD7 pathway via TGFBRAP1 and FOXO3. Life Sci Alliance. 2019;2(3).
81. Zhou Y, He CH, Herzog EL, Peng X, Lee CM, Nguyen TH, et al. Chitinase 3-like-1 and its receptors in Hermansky-Pudlak syndrome-associated lung disease. J Clin Invest. 2015;125(8):3178–92.
82. Lee S-Y, Lee C-M, Ma B, Kamle S, Elias JA, Zhou Y, et al. Targeting Chitinase 1 and Chitinase 3-like 1 as novel therapeutic strategy of pulmonary fibrosis. Front Pharmacol. 2022;13:826471.
83. Lee CG, Elias JA. Role of breast regression protein-39/YKL-40 in asthma and allergic responses. Allergy Asthma Immunol Res. 2010;2(1):20–7.
84. He CH, Lee CG, DelaCruz CS, Lee CM, Zhou Y, Ahangari F, et al. Chitinase 3-like 1 regulates cellular and tissue responses via IL-13 receptor α2. Cell Rep. 2013;4(4):830–41.
85. Cullinane AR, Yeager C, Dorward H, Carmona-Rivera C, Wu HP, Moss J, et al. Dysregulation of galectin-3. Implications for Hermansky-Pudlak syndrome pulmonary fibrosis. Am J Respir Cell Mol Biol. 2014;50(3):605–13.
86. Young LR, Borchers MT, Allen HL, Gibbons RS, McCormack FX. Lung-restricted macrophage activation in the pearl mouse model of Hermansky-Pudlak syndrome. J Immunol. 2006;176(7):4361–8.
87. Furuhashi K, Suda T, Nakamura Y, Inui N, Hashimoto D, Miwa S, et al. Increased expression of YKL-40, a chitinase-like protein, in serum and lung of patients with idiopathic pulmonary fibrosis. Respir Med. 2010;104(8):1204–10.
88. Korthagen NM, Van Moorsel CHM, Barlo NP, Ruven HJT, Kruit A, Heron M, et al. Serum and BALF YKL-40 levels are predictors of survival in idiopathic pulmonary fibrosis. Respir Med. 2011;105(1):106–13.
89. Hozumi H, Fujisawa T, Enomoto N, Nakashima R, Enomoto Y, Suzuki Y, et al. Clinical utility of YKL-40 in Polymyositis/dermatomyositis-associated interstitial lung disease. J Rheumatol. 2017;44(9):1394–401.
90. Jiang L, Wang Y, Peng Q, Shu X, Wang G, Wu X. Serum YKL-40 level is associated with severity of interstitial lung disease and poor prognosis in dermatomyositis with anti-MDA5 antibody. Clin Rheumatol. 2019;38(6):1655–63.
91. Johansen JS, Milman N, Hansen M, Garbarsch C, Price PA, Graudal N. Increased serum YKL-40 in patients with pulmonary sarcoidosis – a potential marker of disease activity? Respir Med. 2005;99(4):396–402.
92. Kruit A, Grutters JC, Ruven HJT, van Moorsel CCM, van den Bosch JMM. A CHI3L1 gene polymorphism is associated with serum levels of YKL-40, a novel sarcoidosis marker. Respir Med. 2007;101(7):1563–71.

93. Korthagen NM, van Moorsel CHM, Zanen P, Ruven HJ, Grutters JC. Evaluation of circulating YKL-40 levels in idiopathic interstitial pneumonias. Lung. 2014;192(6):975–80.
94. Long X, He X, Ohshimo S, Griese M, Sarria R, Guzman J, et al. Serum YKL-40 as predictor of outcome in hypersensitivity pneumonitis. Eur Respir J. 2017;49(2).
95. Väänänen T, Lehtimäki L, Vuolteenaho K, Hämäläinen M, Oksa P, Vierikko T, et al. Glycoprotein YKL-40 levels in plasma are associated with fibrotic changes on HRCT in Asbestos-exposed subjects. Mediat Inflamm. 2017.
96. De Lauretis A, Sestini P, Pantelidis P, Hoyles R, Hansell DM, Goh NSL, et al. Personal non-commercial use only. J Rheumatol. 2016; https://doi.org/10.3899/jrheum.120725.
97. Tsoutsou PG, Gourgoulianis KI, Petinaki E, Germenis A, Tsoutsou AG, Mpaka M, et al. Cytokine levels in the sera of patients with idiopathic pulmonary fibrosis ARTICLE IN PRESS. Respir Med. 2006;100:938–45.
98. Alhamad EH, Cal JG, Shakoor Z, Almogren A, AlBoukai AA. Cytokine gene polymorphisms and serum cytokine levels in patients with idiopathic pulmonary fibrosis. BMC Med Genet. 2013;14(1).
99. Wynn TA. Fibrotic disease and the TH1/TH2 paradigm. Nat Rev Immunol. 2004;4(8):583–94.
100. Hieshima K, Imai T, Baba M, Shoudai K, Ishizuka K, Nakagawa T, Tsuruta J, Takeya M, Sakaki Y, Takatsuki K, Miura R. A novel human CC chemokine PARC that is most homologous to macrophage-inflammatory protein-1 alpha/LD78 alpha and chemotactic for T lymphocytes, but not for monocytes. J Immunol. 1997;159(3):1140–9.
101. Struyf S, Schutyser E, Gouwy M, Gijsbers K, Proost P, Benoit Y, Opdenakker G, Van Damme J, Laureys G. PARC/CCL18 is a plasma CC chemokine with increased levels in childhood acute lymphoblastic leukemia. Am J Pathol. 2003;163(5):2065–75.
102. Günther C, Bello-Fernandez C, Kopp T, Kund J, Carballido-Perrig N, Hinteregger S, et al. CCL18 is expressed in atopic dermatitis and mediates skin homing of human memory T cells. J Immunol. 2005;174(3):1723–8.
103. Prasse A, Pechkovsky DV, Toews GB, Jungraithmayr W, Kollert F, Goldmann T, Vollmer E, et al. A vicious circle of alveolar macrophages and fibroblasts perpetuates pulmonary fibrosis via CCL18. Am J Respir Crit Care Med. 2006;173(7):781–92.
104. Atamas SP, Luzina IG, Choi J, Tsymbalyuk N, Carbonetti NH, Singh IS, Trojanowska M, Jimenez SA, White B. Pulmonary and activation-regulated chemokine stimulates collagen production in lung fibroblasts. Am J Respir Cell Mol Biol. 2003;29(6):743–9.
105. Prasse A, Pechkovsky DV, Toews GB, Schäfer M, Eggeling S, Ludwig C, Germann M, Kollert F, Zissel G, et al. CCL18 as an indicator of pulmonary fibrotic activity in idiopathic interstitial pneumonias and systemic sclerosis. Arthritis Rheum. 2007;56(5):1685–93.
106. Prasse A, Probst C, Bargagli E, Zissel G, Toews GB, Flaherty KR, et al. Serum CC-chemokine ligand 18 concentration predicts outcome in idiopathic pulmonary fibrosis. Am J Respir Crit Care Med. 2009;179(8):717–23.
107. Neighbors M, Cabanski CR, Ramalingam TR, Sheng XR, Tew GW, Gu C, Jia G, Peng K, Ray JM, Ley B, Wolters PJ. Prognostic and predictive biomarkers for patients with idiopathic pulmonary fibrosis treated with pirfenidone: post-hoc assessment of the CAPACITY and ASCEND trials. Lancet Respir Med. 2018;6(8):615–26.
108. Qiu L, Gong G, Wu W, Li N, Li Z, Chen S, Li P, Chen T, Zhao H, Hu C, Fang Z. A novel prognostic signature for idiopathic pulmonary fibrosis based on five-immune-related genes. Ann Trans Med. 2021;9(20):1570.
109. Yang IV, Luna LG, Cotter J, Talbert J, Leach SM. The peripheral blood transcriptome identifies the presence and extent of disease in idiopathic pulmonary fibrosis. PLoS One. 2012;7(6):37708.
110. Sivakumar P, Ammar R, Thompson JR, Luo Y, Streltsov D, Porteous M, et al. Integrated plasma proteomics and lung transcriptomics reveal novel biomarkers in idiopathic pulmonary fibrosis. Respir Res. 2021;22(1).

# Chapter 5
# Bronchoscopy in Precision Diagnosis of Interstitial Lung Disease

**Ramsy Abdelghani, Fahim Pyarali, and Fayez Kheir**

Interstitial lung diseases (ILD) encompass a wide array of inflammatory and fibrotic lung diseases [1]. Affected patients often have similar symptoms including cough and dyspnea. Defining a specific ILD diagnosis can be challenging and currently relies on clinical features, high-resolution chest tomography (HRCT), and histologic data in the setting of a multidisciplinary discussion (MDD) [1]. Although some ILDs share overlapping radiographic and histopathologic features, prognosis and treatment response vary across the ILD spectrum. Delays in diagnosis can lead to missed opportunities to intervene early and potentially prevent progressive pulmonary fibrosis (PPF), which is associated with high morbidity and mortality [1]. MDD is currently considered the "gold standard" method for diagnosing ILD. However, in clinical practice, there may be observer discordance in interpretation of radiology images and pathology, both in the terms of interpretation and terminology, that can impact determinations made by an MDD. The use of bronchoalveolar lavage (BAL) cellular analysis and transbronchial lung biopsy (TBLB) with forceps is of limited value in ILD. BAL cellular analysis lacks specificity for different patterns of ILD and is seldom diagnostic but may help support a specific type of ILD in the proper clinical and radiologic settings [1]. TBLB specimens are small in size and often subject to crush artifacts. They tend to miss the diagnosis when the disease is patchy or larger sample size visualization is required to differentiate ILD patterns [1].While this may initially seem discouraging, the

R. Abdelghani
Division of Pulmonary Diseases, Critical Care and Environmental Medicine, Tulane University Health Sciences Center, New Orleans, LA, USA
e-mail: rabdelgh@tulane.edu

F. Pyarali · F. Kheir (✉)
Division of Pulmonary and Critical Care Medicine, Massachusetts General Hospital, Harvard Medical School, Boston, MA, USA
e-mail: ffp2107@cumc.columbia.edu; fkheir@mgh.harvard.edu



B. F. Collins, S. B. Montesi (eds.), *Precision Medicine in Interstitial Lung Disease*, Respiratory Medicine, https://doi.org/10.1007/978-3-031-87183-2_5

future is promising. Recent investigation into novel diagnostic techniques is causing a paradigm shift toward increased precision, targeted therapeutics, and hopefully improved patient outcomes.

## Cryobiopsy

Diagnosis of ILD requires a MDD approach that includes input from multiple medical teams [1]. Pathology plays an important role in the diagnosis of some patients with ILD. Surgical lung biopsy (SLB) was historically considered the gold standard for obtaining lung tissue for histologic diagnosis [2]. However, despite its high diagnostic yield (approximately 90%), SLB carries significant risks and complications. In patients undergoing elective SLB, risk of short-term (in-hospital) mortality has been estimated at 1.7%, risk of 30-day mortality has been estimated at 1.5–2.4%, and risk of 90-day mortality has been estimated at 2.8–3.9% [3–5]. This necessitates a discussion of the risk-to-benefit ratio between the patient and clinical team. Furthermore, SLB cannot be offered to patients who are not surgical candidates due to ILD severity or comorbidities.

In patients without a typical usual interstitial pneumonia (UIP) pattern on HRCT, current guidelines conditionally recommended bronchoscopic lung cryobiopsy (BLC) as an acceptable alternative to SLB when done at experienced centers [1]. High volume centers have increasingly utilized BLC, as it can provide a comparable diagnostic yield with a lower risk profile when compared to SLB [6, 7]. Specific procedural steps may vary among bronchoscopists. Usually, all BLC (Fig. 5.1) are performed under general anesthesia. The biopsy sites are chosen by the bronchoscopist after considering the HRCT scan appearance. All cryobiopsies are performed under fluoroscopic guidance using a cryoprobe (ERBOKRYO; Erbe USA Inc) [8]. After assessing that the cryoprobe is about 1 cm from the pleura, the cryoprobe is activated for 5–8 s and then removed with bronchoscope en bloc in one quick motion. An endobronchial blocker or Fogarty balloon is immediately inflated in the

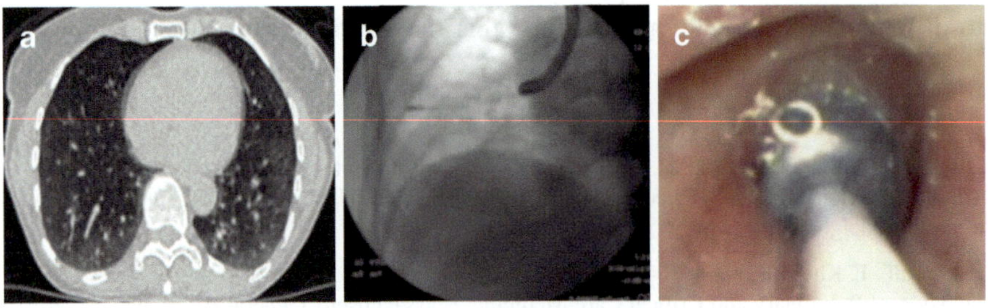


**Fig. 5.1** Images of our procedural technique. (**a**) High-resolution computed tomography with predominant ground-glass opacities in bilateral lower lung zones. (**b**) Cryoprobe in the lateral segment of the right lower lobe. (**c**) Prophylactic Fogarty balloon inflation in lateral segment of right lower lobe

targeted airway to achieve hemostasis. Once the total amount of specimens is collected (typically a total of three to five pieces from two separate sites), attention is turned to achieving hemostasis if significant bleeding has occurred. In addition, lateral airways are preferred so that the cryoprobe intersects with the pleura in a perpendicular manner, allowing for improved visualization of probe to pleural distance on fluoroscopy. Next, a postprocedural chest X-ray is obtained to rule out pneumothorax. Once stable, the patient is discharged home, usually the same day.

There are two types of cryoprobes: single-use and reusable. The reusable cryoprobes are available in 1.9 mm and 2.4 mm sizes and were used in most studies of cryobiopsy. In January 2020, an updated cryosurgical system received United States Food and Drug Administration 510(k) clearance and is compatible with three single-use probe sizes: 1.1 mm, 1.7 mm, and 2.4 mm. The 1.1 mm cryoprobe addressed important limitations of the technique of BLC where en bloc removal of the bronchoscope, cryoprobe, and attached specimen is needed. To address this, the 1.1 mm cryoprobe was paired with a sheath that passes through the working channel of a flexible bronchoscope. This allows the specimen to be removed without extracting the bronchoscope from the airway, thus controlling airway bleeding immediately. A properly performed cryobiopsy should produce a sample with a diameter of at least 5 mm, allowing pathologists to recognize different ILD patterns [9]. Overall, the quality of tissue specimens obtained by cryobiopsy has more favorable histopathologic interpretation as compared to forceps biopsy, improving diagnostic yield in ILD. Potential advantages are bigger tissue size, better preserved specimens, less crush artifact, and minimal hemorrhage on cryobiopsy specimens [9].

In patients undergoing SLB, a definitive diagnosis may not be reached in up to 15% of cases [10]. This compares favorably to cryobiopsy, with pooled diagnostic yield of BLC 77–80% [11, 12]. Diagnostic yield increases with larger sample size, number of samples taken, and when three or more samples are obtained [11, 12]. Furthermore, the COLDICE study, the largest prospective study that performed both BLC and SLB during one procedure, included 65 patients requiring histopathologic evaluation for ILD [6]. Blinded review by three expert pathologists suggested an agreement in histopathologic diagnosis between both BLC and SLB in 70.8% ($\kappa = 0.70$) and consensus diagnosis by multidisciplinary discussion in 76.9% ($\kappa = 0.62$). The final diagnosis was made with high confidence in 60% of cases utilizing BLC, compared to 74% of cases utilizing SLB without reaching statistical significance ($p = 0.09$). Secondary analysis of COLDICE suggested that "predominantly subpleural or paraseptal fibrosis" were infrequently seen on BLC (as samples typically don't include pleura), whereas "patchy fibrosis," "fibroblast foci," and the "absence of alternative diagnostic features" were frequently observed in BLC. The combination of these three features could provide a confident diagnosis of usual interstitial pneumonia (UIP) with odds ratio [OR] of 23.4 as compared to SLB [13].

Localization of the cryoprobe is important in obtaining an optimal biopsy specimen as well as minimizing adverse events. It is recommended to place the tip of the cryoprobe 1 cm from the pleura [14]. This will decrease risk of bleeding by avoiding a biopsy at the more proximal airway with medium-sized vessels and reduce visceral pleural injury causing pneumothorax. Furthermore, it is essential to biopsy active inflammatory disease and avoid densely fibrotic areas to improve diagnostic yield. Fluoroscopy has been commonly used to confirm the distance between tip of the probe and pleura. However, such distance might be difficult to assess if airway is not perpendicular to the fluoroscopy image due to two-dimensional nature of fluoroscopy. Radial endobronchial ultrasound (R-EBUS) is useful for identification of ground-glass opacity lesions (blizzard/mixed blizzard sign) (Fig. 5.2), help identify target lung parenchyma, and avoid large vessels [8, 15]. Advanced imaging techniques such as cone-beam computed tomography (CBCT) have been used to guide BLC and potentially improve diagnostic yield [16–19]. In these studies, CBCT-guided cryobiopsy was associated with a favorable safety profile, with low risks of pneumothorax and moderate-to-severe bleeding with a diagnostic yield ranging between 86 and 100%. However, the use of advanced imaging is limited by the availability and cost. Recently, navigational bronchoscopy has also been used to optimize cryoprobe location in a desired area of interest but remains an area of active investigation [20].

Despite having less morbidity and mortality than SLB, BLC does have procedure-related complications in a recent American Thoracic Society guideline [11]. Bleeding is the most common complication, with 29.9% of cases reporting bleeding as a complication [11]. However, the rate of bleeding is difficult to estimate due to various definitions used in the literature, but the rate of severe bleeding is only 1.6% [11]. Pneumothorax is another significant risk of TBLC, with rate occurring in 7% of procedures [11]. Minor complications reported in recent guidelines are postprocedural respiratory failure or infection and persistent air leak [11].

It is important to note that these safety data in BLC are due to using 1.9 mm and 2.4 mm cryoprobes. Due to differences in probe size and sampling technique, the 1.1 mm cryoprobe may have a more favorable safety profile. In fact, a recent multicenter prospective study of 50 patients undergoing TBCB with the 1.1 mm cryoprobe revealed complication rates similar to those reported with transbronchial forceps biopsy [21]. In this study, pneumothorax occurred in 4%, none of which required chest tube placement, and grade 2 bleeding (defined as requiring wedging of biopsied segment or iced saline) occurred in 4%. There was no bleeding requiring bronchial blocker use or device-related respiratory failure. Despite the fact that

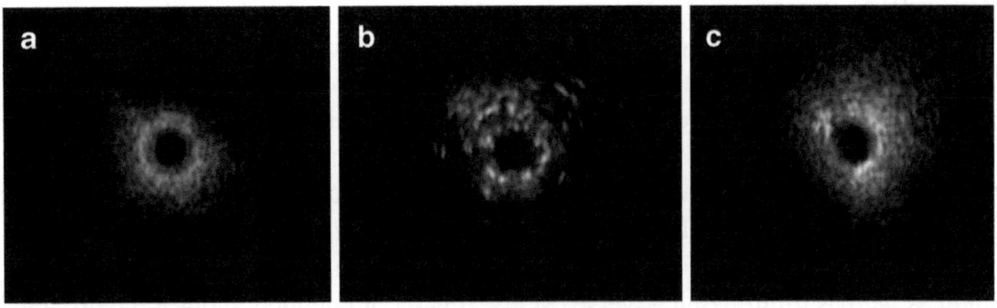


**Fig. 5.2** Radial-EBUS imaging. (**a**) Normal lung pattern on radial-EBUS. (**b**) Subtle homogenous increase in white acoustic shadow (blizzard pattern). (**c**) Heterogeneous white acoustic shadow with hyperechoic dots, linear arcs, and vessels (mixed blizzard pattern)

further studies are needed to verify the safety profile of the 1.1 mm cryoprobe, it seems that such probe may reduce the complication rate of BLC.

Although there is not likely to be one optimal way to perform BLC, standardization of BLC and performance by bronchoscopists with expertise are likely to reduce associated complications [12]. Furthermore, improvement in the interpretation of BLC specimens by expert pathologists comfortable in interpreting relatively small samples is necessary and needs to be further defined to improve clinical utility, since the histopathologic criteria are traditionally based on SLB specimens [13]. Further high-quality prospective trials are needed to evaluate both optimal procedural technique and histopathological interpretation of BLC.

## Genomic Classifier

A genomic classifier has been recently introduced for clinical use [22]. It was developed using machine learning analysis of next-generation RNA sequencing based on genomic data from SLB and quantifies 190 exons to identify a profile predictive of UIP in lung tissue obtained by transbronchial forceps biopsy (3 samples from lower or upper lobes). The classifier distinguishes UIP from non-UIP histopathology, helping clinicians and multidisciplinary teams predict histologic UIP in patients without a definite UIP pattern at chest imaging with a specificity of 92% and sensitivity of 68% [23]. Unlike descriptive pathology reports, the genomic classifier report is binary and reported as positive or negative for UIP.

Studies have demonstrated how the genomic may be incorporated into the diagnostic evaluation of patients with fibrotic ILD to increase diagnostic confidence in the absence of a SLB [22–27]. Genomic classifier may decrease the subjectivity as well as interobserver variability of histopathology interpretation and increases the yield of less invasive testing. In a study by Richeldi and colleagues [26], the genomic classifier identified UIP histopathology with a sensitivity of 60.3% and a specificity 92.1% as compared with SLB or BLC. When genomic classifier results were combined with high-resolution computed tomography (HRCT) reports from local radiologists, the sensitivity increased from 34% to 79.2%, whereas specificity remained almost the same (90.6%). Thus, the integration of radiologic data markedly reduced false-negative results. Another study evaluated the impact of BLC and genomic classifier on the multidisciplinary process in cases where HRCT scan indicated probable UIP with confounding clinical factors or was indeterminate for UIP. There was a significant increase in confidence levels of idiopathic pulmonary fibrosis (IPF) diagnosis when the classifier was added to the BLC [25]. The CATALYST study found 86% agreement between two separate MDDs that were either given histopathology results or the genomic classifier [22]. A prospective randomized decision impact survey found pulmonologists were more likely to diagnose UIP and start antifibrotic treatment when provided with a positive genomic classifier result [27]. There was a 36% increase in antifibrotic recommendation in the pre-/post-genomic classifier cohort when information was given in a staged fashion and 11%

increase in antifibrotic recommendation in an independent cohort when all information was given simultaneously [27].

Chaudhary et al. [28] compared progression-free survival defined as composite outcomes (time to death, lung transplant, or FVC decline ≥10% up to 18 months) in a retrospective, multicenter, US-based cohort study between patients that were genomic classifier positive and negative for UIP. This study did not show a statistically significant association between disease progression and a positive classifier pattern. However, the study was limited by a small sample size and relatively short-term follow-up. Also, treatment of patients who had positive genomic classifier pattern with antifibrotics may have slowed disease progression. These findings indicate the need for larger-scale studies investigating the utility of a genomic classifier in predicting prognosis in such patients. Another study evaluated whether the combined genomic classifier and BLC data were associated with a change of treatment strategy and evaluated the disease progression in patients with a positive genomic classifier result compared with patients who had negative genomic classifier [29]. Combined genomic classifier and histopathologic data were associated with change of therapeutic strategy in 59.5% of patients, and this increased to 76.2% when the genomic classifier was positive for UIP and the BLC was indeterminate. This 16.7% increase in initiation of antifibrotics could potentially increase appropriate antifibrotic prescriptions and reduce the risk of initiating harmful immunosuppressive therapies in patients with IPF. Furthermore, the study did not show a statistically significant difference in disease progression in patients that had positive genomic classifier as compared with UIP negative. However, there was a trend toward statistical significance among patients who were positive for UIP by genomic classifier and not treated with antifibrotics compared to patients with genomic classifier-negative results [29].

Recently, there has been a paradigm shift by some experts proposing that UIP can represent a single diagnostic entity whether due to primary (IPF) or secondary (non-IPF) etiology. This is due to similarities in disease behavior, pathogenic profile, progression, and possible treatment response to antifibrotic therapy [30–32]. This could represent diagnostic simplification where UIP identified at cryobiopsy or genomic classifier could facilitate earlier treatment with currently approved antifibrotics or antifibrotic trials for specific secondary UIP or trials of novel agents. However, the distinction of a UIP pattern remains important when trying to determine the underlying ILD. Non-IPF UIP has implications for other important aspects of management such as antigen identification and avoidance in hypersensitivity pneumonitis or monitoring as well as management of extrapulmonary involvement in connective tissue diseases.

As current guidelines recommend a MDD to review radiographical and tissue data to reach a consensus in the diagnosis of ILD, the genomic classifier may be of a beneficial addition to the process. Genomic classifier may serve as a surrogate for, or addition to, the BLC. It is useful to the diagnostic armamentarium in patients with unclassifiable ILD who need further testing for a confident diagnosis and may serve as a biomarker for disease progression. Also, the genomic classifier may be particularly useful for patients with disease too advanced to tolerate surgical biopsy.

## Confocal Laser Endomicroscopy

Confocal laser endomicroscopy (CLE) is an optical imaging technology that can provide real-time images of the alveolar compartment, pulmonary microvessels, terminal bronchioles, as well as pleura. CLE can aid in direct visualization of ILD and also guide selection of biopsy site. It has a resolution up to 3.5 μm, with a maximum depth of 70 μm and a maximum field of view of 600 μm [33–35]. A probe (Alveoflex™) with an outer diameter of 1.4 mm is advanced through the working channel of a bronchoscope and directed to the area of interest under fluoroscopic guidance. The probe illuminates tissue with laser light (wavelength 488 nm) utilizing the principle that the elastin present in the alveolar compartment and pleura emits autofluorescence under excitation. These reflections are captured through a pinhole detector that is on the same plane (i.e., confocal) as the laser [33–35]. This results in dynamic real-time high-resolution images (Fig. 5.3). Imaging the bronchi and alveolar compartment with CLE does not require a contrast agent, such as fluorescein, since elastin fibers are partially autofluorescent [33–35].

Using endoscopic visualization and fluoroscopy, the CLE probe can gently be advanced from the working channel of the bronchoscope to the alveolar compartment until the pleura is reached. During the procedure, video recording and image capture can be performed by a confocal microprobe imager (Cellvizio) and stored for revision or further analysis. Multiple airway segments (up to eight bronchoalveolar areas) should be visualized to assess ILD pattern and possible site for biopsy. Although the etiologies of ILD are varied, studies have shown that these subtypes reliably show abnormal elastin fibers using CLE. Multiple patterns of CLE imaging can be recognized during bronchoscopy [36–38]. Normal alveolar compartment images typically show thin, single-fibered elastin fiber network and dark alveolar air spaces. Mild increase of elastin fibers and preserved alveolar architecture can be seen in areas with mild lung fibrosis and may aid in identifying a suitable area for biopsy. Areas of dense fibrotic lung can demonstrate destruction of alveolar architecture and dramatic increase of the elastin fibers with loss of normal architecture

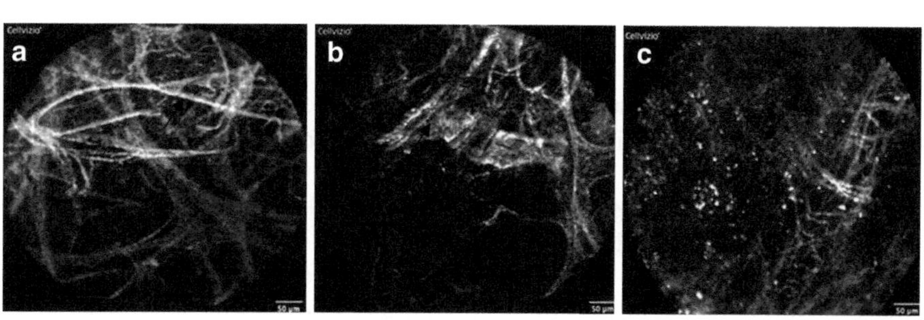


**Fig. 5.3** Bronchoscopic confocal laser endomicroscopy imaging in interstitial lung disease. (**a**) mild increase of elastin fibers (arrow) with preserved alveolar architecture. (**b**) Dramatic increase of elastin fibers (arrow) with destruction alveolar architecture. (**c**) Hypercellular patterns with filling of the alveolar space with auto fluorescent cells

on CLE imaging. These areas are considered less optimal sites for biopsy. Biopsy should be avoided in areas where there is pulmonary microvasculature. This appears as a strip-like microvascular sheath, typically thicker than alveolar septae, and may have branches. Pleural CLE imaging is shown as a dense cross-fiber pattern or linearly arranged fiber bundles, without alveolar and microvascular sheath structures, and biopsy should also be avoided here to reduce risk of pneumothorax.

Although CLE's ability to differentiate normal from abnormal tissue appears promising, its role in identifying specific subtypes of ILD remains to be established. Meng et al. identified six different patterns in ILD [36]. Salaün et al. identified nine specific CLE characteristics which can discriminate normal from diseased lung [37]. Furthermore, they were able to show that certain ILDs were associated with a cellular CLE pattern (fluorescent bronchial and alveolar cells), while others were associated with a fibrotic CLE pattern (small alveolar mouths, disorganized dense elastin fiber network with thickened septae) [37]. Another study showed that bronchoscopic CLE provided real-time imaging of ILD features in fibrotic (increased alveolar elastin fibers) and nonfibrotic ILDs (alveolar cells filled with auto fluorescent cells), with higher resolution than HRCT scan [38]. Thus, it seems that CLE can differentiate cellular from fibrotic ILDs; however, whether CLE can differentiate between specific subgroups of ILDs remains to be established, as does application in clinical practice.

As alluded to above, CLE imaging can be utilized as a high-resolution guidance tool for bronchoscopic lung cryobiopsies. Wijmans et al. evaluated the feasibility of using CLE to guide cryobiopsy in 14 patients with fibrotic ILD [39]. CLE imaging was able to identify key information to influence both diagnostic yield (avoid targeting dense fibrotic areas) and complication rate (pleura and subpleural space) with a diagnostic yield of 83%. Another prospective, observational, single-center study evaluated the feasibility and safety of only CLE-guided transbronchial lung cryobiopsy in 17 patients with ILD [40]. Similar to Wijmans et al., they concluded that using CLE to guide biopsy can improve diagnostic yield reported as 94% and reduce complications. Recently, results were published from a randomized controlled study comparing efficacy and safety of cryobiopsy combined with CLE or fluoroscopy in the diagnosis of fibrotic ILD [41]. A total of 60 patients were included. The diagnostic yield in the CLE group was significantly higher than that in the fluoroscopy group (95.0% vs. 80.0%, $p < 0.05$) without difference in the maximum cross-sectional area of the specimens obtained. Also, the incidence of pneumothorax in the CLE group was significantly lower than that in the fluoroscopy group (0 vs. 25.0%, $p < 0.001$).

The use of CLE imaging in diagnosis of ILD is still evolving and remains to be determined in large clinical studies. Although imaging from CLE is typically interpreted by expert observers, there have been efforts made to automate this interpretation using machine learning algorithm [42]. Further work may facilitate consistency in the identification of pathology among patients with interstitial lung disease. There is not much data to guide decisions surrounding initiation of immunosuppression or antifibrotic therapy for patients with non-IPF progressive fibrotic lung disease. As our understanding of hypercellular or fibrotic patterns seen on CLE evolves, this may allow clinicians to be better informed about starting such medications and delivers personalized treatment.

## Optical Coherence Tomography

Optical coherence tomography (OCT) is a nonionizing imaging technology that employs low coherence light waves to capture high resolution of soft tissues to a resolution of <10 μm and imaging depth of 2–3 mm [43, 44] . This technology can be used to image the alveolar space, which may help identify early ILD although thus far has only been used in the research setting [43–45]. OCT is performed by passing an OCT probe (1.65 mm) through the working channel of a flexible bronchoscope to evaluate peripheral and subpleural lung tissue in vivo, similar to a traditional bronchoscopic airway exam. Once position is confirmed, real-time imaging of the lung parenchyma and airways is performed by generating pullbacks from distal to proximal. Helical cross-sectional scans can be reconstructed into a three-dimensional overview and are reviewed for adequacy in real time. Next, the images are reconstructed in three dimensions along the airway path and sent for interpretation by trained pathologists or pulmonologists who can recognize different patterns [43]. Polarization-sensitive OCT is an extension of conventional OCT that adds tissue-specific contrast by assessing the presence of birefringence [46]. Since pulmonary fibrosis is characterized by an increase in collagen, polarization-sensitive OCT can visualize pulmonary fibrosis [46]. OCT can identify subpleural fibrosis with and without associated architectural distortion, spatial heterogeneity, microscopic honeycombing (which may allow for a diagnosis of ILD sooner), and airway-centered fibrosis without the need for tissue sampling [47].

A prospective diagnostic accuracy study compared OCT to SLB in a small cohort of patients with unclassifiable or low confidence fibrotic ILD diagnoses [43]. OCT had sensitivity of 100% (95% CI 75.8–100%) and specificity of 100% (95% CI 79.6–100%) for both histopathologic diagnosis of UIP and clinical diagnosis of IPF. Furthermore, high agreement was also demonstrated between OCT (interpreted by both OCT expert pathologist and novice pathologists who were trained in interpretation during the study) and histopathologic ILD pattern (weighted k:0.87 [0.72–1.0]). Recently, two small studies investigated polarization-sensitive OCT (able to detect tissue endogenous birefringence) to quantify microscopic fibrosis in ILD. One found that polarization-sensitive OCT could use quantitative birefringence to differentiate between types of fibrosis. The other noted that identification of microscopic definite fibrosis by OCT was associated with high risk of progression to pulmonary fibrosis among patients' interstitial lung abnormalities. While these data are promising, larger studies are needed to continue to explore clinical utility in diagnosis, prognosis, and monitoring [48, 49].

Although these results are certainly very promising and propose OCT as both a novel diagnostic tool and means of monitoring treatment response and/or disease progression, larger multicenter studies are needed before OCT is ready for implementation in routine clinical practice. Whether OCT will complement histopathology, guide biopsies, or eventually replace invasive diagnostic procedures remains to be determined.

## Conclusion

In summary, there is considerable research to advance our ability to diagnose and classify ILDs in a safe, minimally invasive, and accurate manner. The growing body of literature for BLC reflects a diagnostic yield approaching that of SLB with a favorable safety profile, especially in the context of MDD. Promising strategies that could further improve diagnostic yield include combining BLC with genomic classifier and advanced imaging modalities such as R-EBUS, CBCT, OCT, and/or CLE.

## References

1. Raghu G, Remy-Jardin M, Richeldi L, Thomson CC, Inoue Y, Johkoh T, Kreuter M, Lynch DA, Maher TM, Martinez FJ, Molina-Molina M, Myers JL, Nicholson AG, Ryerson CJ, Strek ME, Troy LK, Wijsenbeek M, Mammen MJ, Hossain T, Bissell BD, Herman DD, Hon SM, Kheir F, Khor YH, Macrea M, Antoniou KM, Bouros D, Buendia-Roldan I, Caro F, Crestani B, Ho L, Morisset J, Olson AL, Podolanczuk A, Poletti V, Selman M, Ewing T, Jones S, Knight SL, Ghazipura M, Wilson KC. Idiopathic pulmonary fibrosis (an update) and progressive pulmonary fibrosis in adults: an official ATS/ERS/JRS/ALAT clinical practice guideline. Am J Respir Crit Care Med. 2022;205(9):e18–47.
2. Hariri LP, Roden AC, Chung JH, Danoff SK, Gomez Manjarres DC, Hartwig M, Kheir F, King C, Kreider M, Lynch DA, Mooney J, Muniappan A, Myers JL, Paoletti L, Raj R, Safdar Z, Suliman S, Thavarajah K, Lederer DJ, Rudell FL, Bianchi P, Shea BS, Ley B. The role of surgical lung biopsy in the diagnosis of fibrotic interstitial lung disease: perspective from the Pulmonary Fibrosis Foundation. Ann Am Thorac Soc. 2021;18(10):1601–9.
3. Hutchinson JP, Fogarty AW, McKeever TM, Hubbard RB. In-hospital mortality after surgical lung biopsy for interstitial lung disease in the United States: 2000 to 2011. Am J Respir Crit Care Med. 2016;193:1161–7.
4. Hutchinson JP, McKeever TM, Fogarty AW, Navaratnam V, Hubbard RB. Surgical lung biopsy for the diagnosis of interstitial lung disease in England: 1997-2008. Eur Respir J. 2016;48:1453–61.
5. Nguyen W, Meyer KC. Surgical lung biopsy for the diagnosis of interstitial lung disease: a review of the literature and recommendations for optimizing safety and efficacy. Sarcoidosis Vasc Diffuse Lung Dis. 2013;30:3–16.
6. Troy LK, Grainge C, Corte TJ, Williamson JP, Vallely MP, Cooper WA, Mahar A, Myers JL, Lai S, Mulyadi E, Torzillo PJ, Phillips MJ, Jo HE, Webster SE, Lin QT, Rhodes JE, Salamonsen M, Wrobel JP, Harris B, Don G, Wu PJC, Ng BJ, Oldmeadow C, Raghu G, Lau EMT. Cryobiopsy versus open lung biopsy in the diagnosis of interstitial lung disease alliance (COLDICE) investigators. Diagnostic accuracy of transbronchial lung cryobiopsy for interstitial lung disease diagnosis (COLDICE): a prospective, comparative study. Lancet Respir Med. 2020;8(2):171–81.
7. Ravaglia C, Poletti V. Transbronchial lung cryobiopsy for the diagnosis of interstitial lung diseases. Curr Opin Pulm Med. 2022;28(1):9–16.

8. Abdelghani R, Thakore S, Kaphle U, Lasky JA, Kheir F. Radial endobronchial ultrasound-guided transbronchial cryobiopsy. J Bronchol Interv Pulmonol. 2019;26(4):245–9.
9. Colby TV, Tomassetti S, Cavazza A, et al. Transbronchial cryobiopsy in diffuse lung disease: update for the pathologist. Arch Pathol Lab Med. 2017;141(7):891–900.
10. Raghu G, Remy-Jardin M, Myers JL, et al. Diagnosis of idiopathic pulmonary fibrosis. An official ATS/ERS/JRS/ALAT clinical practice guideline. Am J Respir Crit Care Med. 2018;198(5):e44–68.
11. Kheir F, Uribe Becerra JP, Bissell B, Ghazipura M, Herman D, Hon SM, Hossain T, Khor YH, Knight SL, Kreuter M, Macrea M, Mammen MJ, Martinez FJ, Poletti V, Troy L, Raghu G, Wilson KC. Transbronchial lung cryobiopsy in patients with interstitial lung disease: a systematic review. Ann Am Thorac Soc. 2022;19(7):1193–202.
12. Rodrigues I, Estêvão Gomes R, Coutinho LM, Rego MT, Machado F, Morais A, Novais BH. Diagnostic yield and safety of transbronchial lung cryobiopsy and surgical lung biopsy in interstitial lung diseases: a systematic review and meta-analysis. Eur Respir Rev. 2022;31(166):210280.
13. Cooper WA, Mahar A, Myers JL, et al. Cryobiopsy for identification of usual interstitial pneumonia and other interstitial lung disease features. Further lessons from coldice, a prospective multicenter clinical trial. Am J Respir Crit Care Med. 2021;203(10):1306–13.
14. Maldonado F, Danoff SK, Wells AU, et al. Transbronchial cryobiopsy for the diagnosis of interstitial lung diseases: CHEST guideline and expert panel report. Chest. 2020;157(4):1030–42.
15. Inomata M, Kuse N, Awano N, Tone M, Yoshimura H, Jo T, Minami J, Takada K, Muto Y, Fujimoto K, Harada A, Bae Y, Kumasaka T, Yamakawa H, Sato S, Tobino K, Matsushima H, Takemura T, Izumo T. Utility of radial endobronchial ultrasonography combined with transbronchial lung cryobiopsy in patients with diffuse parenchymal lung diseases: a multicentre prospective study. BMJ Open Respir Res. 2021;8(1):e000826.
16. Steinfort DP, D'Agostino RD, Vrjlic I, Einsiedel P, Prasad JD, Jennings BR, Heinze S, Irving LB. CT-fluoroscopic guidance for performance of targeted transbronchial cryobiopsy: a preliminary report. Respiration. 2018;96(5):472–9.
17. Benn BS, Romero AO, Bawaadam H, Ivanick N, Lum M, Krishna G. Cone beam CT guidance improves Transbronchial lung Cryobiopsy safety. Lung. 2021;199(5):485–92.
18. Zhou G, Ren Y, Li J, Yang T, Su N, Zhao L, Wang D, Li Y, Tian Z, Liu R, Dai H, Wang C. Safety, and diagnostic efficacy of cone beam computed tomography-guided transbronchial cryobiopsy for interstitial lung disease: a cohort study. Eur Respir J. 2020;56(2):2000724.
19. Ali SO, Castellani C, Benn BS. Transbronchial lung cryobiopsy performed with cone beam computed tomography guidance versus fluoroscopy: a retrospective cohort review. Lung. 2024;202(1):73–81.
20. Kronborg-White S, Bendstrup E, Gori L, Luzzi V, Madsen LB, Poletti V, Rasmussen TR, Trigiani M, Vezzosi S, Tomassetti S. A pilot study on the use of the super dimension navigation system for optimal cryobiopsy location in interstitial lung disease diagnostics. Pulmonology. 2023;29(2):119–23.
21. Thiboutot J, Illei PB, et al. Safety and feasibility of a sheath cryoprobe for bronchoscopic transbronchial biopsy: the FROSTBITE trial. Respiration. 2022;101(12):1131–8.
22. Raghu G, Flaherty KR, Lederer DJ, Lynch DA, Colby TV, Myers JL, Groshong SD, Larsen BT, Chung JH, Steele MP, Benzaquen S, Calero K, Case AH, Criner GJ, Nathan SD, Rai NS, Ramaswamy M, Hagmeyer L, Davis JR, Gauhar UA, Pankratz DG, Choi Y, Huang J, Walsh PS, Neville H, Lofaro LR, Barth NM, Kennedy GC, Brown KK, Martinez FJ. Use of a molecular classifier to identify usual interstitial pneumonia in conventional transbronchial lung biopsy samples: a prospective validation study. Lancet Respir Med. 2019;7(6):487–96.
23. Kheir F, Uribe Becerra JP, Bissell B, Ghazipura M, Herman D, Hon SM, Hossain T, Khor YH, Knight SL, Kreuter M, Macrea M, Mammen MJ, Martinez FJ, Poletti V, Troy L, Raghu G, Wilson KC. Use of a genomic classifier in patients with interstitial lung disease: a systematic review and meta-analysis. Ann Am Thorac Soc. 2022;19(5):827–32.

24. Pankratz DG, Choi Y, Imtiaz U, Fedorowicz GM, Anderson JD, Colby TV, Myers JL, Lynch DA, Brown KK, Flaherty KR, Steele MP, Groshong SD, Raghu G, Barth NM, Walsh PS, Huang J, Kennedy GC, Martinez FJ. Usual interstitial pneumonia can be detected in transbronchial biopsies using machine learning. Ann Am Thorac Soc. 2017;14(11):1646–54.
25. Kheir F, Alkhatib A, Berry GJ, Daroca P, Diethelm L, Rampolla R, Saito S, Smith DL, Weill D, Bateman M, Abdelghani R, Lasky JA. Using bronchoscopic lung cryobiopsy and a genomic classifier in the multidisciplinary diagnosis of diffuse interstitial lung diseases. Chest. 2020;158(5):2015–25.
26. Richeldi L, Scholand MB, Lynch DA, Colby TV, Myers JL, Groshong SD, Chung JH, Benzaquen S, Nathan SD, Davis JR, Schmidt SL, Hagmeyer L, Sonetti D, Hetzel J, Criner GJ, Case AH, Ramaswamy M, Calero K, Gauhar UA, Patel NM, Lancaster L, Choi Y, Pankratz DG, Walsh PS, Lofaro LR, Huang J, Bhorade SM, Kennedy GC, Martinez FJ, Raghu G. Utility of a molecular classifier as a complement to high-resolution computed tomography to identify usual interstitial pneumonia. Am J Respir Crit Care Med. 2021;203(2):211–20.
27. Lasky JA, Case A, Unterman A, Kreuter M, Scholand MB, Chaudhary S, Lofaro LR, Johnson M, Huang J, Bhorade SM, Kennedy GC. The impact of the Envisia genomic classifier in the diagnosis and management of patients with idiopathic pulmonary fibrosis. Ann Am Thorac Soc. 2022;19(6):916–24.
28. Chaudhary S, Weigt SS, Ribeiro Neto ML, Benn BS, Pugashetti JV, Keith R, Chand A, Oh S, Kheir F, Ramalingam V, Solomon JJ, Harper R, Lasky JA, Oldham JM. Interstitial lung disease progression after genomic usual interstitial pneumonia testing. Eur Respir J. 2023;61(4):2201245.
29. Kheir F, Abdelghani R, Espinoza D, Villalobos R, Becnel D, Herr R, Aragaki A, Uribe Becerra JP, Oldham J, Lasky J. Employment of the Envisia genomic classifier in conjunction with cryobiopsy in patients with undiagnosed interstitial lung disease. CHEST Pulmonary. 2024;2:100034.
30. Selman M, Pardo A, Wells AU. Usual interstitial pneumonia as a stand-alone diagnostic entity: the case for a paradigm shift? Lancet Respir Med. 2023;11(2):188–96.
31. Flaherty KR, Wells AU, Cottin V, Devaraj A, Walsh SLF, Inoue Y, Richeldi L, Kolb M, Tetzlaff K, Stowasser S, Coeck C, Clerisme-Beaty E, Rosenstock B, Quaresma M, Haeufel T, Goeldner RG, Schlenker-Herceg R, Brown KK. INBUILD trial investigators. Nintedanib in progressive fibrosing interstitial lung diseases. N Engl J Med. 2019;381(18):1718–27.
32. Maher TM, Corte TJ, Fischer A, Kreuter M, Lederer DJ, Molina-Molina M, Axmann J, Kirchgaessler KU, Samara K, Gilberg F, Cottin V. Pirfenidone in patients with unclassifiable progressive fibrosing interstitial lung disease: a double-blind, randomised, placebo-controlled, phase 2 trial. Lancet Respir Med. 2020;8(2):147–57.
33. Thiberville L, Moreno-Swirc S, Vercauteren T, Peltier E, Cavé C, Bourg HG. In vivo imaging of the bronchial wall microstructure using fibered confocal fluorescence microscopy. Am J Respir Crit Care Med. 2007;175(1):22–31.
34. Yick CY, von der Thüsen JH, Bel EH, Sterk PJ, Kunst PW. In vivo imaging of the airway wall in asthma: fibered confocal fluorescence microscopy in relation to histology and lung function. Respir Res. 2011;12(1):85.
35. Thiberville L, Salaün M, Lachkar S, Dominique S, Moreno-Swirc S, Vever-Bizet C, Bourg-Heckly G. Human in vivo fluorescence microimaging of the alveolar ducts and sacs during bronchoscopy. Eur Respir J. 2009;33(5):974–85.
36. Meng P, Tan GL, Low SY, Takano A, Ng YL, Anantham D. Fibred confocal fluorescence microscopy in the diagnosis of interstitial lung diseases. J Thorac Dis. 2016;8(12):3505–14.
37. Salaün M, Guisier F, Dominique S, Genevois A, Jounieaux V, Bergot E, Thill C, Piton N, Thiberville L. In vivo probe-based confocal laser endomicroscopy in chronic interstitial lung diseases: specific descriptors and correlation with chest CT. Respirology. 2019;24(8):783–91.
38. Wijmans L, Kalverda K, de Bruin D, Brinkman P, van den Berk I, Roelofs JJTH, Jonkers R, Bonta PI, Annema J. Bronchoscopic journey of in vivo real-time microscopic imaging in ILD: a case series. Respiration. 2022;101(11):1006–14.

39. Wijmans L, Bonta PI, Rocha-Pinto R, de Bruin DM, Brinkman P, Jonkers RE, Roelofs JJTH, Poletti V, Hetzel J, Annema JT. Confocal laser endomicroscopy as a guidance tool for transbronchial lung cryobiopsies in interstitial lung disorder. Respiration. 2019;97(3):259–63.
40. Zheng Y, Zhang L, Lou Y, Fan B, Cui Y, Wu X, Tan X. The cryobiopsy in interstitial lung diseases guided by probe-based confocal laser endomicroscopy is feasible. Clin Respir J. 2023;17(10):998–1005.
41. Zuo C, Xue K, Yang H, Huang R, Yong Z, Zhang M, Lin Y, Tian X, Gu Y, Ke M. Clinical application of confocal laser endomircoscopy combined with cryobiopsy in the diagnosis of interstitial lung disease. Respiration. 2023;102(10):891–8.
42. Bondesson D, Schneider MJ, Silbernagel E, Behr J, Reichenberger F, Dinkel J. Automated evaluation of probe-based confocal laser endomicroscopy in the lung. PLoS One. 2020;15(5):e0232847.
43. Nandy S, Raphaely RA, Muniappan A, Shih A, Roop BW, Sharma A, Keyes CM, Colby TV, Auchincloss HG, Gaissert HA, Lanuti M, Morse CR, Ott HC, Wain JC, Wright CD, Garcia-Moliner ML, Smith ML, VanderLaan PA, Berigei SR, Mino-Kenudson M, Horick NK, Liang LL, Davies DL, Szabari MV, Caravan P, Medoff BD, Tager AM, Suter MJ, Hariri LP. Diagnostic accuracy of endobronchial optical coherence tomography for the microscopic diagnosis of usual interstitial pneumonia. Am J Respir Crit Care Med. 2021;204(10):1164–79.
44. Popescu DP, Choo-Smith LP, Flueraru C, Mao Y, Chang S, Disano J, Sherif S, Sowa MG. Optical coherence tomography: fundamental principles, instrumental designs and biomedical applications. Biophys Rev. 2011;3(3):155.
45. Wijmans L, de Bruin DM, Bonta PI, Jonkers RE, Poletti V, Annema JT. Optical coherence tomography: a valuable novel tool for assessing the alveolar compartment in interstitial lung disease? Am J Respir Crit Care Med. 2018;197(9):1231–2.
46. Vaselli M, Kalverda-Mooij K, Thunnissen E, Tanck MWT, Mets OM, van den Berk IAH, Annema JT, Bonta PI, de Boer JF. In vivo polarisation sensitive optical coherence tomography for fibrosis assessment in interstitial lung disease: a prospective, exploratory, observational study. BMJ Open Respir Res. 2023;10(1):e001628.
47. Hariri LP, Adams DC, Wain JC, Lanuti M, Muniappan A, Sharma A, Colby TV, Mino-Kenudson M, Mark EJ, Kradin RL, Goulart H, Tager AM, Suter MJ. Endobronchial optical coherence tomography for Low-risk microscopic assessment and diagnosis of idiopathic pulmonary fibrosis in vivo. Am J Respir Crit Care Med. 2018;197(7):949–52.
48. Nandy S, Berigei SR, Keyes CM, Muniappan A, Auchincloss HG, Lanuti M, Roop BW, Shih AR, Colby TV, Medoff BD, Suter MJ, Villiger M, Hariri LP. Polarization-sensitive endobronchial optical coherence tomography for microscopic imaging of fibrosis in interstitial lung disease. Am J Respir Crit Care Med. 2022;206(7):905–10.
49. Hariri LP, Sharma A, Nandy S, Berigei SR, Yamamoto S, Raphaely RA, Flashner BM, Muniappan A, Auchincloss HG, Lanuti M, Hallowell RW, Shea BS, Keyes CM. Endobronchial optical coherence tomography as a novel method for in vivo microscopic assessment of interstitial lung abnormalities. Am J Respir Crit Care Med. 2024.

# Chapter 6
# Environmental Influences on ILD Development and Clinical Course

**Hayley Barnes and Christopher Barber**

## Introduction

Interstitial lung diseases (ILDs) are a group of similarly related parenchymal lung diseases which result from an inflammatory and/or fibrotic process. Their subclassification relates in part to their associated risk factors and pathogenesis, and the most common include idiopathic pulmonary fibrosis (IPF), connective tissue disease-associated interstitial lung disease (CTD-ILD), and hypersensitivity pneumonitis (HP) [1]. Their development results in impairment of gas exchange across the lung interstitium, breathlessness, cough, fatigue, increased susceptibility to infections, and in some cases respiratory failure [2]. Management is focused on reducing inciting exposures and immunosuppression and/or antifibrotic therapy where appropriate. However, effective treatment is limited, and prognosis is often poor.

H. Barnes (✉)
Department of Respiratory Medicine, Alfred Health, Melbourne, Australia

Monash Centre for Occupational and Environmental Health, Monash University, Melbourne, Australia

School of Translational Medicine, Monash University, Melbourne, Australia
e-mail: Hayley.Barnes@monash.edu

C. Barber
Centre for Workplace Health, Science Division, Health and Safety Executive, Buxton, UK

Department of Respiratory Medicine, Northern General Hospital, Sheffield, UK
e-mail: chris.barber4@nhs.net



B. F. Collins, S. B. Montesi (eds.), *Precision Medicine in Interstitial Lung Disease*, Respiratory Medicine, https://doi.org/10.1007/978-3-031-87183-2_6

## Environmental Risk Factors in ILD

Multiple occupational and environmental triggers have been identified in ILD, some specific to certain ILDs (e.g., silica dust exposure leading to silicosis) and others partly contributory (e.g., tobacco smoke, air pollution) to many ILDs across the spectrum.

### *Tobacco Smoke*

Tobacco smoke greatly increases the development of many ILDs including interstitial lung abnormalities (ILAs), IPF, asbestosis, possibly some CTD-ILDs, and smoking-related ILDs including respiratory bronchiolitis-interstitial lung disease (RB-ILD), desquamative interstitial pneumonia (DIP), Langerhans cell histiocytosis (LCH), and combined pulmonary fibrosis and emphysema (CPFE) [3–5]. Smoking history is also associated with poorer prognosis in those with IPF [6, 7] and HP [8, 9], with conflicting evidence in other ILDs.

Tobacco smoke induces a variety of inflammatory, genotoxic, and epigenetic changes in the lungs. Tobacco smoke impairs mucociliary clearance, which increases the risk of retained inhaled asbestos fibers and other dusts [10]. It causes oxidative stress via the production of free radicals, which leads to DNA damage, and affects the posttranslational modification of histone proteins in the epigenetic regulation of gene transcription, specifically histone deacetylase (HDAC-2) and IP-10 expression [11, 12]. Tobacco smoke also induces cellular senescence and increases pro-inflammatory and profibrotic cytokines including TGF-β1 and platelet-derived growth factor (PDGF)-A and (PDGF)-B, inducing extracellular matrix as well as fibroblast and myofibroblast proliferation [13]. Smoking also induces a M2-type macrophage response and production of osteopontin, which is involved in antigen-presenting cell trafficking, and increases a Th17 response pathway, which leads to fibrosis [14]. Conversely, history of smoking is associated with a reduced incidence of HP, likely due to the nicotine inhibitory effects on IL-1, TNF, and impairment of macrophage phagocytosis. However, once HP develops, there is a greater chance of developing fibrosis with ongoing smoking and history of smoking has been associated with higher risk of mortality in some cohorts [8, 15].

### *Air Pollution*

Particulate matter from air pollution is also associated with increased risk of development of ILD. Air pollution results from suspended particulates in ambient air, which includes an accumulation of organic, inorganic, and biologic matter with or without toxic gases (ozone, sulfur dioxide, nitrogen dioxide) [16]. Respirable particulate matter is usually <2.5um in diameter. $PM_{2.5}$ has been associated with increased risk of IPF [17–19], HP [20] and other ILDs [21]. Specific pollutants including nitrogen oxide and elemental carbon exposure have been associated with increased risk of developing interstitial lung abnormalities [21]. Airborne pollutants affect ciliary and macrophage clearance mechanisms, induce oxidative stress, and induce epigenetic mechanisms including histone modifications and DNA methylation [22].

## *Inorganic Dust Exposure*

Exposure to high concentrations of specific particulate matter through occupational sources also contributes to the risk of ILD. Construction, mining, foundry work, and stone processing increase the risk of inhalation of silica dust, iron, metalloids, asbestos fibers, and other heavy metals. Inhalation of these dusts is directly associated with specific ILDs including silicosis, coal-workers pneumoconiosis, asbestosis, and hard metal lung disease [23–25]. Occupational and environmental exposures also increase the risk of other ILDs; a large meta-analysis found that occupational exposures contributed to at least 26% of IPF, 19% of HP, and 30% of sarcoidosis cases [26].

## *Silica and Coal Dust*

Silicosis is a parenchymal lung disease resulting from the inhalation and deposition of respirable crystalline silica. There has been an increase in diagnosis due to the development of newer industries (artificial stone benchtop fabrication [27], denim jean sandblasting [28], and jewelry polishing [29], where silica has been introduced without recognition or control of its hazards. Rates have also increased in Central Appalachian coal miners, possibly reflecting increased mechanization in mining practices [30]. When silica particles are inhaled in the lungs, they are engulfed by alveolar macrophages, which stimulate pro-inflammatory and pro-fibrotic pathways [31]. Freshly fractured silica also penetrates the epithelium directly to cause interstitial damage. Silica particles generate free radicals, leading to oxidative stress and stimulation of cytokine transcription factors [32, 33]. Persistent silica uptake leads to the formation of parenchymal silicotic nodules, which over time conglomerate and obliterate the surrounding small airways and pulmonary vessels, resulting in progressive massive fibrosis (PMF) [34, 35]. The intensity and duration of previous silica exposure are associated with its likelihood of disease and risk of progression [27]. The mainstay of management is reduction or elimination of exposure, as persistent exposure is associated with increased risk of disease progression.

Coal worker's pneumoconiosis (CWP) results from chronic inhalation of mixed coal dust. Most fibrogenic is respirable crystalline silica, although other compounds including pure carbon, iron, cadmium, lead, and polycyclic aromatic hydrocarbons may contribute to alveolar damage [25]. The mechanism of disease is similar to that described in silicosis. Disease progression is dependent on the level of exposure, profusion of nodules, presence of PMF, and concomitant risk factors including advancing age and smoking. Avoidance of further dust exposure may reduce risk of progression [36].

## *Asbestos Fibers*

Asbestosis is an interstitial lung disease caused specifically by exposure to asbestos fibers. Unlike asbestos-associated malignancies, there is no clear evidence that different asbestos fiber types confer different risks for asbestosis [37]. Asbestos fibers are inhaled and engulfed by alveolar macrophages, which subsequently lyse, releasing cytokines that attract further macrophages, CD4+ T lymphocytes, and mast cells. Ingestion of asbestos fibers by alveolar macrophages also stimulates the NALP3 inflammasome which stimulates a pro-inflammatory and pro-fibrotic response. Hypertrophy and hyperplasia of type II epithelial cells promote fibrogenesis, and the upregulation of proto-oncogenes, leading not only to fibrosis but an increase in the risk of lung cancer [38, 39]. Asbestosis tends to be less rapidly progressive than untreated IPF, although cases of progressive asbestosis do occur [40]. Treatment of progressive asbestosis is no different to that of other progressive-fibrosing ILDs; nintedanib may be considered [41, 42]. Avoidance of ongoing exposure is essential to reduce further progression, although this may be difficult to implement given the long latency of the disease, with many patients reporting historical rather than current exposure. Monitoring for mesothelioma and lung cancer is also important in exposed individuals.

## *Metal Dust Exposure*

Inhalation of certain metals can cause granulomatous lung disease, the most common of which is chronic beryllium disease. Workers with potential beryllium exposure include those employed in the aerospace, defense, nuclear energy, computer, and electronics industries [43]. Histopathology demonstrates noncaseating granulomas which can subsequently lead to parenchymal destruction and fibrosis. Increased risk of chronic beryllium disease has been associated with genetic variants located in the HLA-DPB1 region [44]. Hard metal lung disease is another type of granulomatous ILD, caused by a specific type of metal alloy produced by sintering (heat and pressure treating) cobalt with tungsten carbide; exposure may occur during manufacturing the alloy, or the use of carbide tipped drilling and cutting tools. Histopathology demonstrates a hypersensitivity reaction with formation of giant cells [45, 46].

## *Organic Dust Exposure*

Exposure to respirable organic dust is commonly implicated in HP but also associated with increased risk of IPF, CTD-ILD, and other ILDs [47, 48]. Commonly implicated antigens include mold due to water damage and microbial and bacterial contamination of ventilation systems, microbial and fungal species associated with farming (hay) and other agricultural roles, and bird antigen from bloom feathers and mucin from bird droppings. Additional risk factors including occupational exposure to pesticides [49] and previous viral infections [50] also increase risk. These antigens induce a macrophage response and upregulate a Th1 and subsequently Th2 and Th17 response, which stimulates further inflammation, epithelial damage, and destruction of the alveolar-capillary membrane. Profibrotic cytokines stimulate fibroblasts, differentiation into myofibroblasts, and lead to extracellular matrix production, and lung tissue remodeling, which perpetuates fibrosis [51]. Similar to other occupational and environmental ILDs, identification and cessation of the exposure significantly reduce the risk of progression of HP, and in some cases, complete remission is possible with exposure removal in non-fibrotic HP [52].

## Interplay Between Genetics and Environmental Factors

The development of ILD requires multiple "hits" not only genetic polymorphisms but also environmental factors to develop and perpetuate disease (Fig. 6.1). Many of the genetic polymorphisms identified thus far increase susceptibility and cause a maladaptive response to environmental triggers. Epigenetics describes the effect from which environmental factors might influence the expression of certain genes (epigenetics) or certain genomes (epigenomics) [54]. In ILD, epigenetic changes including DNA methylation, histone modifications, and microRNAs have been the most well studied. DNA methylation involves the addition of a methyl group to the fifth position of CpG islands, mediated by DNA methyltransferases. DNA methylation has been associated with cell adhesion, molecule binding, surfactant homeostasis, extracellular matrix differentiation, and receptor binding in IPF [55]. Some case-control studies also demonstrate a difference in methylation and expressed genes previously implicated in ILD disease pathogenesis, including TOLLIP, NOTCH1, HDAC4, PDGF, SERPINF, and collagen [56, 57]. Histone modification includes acetylation and methylation and plays an essential role in the response to DNA damage, transcription regulation, and apoptosis. MicroRNA (miRNAs) are noncoding RNAs that can silence or degrade gene expression [54, 55]. miRNA dysregulation has been demonstrated in the lungs of some patients with ILD and may play a role in disease development and progression.

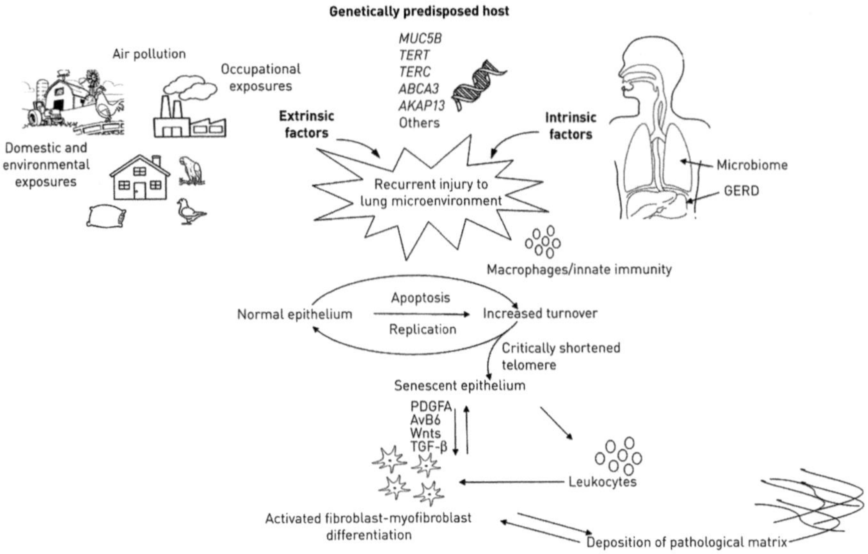


**Fig. 6.1** Proposed model for the pathogenesis of idiopathic pulmonary fibrosis. Extrinsic and intrinsic environmental exposures to the lung microenvironment cause recurrent airway injury. In the genetically predisposed host (mutations in mucin 5B (*MUC5B*), telomerase reverse transcriptase (*TERT*), telomerase RNA component (*TERC*), ATP-binding cassette sub-family A3 (*ABCA3*), A-kinase anchor protein 13 (*AKAP13*), etc.), this cycle of increased epithelial turnover eventually leads to reprogramming to senescent epithelium. Fibroblasts are activated via pro-fibrotic mediators (platelet-derived growth factor subunit A (PDGFA), activating integrin B6 (avB6), Wnts, transforming growth factor-β (TGF-β)) that are released directly from abnormal epithelium, the activated innate immune system, and leukocytes. Once activated, fibroblasts deposit pathological matrix, which leads to myofibroblast differentiation and progressive fibrosis. GERD: gastro-oesophageal reflux disease. From Sack and Raghu [48]. (Adapted from Wolters et al. [53] and reproduced with permission)

## Genetic Risk Factors in ILD

There are a multitude of identified genetic variants which contribute to the pathogenesis of pulmonary fibrosis. These have been best studied in idiopathic pulmonary fibrosis (IPF) and subsequently translated to other ILDs. The most strongly associated variants relate to the subsequent response to noxious stimuli, including host defense, cellular senescence, and antigen processing (Table 6.1).

### *Host Defense*

Inflammation and fibrosis are an essential response of the body against pathogens and in normal wound healing [58]. In ILD, various and disease-specific triggers stimulate aberrant and exaggerated cascades of inflammatory and fibrotic responses.

**Table 6.1** Genetic risk factors in ILD

| Genetic polymorphism | Role in ILD | Role in precision medicine |
|---|---|---|
| MUC5B single-nucleotide polymorphism (SNP) rs35705950 | Chronic mucous production, impaired mucociliary transport, chronic inflammation, and injury; impairment of the differentiation of progenitor type 2 alveolar epithelial cells (AECs) | T allele of the rs35705950 SNP increases risk of development of sporadic and familial IPF, asbestosis, fibrotic HP, RA-ILD<br>Increased cough severity<br>Conflicting evidence for prognosis<br>Increased risk of IPF in those with a smoking history and asbestos exposure |
| TOLLIP | Regulates the innate immune response by inhibiting toll-like receptor signaling | The genetic variant rs5743890 T allele is associated with increased IPF, HP susceptibility but increased IPF survival<br>TT genotype associated with response to n-acetylcysteine, but the CC genotype associated with a trend toward harm in PANTHER-IPF; now being studied in the PRECISIONS trial |
| Short telomere length<br>Telomere mutations (TERT, TERC, PARN, RTEL1, DKCI, NAF1, TINF2, ACD) | Activates DNA damage response pathways which initiates and maintains cellular senescence, proliferative arrest, apoptosis, and autophagy | Short telomere length increases the risk of pulmonary fibrosis by approximately 3.6-fold; is associated with worse survival; effect is consistent across other non-IPF-ILDs including HP, unclassifiable ILD, and possibly CTD-ILD<br>Poor response to immunosuppression in IPF (PANTHER-IPF) and in HP. possible therapeutic targets with medications which aim to restore telomere length (e.g., danazol) |
| HLA-DR3 | Increased affinity for antigen presentation and processing | Increased risk of bird-related HP |
| HLA-DQ3 | Increased affinity for antigen presentation and processing | Increased risk of summer-type HP |
| HLA-A, -B, -C, and tumor necrosis factor (TNF)-gene promoter region variants | Increased affinity for antigen presentation and processing | Increased risk of HP |
| HLA-DRB1*04 | Increased affinity for antigen presentation and processing | Increased risk of RA, multiplicative in smokers |
| HLA-DRB1*11 | Increased affinity for antigen presentation and processing | Increased risk of scleroderma-related ILD |

Genetic variations in host defense increase the risk of damage to these triggers. MUC5B overexpression results in chronic mucous production, inflammation, and injury [59–64]. In a UK case-control study, the odds of IPF were increased with the combination of the MUC5B rs35705950 minor allele variant plus smoking and asbestos exposure, compared to these environmental risk factors alone [65]. In animal studies, addition $PM_{2.5}$ resulted in a significant increase in inflammation and fibrosis in MUC5B-overexpressed rats [66].

TOLLIP is expressed in lung macrophages and epithelial cells and regulates the innate immune response by inhibiting toll-like receptor signaling, leading to impaired wound healing and fibrosis [67–72]. In vitro studies demonstrate an interaction effect between nitrogen oxide exposure and diesel particulate matter in TOLLIP polymorphisms [73]. Other rarer genetic variants associated with host defense encode for surfactant proteins SP-A, SB-B, SP-C, and SP-D, and SFTPA1, SFTPA2, SFTPC, and ABCA3, all of which have been associated with a greater risk of the development of IPF [74–79]. These mutations result in abnormal surfactant processing, protein misfolding, and endoplasmic reticulum stress, all of which can decrease the host lung's mucociliary defense mechanisms and increase the risk of exposure to noxious stimuli and subsequent damage.

## *Cellular Senescence and Telomere Biology*

Germline mutations in the molecules involved in telomere biology also contribute to the development of pulmonary fibrosis. Telomeres are the genomic caps on the end of linear chromosomes which protect genomic integrity upon cell division. As the DNA replication machinery is not capable of completely copying DNA at the very ends of chromosomes, it relies on telomerases to add a small repeat sequence to compensate (composed of a catalytic subunit, the telomerase reverse transcriptase, the telomere RNA component, and other protein regulators) [80]. In the absence of functioning telomerases, DNA replication results in progressively shortened telomeres, and exposed DNA ends activate DNA damage response pathways which initiates and maintains cellular senescence, proliferative arrest, apoptosis, and autophagy. Senescent cells secrete pro-inflammatory cytokines which affects the extracellular matrix and promotes cell transdifferentiation [81]. Exposure to environmental pollutants, radiation, infections, reactive oxygen species, and heavy metal exposure has been associated with shortened telomere length and telomerase activity [82]. Short telomere length (<tenth percentile of the general population) and specific telomere mutations have been identified as strongly associated with the development of and poor prognosis of pulmonary fibrosis [70, 76, 83–95].

## *Antigen Presentation and Processing*

Genetic polymorphisms in antigen presentation and processing have also been associated with ILD, including HP and CTD-ILD [96–98]. These mutations lead to a greater affinity for antigen processing and stimulation of the adaptive immune response and increased production of pro-inflammatory cytokines including TNF-$\alpha$. Gene variants encoding MHC have also been demonstrated in CTD-ILD, including

HLA-DRB alleles (Table 6.1); multiplicative risk has been associated with smoking in some cases [99].

## Management of Noxious Environmental Factors in ILD: A Precision Medicine Approach

Management of ILDs is dependent on the specific ILD diagnosis, as well as phenotypes shared across the ILD spectrum. For many ILDs, the first step in management includes identification and mitigation of environmental risk factors, and in some cases (e.g., non-fibrotic HP), this can result in complete remission or disease stability. Other pharmacological and non-pharmacological approaches are discussed in Chap. 10.

Identification of implicated environmental exposures begins with a comprehensive clinical history, including a thorough occupational history (current and historical roles) and any relevant avocational and environmental exposures [100, 101]. A thorough clinical history alongside relevant investigations is often sufficient to identify causative exposures (e.g., history of construction work with relevant CT findings indicating silicosis, history of smoking with CT findings indicating RB-ILD). However, in some conditions, such as HP, the implicated exposure is difficult to ascertain, or multiple exposures are elicited, and it is unclear which are potentially causative. Precision medicine approaches can aid in determination of potentially causative exposures. Antigen panels which test for IgG antibodies to preformed antigens in a patient's serum can be useful not only in supporting diagnosis but also identification of possible relevant exposures [101] [102]. In some studies, individualized testing combining home/site visits to collect antigens with personalized antibody testing can reduce the incidence of antigen-indeterminate HP and clarify whether the relevant exposures are related to workplace or home [103].

Where relevant, exposure avoidance is an essential component of ILD management, as persistent exposure can be associated with poorer prognosis [27] [6, 7]. Exposure avoidance often requires a personalized approach, dependent on the source of exposure, and ideally follows the hierarchy of controls. For example, avoidance of silica dust requires workplaces to completely eliminate sources, such as removal of engineered stone, or substitution with safer products. Where that is not possible, engineering controls including wet cutting alongside personal protective equipment can reduce exposure [104]. Individual management plans may be required depending on the disease severity, financial constraints, workplace policies and practices, and possibility for workplace adaptation. Personalized dust disease monitoring and site visits can be used to assess adherence to exposure reduction.

Individualized management plans are also required for home- or avocational-related exposures. Remediation of these exposures can be difficult, in part because there is lack of guidance on how to perform remediation appropriately. Also, patients may be unable or reluctant to eliminate exposures [101]. Patients with fibrotic HP experience more impaired quality of life compared to other ILD counterparts, and qualitative research suggests this is in part associated with uncertainty of implicated exposures and complex psychosocial problems associated with antigen identification and avoidance [105].

## Conclusions

ILDs arise from a complex interplay of intrinsic genetic factors and occupational and environmental triggers. The contribution and pathogenetic pathways of each are often studied in isolation, but future research needs to consider the interaction between multiple contributing factors. Large-scale registries incorporating well-phenotyped occupational and environmental histories paired with bioregistry data utilizing epigenetic and epigenomic studies will aid in understanding the contribution of multiple factors. It remains imperative to reduce and ultimately prevent known noxious environmental and occupational exposures for all. Identification of biomarkers which indicate increased susceptibility to and progression from ILDs will also aid in risk stratification for prognosis and return to work strategies and may ultimately lead to more precision-based treatment approaches.

## References

1. Kaul B, Cottin V, Collard HR, Valenzuela C. Variability in global prevalence of interstitial lung disease. Front Med (Lausanne). 2021;8:751181. https://doi.org/10.3389/fmed.2021.751181.
2. Cottin V, Hirani NA, Hotchkin DL, Nambiar AM, Ogura T, Otaola M, Skowasch D, Park JS, Poonyagariyagorn HK, Wuyts W, Wells AU. Presentation, diagnosis and clinical course of the spectrum of progressive-fibrosing interstitial lung diseases. Eur Respir Rev. 2018;27(150):180076. https://doi.org/10.1183/16000617.0076-2018.
3. Brims FJH, Kong K, Harris EJA, Sodhi-Berry N, Reid A, Murray CP, Franklin PJ, Musk AB, de Klerk NH. Pleural plaques and the risk of lung cancer in asbestos-exposed subjects. Am J Respir Crit Care Med. 2020;201(1):57–62. https://doi.org/10.1164/rccm.201901-0096OC.
4. George AM, Eirini V, Joseph J, Athol UW, Katerina MA. Smoking and interstitial lung diseases. Eur Respir Rev. 2015;24(137):428. https://doi.org/10.1183/16000617.0050-2015.
5. Hoyer N, Wille MMW, Thomsen LH, Wilcke T, Dirksen A, Pedersen JH, Saghir Z, Ashraf H, Shaker SB. Interstitial lung abnormalities are associated with increased mortality in smokers. Respir Med. 2018;136:77–82. https://doi.org/10.1016/j.rmed.2018.02.001.
6. Ekstrom M, Gustafson T, Boman K, Nilsson K, Tornling G, Murgia N, Toren K. Effects of smoking, gender and occupational exposure on the risk of severe pulmonary fibrosis: a population-based case-control study. BMJ Open. 2014;4(1):e004018. https://doi.org/10.1136/bmjopen-2013-004018.
7. Karkkainen M, Kettunen HP, Nurmi H, Selander T, Purokivi M, Kaarteenaho R. Effect of smoking and comorbidities on survival in idiopathic pulmonary fibrosis. Respir Res. 2017;18(1):160. https://doi.org/10.1186/s12931-017-0642-6.
8. Mooney JJ, Elicker BM, Urbania TH, Agarwal MR, Ryerson CJ, Nguyen MLT, Woodruff PG, Jones KD, Collard HR, King TE Jr, Koth LL. Radiographic fibrosis score predicts survival

in hypersensitivity pneumonitis. Chest. 2013;144(2):586–92. https://doi.org/10.1378/chest.12-2623.
9. Ohtsuka Y, Munakata M, Tanimura K, Ukita H, Kusaka H, Masaki Y, Doi I, Ohe M, Amishima M, Homma Y, et al. Smoking promotes insidious and chronic farmer's lung disease, and deteriorates the clinical outcome. Intern Med. 1995;34(10):966–71. https://doi.org/10.2169/internalmedicine.34.966.
10. Churg A, Wright JL, Hobson J, Stevens B. Effects of cigarette smoke on the clearance of short asbestos fibres from the lung and a comparison with the clearance of long asbestos fibres. Int J Exp Pathol. 1992;73(3):287–97.
11. Barnes PJ, Adcock IM, Ito K. Histone acetylation and deacetylation: importance in inflammatory lung diseases. Eur Respir J. 2005;25(3):552–63. https://doi.org/10.1183/09031936.05.00117504.
12. Coward WR, Watts K, Feghali-Bostwick CA, Jenkins G, Pang L. Repression of IP-10 by interactions between histone deacetylation and hypermethylation in idiopathic pulmonary fibrosis. Mol Cell Biol. 2010;30(12):2874–86. https://doi.org/10.1128/MCB.01527-09.
13. Checa M, Hagood JS, Velazquez-Cruz R, Ruiz V, Garcia-De-Alba C, Rangel-Escareno C, Urrea F, Becerril C, Montano M, Garcia-Trejo S, Cisneros Lira J, Aquino-Galvez A, Pardo A, Selman M. Cigarette smoke enhances the expression of profibrotic molecules in alveolar epithelial cells. PLoS One. 2016;11(3):e0150383. https://doi.org/10.1371/journal.pone.0150383.
14. Shan M, Yuan X, Song LZ, Roberts L, Zarinkamar N, Seryshev A, Zhang Y, Hilsenbeck S, Chang SH, Dong C, Corry DB, Kheradmand F. Cigarette smoke induction of osteopontin (SPP1) mediates T(H)17 inflammation in human and experimental emphysema. Sci Transl Med. 2012;4(117):117ra119. https://doi.org/10.1126/scitranslmed.3003041.
15. Blanchet MR, Israël-Assayag E, Cormier Y. Inhibitory effect of nicotine on experimental hypersensitivity pneumonitis in vivo and in vitro. Am J Respir Crit Care Med. 2004;169(8):903–9. https://doi.org/10.1164/rccm.200210-1154OC.
16. Di Q, Wang Y, Zanobetti A, Wang Y, Koutrakis P, Choirat C, Dominici F, Schwartz JD. Air pollution and mortality in the Medicare population. N Engl J Med. 2017;376(26):2513–22. https://doi.org/10.1056/NEJMoa1702747.
17. Johannson KA, Vittinghoff E, Lee K, Balmes JR, Ji W, Kaplan GG, Kim DS, Collard HR. Acute exacerbation of idiopathic pulmonary fibrosis associated with air pollution exposure. Eur Respir J. 2014;43(4):1124–31. https://doi.org/10.1183/09031936.00122213.
18. Johannson KA, Vittinghoff E, Morisset J, Wolters PJ, Noth EM, Balmes JR, Collard HR. Air pollution exposure is associated with lower lung function, but not changes in lung function, in patients with idiopathic pulmonary fibrosis. Chest. 2018;154(1):119–25. https://doi.org/10.1016/j.chest.2018.01.015.
19. Sese L, Nunes H, Cottin V, Sanyal S, Didier M, Carton Z, Israel-Biet D, Crestani B, Cadranel J, Wallaert B, Tazi A, Maitre B, Prevot G, Marchand-Adam S, Guillot-Dudoret S, Nardi A, Dury S, Giraud V, Gondouin A, Juvin K, Borie R, Wislez M, Valeyre D, Annesi-Maesano I. Role of atmospheric pollution on the natural history of idiopathic pulmonary fibrosis. Thorax. 2018;73(2):145–50. https://doi.org/10.1136/thoraxjnl-2017-209967.
20. Singh S, Collins BF, Bairwa M, Joshi JM, Talwar D, Singh N, Samaria JK, Mangal DK, Singh V, Raghu G. Hypersensitivity pneumonitis and its correlation with ambient air pollution in urban India. Eur Respir J. 2019;53(2):1801563. https://doi.org/10.1183/13993003.01563-2018.
21. Sack C, Vedal S, Sheppard L, Raghu G, Barr RG, Podolanczuk A, Doney B, Hoffman EA, Gassett A, Hinckley-Stukovsky K, Williams K, Kawut S, Lederer DJ, Kaufman JD. Air pollution and subclinical interstitial lung disease: the multi-ethnic study of atherosclerosis (MESA) air-lung study. Eur Respir J. 2017;50(6):1700559. https://doi.org/10.1183/13993003.00559-2017.

22. Goobie GC, Nouraie M, Zhang Y, Kass DJ, Ryerson CJ, Carlsten C, Johannson KA. Air pollution and interstitial lung diseases: defining epigenomic effects. Am J Respir Crit Care Med. 2020;202(9):1217–24. https://doi.org/10.1164/rccm.202003-0836PP.
23. Vanka KS, Shukla S, Gomez HM, James C, Palanisami T, Williams K, Chambers DC, Britton WJ, Ilic D, Hansbro PM, Horvat JC. Understanding the pathogenesis of occupational coal and silica dust-associated lung disease. Eur Respir Rev. 2022;31(165):210250. https://doi.org/10.1183/16000617.0250-2021.
24. Zheng M, Marron R, Sehgal S. Hard metal lung disease: update in diagnosis and management. Curr Pulmonol Rep. 2020;9:37. https://doi.org/10.1007/s13665-020-00247-x.
25. Zosky GR, Hoy RF, Silverstone EJ, Brims FJ, Miles S, Johnson AR, Gibson PG, Yates DH. Coal workers' pneumoconiosis: an Australian perspective. Med J Aust. 2016;204(11):414–8. https://doi.org/10.5694/mja16.00357.
26. Blanc PD, Annesi-Maesano I, Balmes JR, Cummings KJ, Fishwick D, Miedinger D, Murgia N, Naidoo RN, Reynolds CJ, Sigsgaard T, Toren K, Vinnikov D, Redlich CA. The occupational burden of nonmalignant respiratory diseases. An official American Thoracic Society and European Respiratory Society statement. Am J Respir Crit Care Med. 2019;199(11):1312–34. https://doi.org/10.1164/rccm.201904-0717ST.
27. Hoy RF, Dimitriadis C, Abramson M, Glass DC, Gwini S, Hore-Lacy F, Jimenez-Martin J, Walker-Bone K, Sim MR. Prevalence and risk factors for silicosis among a large cohort of stone benchtop industry workers. Occup Environ Med. 2023;80(8):439–46. https://doi.org/10.1136/oemed-2023-108892.
28. Akgun M, Araz O, Ucar EY, Karaman A, Alper F, Gorguner M, Kreiss K. Silicosis appears inevitable among former denim sandblasters: a 4-year follow-up study. Chest. 2015;148(3):647–54.
29. Jiang CQ, Xiao LW, Lam TH, Xie NW, Zhu CQ. Accelerated silicosis in workers exposed to agate dust in Guangzhou, China. Am J Ind Med. 2001;40(1):87–91.
30. Antao VC, Petsonk EL, Sokolow LZ, Wolfe AL, Pinheiro GA, Hale JM, Attfield MD. Rapidly progressive coal workers' pneumoconiosis in the United States: geographic clustering and other factors. Occup Environ Med. 2005;62(10):670–4. https://doi.org/10.1136/oem.2004.019679.
31. Barnes H, Goh NSL, Leong TL, Hoy R. Silica-associated lung disease: an old-world exposure in modern industries. Respirology. 2019;24(12):1165–75. https://doi.org/10.1111/resp.13695.
32. Greenberg MI, Waksman J, Curtis J. Silicosis: a review. Dis Mon. 2007;53(8):394–416. https://doi.org/10.1016/j.disamonth.2007.09.020.
33. Leung CC, Yu IT, Chen W. Silicosis. Lancet. 2018;379(9830):2008.
34. Kramer MR, Blanc PD, Fireman E, Amital A, Guber A, Rhahman NA, Shitrit D. Artificial stone silicosis [corrected]: disease resurgence among artificial stone workers. Chest. 2012;142(2):419–24. https://doi.org/10.1378/chest.11-1321.
35. Perez-Alonso A, Cordoba-Dona JA, Millares-Lorenzo JL, Figueroa-Murillo E, Garcia-Vadillo C, Romero-Morillos J. Outbreak of silicosis in Spanish quartz conglomerate workers. Int J Occup Environ Health. 2014;20(1):26–32.
36. Go LHT, Cohen RA. Coal workers' pneumoconiosis and other mining-related lung disease: new manifestations of illness in an age-old occupation. Clin Chest Med. 2020;41(4):687–96. https://doi.org/10.1016/j.ccm.2020.08.002.
37. Bennett K, Brims FJ. Asbestosis. In: Feary J, Suojalehto H, Cullinan P, editors. Occupational and environmental lung disease. European Respiratory Society; 2020. p. 347. https://doi.org/10.1183/2312508X.erm8920.
38. Matsuzaki H, Maeda M, Lee S, Nishimura Y, Kumagai-Takei N, Hayashi H, Yamamoto S, Hatayama T, Kojima Y, Tabata R, Kishimoto T, Hiratsuka J, Otsuki T. Asbestos-induced cellular and molecular alteration of immunocompetent cells and their relationship with chronic inflammation and carcinogenesis. J Biomed Biotechnol. 2012;2012:492608. https://doi.org/10.1155/2012/492608.

39. Mossman BT, Churg A. Mechanisms in the pathogenesis of asbestosis and silicosis. Am J Respir Crit Care Med. 1998;157(5 Pt 1):1666–80. https://doi.org/10.1164/ajrccm.157.5.9707141.
40. Keskitalo E, Salonen J, Vahanikkila H, Kaarteenaho R. Survival of patients with asbestosis can be assessed by risk-predicting models. Occup Environ Med. 2021;78(7):516. https://doi.org/10.1136/oemed-2020-106819.
41. Flaherty KR, Wells AU, Cottin V, Devaraj A, Walsh SLF, Inoue Y, Richeldi L, Kolb M, Tetzlaff K, Stowasser S, Coeck C, Clerisme-Beaty E, Rosenstock B, Quaresma M, Haeufel T, Goeldner RG, Schlenker-Herceg R, Brown KK, Investigators IT. Nintedanib in progressive fibrosing interstitial lung diseases. N Engl J Med. 2019;381(18):1718–27. https://doi.org/10.1056/NEJMoa1908681.
42. Raghu G, Remy-Jardin M, Richeldi L, Thomson CC, Inoue Y, Johkoh T, Kreuter M, Lynch DA, Maher TM, Martinez FJ, Molina-Molina M, Myers JL, Nicholson AG, Ryerson CJ, Strek ME, Troy LK, Wijsenbeek M, Mammen MJ, Hossain T, Bissell BD, Herman DD, Hon SM, Kheir F, Khor YH, Macrea M, Antoniou KM, Bouros D, Buendia-Roldan I, Caro F, Crestani B, Ho L, Morisset J, Olson AL, Podolanczuk A, Poletti V, Selman M, Ewing T, Jones S, Knight SL, Ghazipura M, Wilson KC. Idiopathic pulmonary fibrosis (an update) and progressive pulmonary fibrosis in adults: an official ATS/ERS/JRS/ALAT clinical practice guideline. Am J Respir Crit Care Med. 2022;205(9):e18–47. https://doi.org/10.1164/rccm.202202-0399ST.
43. Balmes JR, Abraham JL, Dweik RA, Fireman E, Fontenot AP, Maier LA, Muller-Quernheim J, Ostiguy G, Pepper LD, Saltini C, Schuler CR, Takaro TK, Wambach PF. An official American thoracic society statement: diagnosis and management of beryllium sensitivity and chronic beryllium disease. Am J Respir Crit Care Med. 2014;190(10):e34–59. https://doi.org/10.1164/rccm.201409-1722ST.
44. McCanlies EC, Kreiss K, Andrew M, Weston A. HLA-DPB1 and chronic beryllium disease: a HuGE review. Am J Epidemiol. 2003;157(5):388–98. https://doi.org/10.1093/aje/kwg001.
45. Nemery B, Abraham JL. Hard metal lung disease: still hard to understand. Am J Respir Crit Care Med. 2007;176(1):2–3. https://doi.org/10.1164/rccm.200704-527ED.
46. Tanaka J, Moriyama H, Terada M, Takada T, Suzuki E, Narita I, Kawabata Y, Yamaguchi T, Hebisawa A, Sakai F, Arakawa H. An observational study of giant cell interstitial pneumonia and lung fibrosis in hard metal lung disease. BMJ Open. 2014;4(3):e004407. https://doi.org/10.1136/bmjopen-2013-004407.
47. Lee CT, Strek ME, Adegunsoye A, Wong AW, Assayag D, Cox G, Fell CD, Fisher JH, Gershon AS, Halayko AJ, Hambly N, Khalil N, Kolb M, Lok SD, Manganas H, Marcoux V, Morisset J, Sadatsafavi M, Shapera S, et al. Inhalational exposures in patients with fibrotic interstitial lung disease: presentation, pulmonary function and survival in the Canadian registry for pulmonary fibrosis. Respirology. 2022;27(8):635–44. https://doi.org/10.1111/resp.14267.
48. Sack C, Raghu G. Idiopathic pulmonary fibrosis: unmasking cryptogenic environmental factors. Eur Respir J. 2019;53(2):1801699. https://doi.org/10.1183/13993003.01699-2018.
49. Hoppin JA, Umbach DM, Kullman GJ, Henneberger PK, London SJ, Alavanja MC, Sandler DP. Pesticides and other agricultural factors associated with self-reported farmer's lung among farm residents in the agricultural health study. Occup Environ Med. 2007;64(5):334–41. https://doi.org/10.1136/oem.2006.028480.
50. Wuyts WA, Agostini C, Antoniou KM, Bouros D, Chambers RC, Cottin V, Egan JJ, Lambrecht BN, Lories R, Parfrey H, Prasse A, Robalo-Cordeiro C, Verbeken E, Verschakelen JA, Wells AU, Verleden GM. The pathogenesis of pulmonary fibrosis: a moving target. Eur Respir J. 2013;41(5):1207–18. https://doi.org/10.1183/09031936.00073012.
51. Barnes H, Troy L, Lee CT, Sperling A, Strek M, Glaspole I. Hypersensitivity pneumonitis: current concepts in pathogenesis, diagnosis, and treatment. Allergy. 2022;77(2):442–53. https://doi.org/10.1111/all.15017.
52. Gimenez A, Storrer K, Kuranishi L, Soares MR, Ferreira RG, Pereira CAC. Change in FVC and survival in chronic fibrotic hypersensitivity pneumonitis. Thorax. 2018;73(4):391–2. https://doi.org/10.1136/thoraxjnl-2017-210035.

53. Wolters PJ, Blackwell TS, Eickelberg O, Loyd JE, Kaminski N, Jenkins G, Maher TM, Molina-Molina M, Noble PW, Raghu G, Richeldi L, Schwarz MI, Selman M, Wuyts WA, Schwartz DA. Time for a change: is idiopathic pulmonary fibrosis still idiopathic and only fibrotic? Lancet Respir Med. 2018;6(2):154–60. https://doi.org/10.1016/S2213-2600(18)30007-9.
54. Effendi WI, Nagano T. Epigenetics approaches toward precision medicine for idiopathic pulmonary fibrosis: focus on DNA methylation. Biomedicines. 2023;11(4) https://doi.org/10.3390/biomedicines11041047.
55. Tzouvelekis A, Kaminski N. Epigenetics in idiopathic pulmonary fibrosis. Biochem Cell Biol. 2015;93(2):159–70. https://doi.org/10.1139/bcb-2014-0126.
56. Rabinovich EI, Kapetanaki MG, Steinfeld I, Gibson KF, Pandit KV, Yu G, Yakhini Z, Kaminski N. Global methylation patterns in idiopathic pulmonary fibrosis. PLoS One. 2012;7(4):e33770. https://doi.org/10.1371/journal.pone.0033770.
57. Sanders YY, Ambalavanan N, Halloran B, Zhang X, Liu H, Crossman DK, Bray M, Zhang K, Thannickal VJ, Hagood JS. Altered DNA methylation profile in idiopathic pulmonary fibrosis. Am J Respir Crit Care Med. 2012;186(6):525–35. https://doi.org/10.1164/rccm.201201-0077OC.
58. Wijsenbeek M, Cottin V. Spectrum of fibrotic lung diseases. N Engl J Med. 2020;383(10):958–68. https://doi.org/10.1056/NEJMra2005230.
59. Biondini D, Cocconcelli E, Bernardinello N, Lorenzoni G, Rigobello C, Lococo S, Castelli G, Baraldo S, Cosio MG, Gregori D, Saetta M, Balestro E, Spagnolo P. Prognostic role of MUC5B rs35705950 genotype in patients with idiopathic pulmonary fibrosis (IPF) on anti-fibrotic treatment. Respir Res. 2021;22(1):98. https://doi.org/10.1186/s12931-021-01694-z.
60. Juge PA, Lee JS, Ebstein E, Furukawa H, Dobrinskikh E, Gazal S, Kannengiesser C, Ottaviani S, Oka S, Tohma S, Tsuchiya N, Rojas-Serrano J, Gonzalez-Perez MI, Mejia M, Buendia-Roldan I, Falfan-Valencia R, Ambrocio-Ortiz E, Manali E, Papiris SA, Karageorgas T, Boumpas D, Antoniou K, van Moorsel CHM, van der Vis J, de Man YA, Grutters JC, Wang Y, Borie R, Wemeau-Stervinou L, Wallaert B, Flipo RM, Nunes H, Valeyre D, Saidenberg-Kermanac'h N, Boissier MC, Marchand-Adam S, Frazier A, Richette P, Allanore Y, Sibilia J, Dromer C, Richez C, Schaeverbeke T, Liote H, Thabut G, Nathan N, Amselem S, Soubrier M, Cottin V, Clement A, Deane K, Walts AD, Fingerlin T, Fischer A, Ryu JH, Matteson EL, Niewold TB, Assayag D, Gross A, Wolters P, Schwarz MI, Holers M, Solomon JJ, Doyle T, Rosas IO, Blauwendraat C, Nalls MA, Debray MP, Boileau C, Crestani B, Schwartz DA, Dieude P. MUC5B promoter variant and rheumatoid arthritis with interstitial lung disease. N Engl J Med. 2018;379(23):2209–19. https://doi.org/10.1056/NEJMoa1801562.
61. Ley B, Newton CA, Arnould I, Elicker BM, Henry TS, Vittinghoff E, Golden JA, Jones KD, Batra K, Torrealba J, Garcia CK, Wolters PJ. The MUC5B promoter polymorphism and telomere length in patients with chronic hypersensitivity pneumonitis: an observational cohort-control study. Lancet Respir Med. 2017;5(8):639–47. https://doi.org/10.1016/S2213-2600(17)30216-3.
62. Pardo A, Selman M. The interplay of the genetic architecture, aging, and environmental factors in the pathogenesis of idiopathic pulmonary fibrosis. Am J Respir Cell Mol Biol. 2021;64(2):163–72. https://doi.org/10.1165/rcmb.2020-0373PS.
63. Platenburg M, Wiertz IA, van der Vis JJ, Crestani B, Borie R, Dieude P, Kannengiesser C, Burgers JA, Grutters JC, van Moorsel CHM. The MUC5B promoter risk allele for idiopathic pulmonary fibrosis predisposes to asbestosis. Eur Respir J. 2020;55(4):1902361. https://doi.org/10.1183/13993003.02361-2019.
64. Seibold MA, Wise AL, Speer MC, Steele MP, Brown KK, Loyd JE, Fingerlin TE, Zhang W, Gudmundsson G, Groshong SD, Evans CM, Garantziotis S, Adler KB, Dickey BF, du Bois RM, Yang IV, Herron A, Kervitsky D, Talbert JL, Markin C, Park J, Crews AL, Slifer SH, Auerbach S, Roy MG, Lin J, Hennessy CE, Schwarz MI, Schwartz DA. A common MUC5B promoter polymorphism and pulmonary fibrosis. N Engl J Med. 2011;364(16):1503–12. https://doi.org/10.1056/NEJMoa1013660.

65. Reynolds CJ, Sisodia R, Barber C, Moffatt M, Minelli C, De Matteis S, Cherrie JW, Newman Taylor A, Cullinan P. What role for asbestos in idiopathic pulmonary fibrosis? Findings from the IPF job exposures case-control study. Occup Environ Med. 2023;80(2):97–103. https://doi.org/10.1136/oemed-2022-108404.
66. Zhou L, Liu H, Zhang R, Yin J, Huo C, WangMo K, Hua S, Ye L. MUC5B regulates the airway inflammation induced by atmospheric PM(2.5) in rats and A549 cells. Ecotoxicol Environ Saf. 2021;221:112448. https://doi.org/10.1016/j.ecoenv.2021.112448.
67. Isshiki T, Koyama K, Homma S, Sakamoto S, Yamasaki A, Shimizu H, Miyoshi S, Nakamura Y, Kishi K. Association of rs3750920 polymorphism in TOLLIP with clinical characteristics of fibrosing interstitial lung diseases in Japanese. Sci Rep. 2021;11(1):16250. https://doi.org/10.1038/s41598-021-95869-9.
68. Mota PC, Soares ML, Ferreira AC, Santos RF, Rufo JC, Vasconcelos D, Carvalho A, Guimaraes S, Vasques-Novoa F, Cardoso C, Melo N, Alexandre AT, Coelho D, Novais-Bastos H, Morais A. Polymorphisms and haplotypes of TOLLIP and MUC5B are associated with susceptibility and survival in patients with fibrotic hypersensitivity pneumonitis. Pulmonology. 2024;31:2416788. https://doi.org/10.1016/j.pulmoe.2024.01.002.
69. Noth I, Zhang Y, Ma SF, Flores C, Barber M, Huang Y, Broderick SM, Wade MS, Hysi P, Scuirba J, Richards TJ, Juan-Guardela BM, Vij R, Han MK, Martinez FJ, Kossen K, Seiwert SD, Christie JD, Nicolae D, Kaminski N, Garcia JGN. Genetic variants associated with idiopathic pulmonary fibrosis susceptibility and mortality: a genome-wide association study. Lancet Respir Med. 2013;1(4):309–17. https://doi.org/10.1016/S2213-2600(13)70045-6.
70. Oldham JM, Ma SF, Martinez FJ, Anstrom KJ, Raghu G, Schwartz DA, Valenzi E, Witt L, Lee C, Vij R, Huang Y, Strek ME, Noth I, Investigators IP. TOLLIP, MUC5B, and the response to N-Acetylcysteine among individuals with idiopathic pulmonary fibrosis. Am J Respir Crit Care Med. 2015;192(12):1475–82. https://doi.org/10.1164/rccm.201505-1010OC.
71. Podolanczuk AJ, Kim JS, Cooper CB, et al. Design and rationale for the prospective treatment efficacy in IPF using genotype for NAC selection (PRECISIONS) clinical trial. BMC Pulm Med. 2022;22(1):475. https://doi.org/10.1186/s12890-022-02281-8.
72. Zhang G, Ghosh S. Negative regulation of toll-like receptor-mediated signaling by Tollip. J Biol Chem. 2002;277(9):7059–65. https://doi.org/10.1074/jbc.M109537200.
73. Frey U, Gorlanova O, Rüttimann C, Röösli M, Soti A, Hoogh Kd, Vienneau D, Künstle N, Sena CRDS, Steinberg R, Bovermann X, Schulzke S, Latzin P, Müller L (2024) Tollip and Muc5b modulate the effect of ambient No2 on respiratory symptoms in infancy. Available at SSRN: https://ssrn.com/abstract=4777074 or https://doi.org/10.2139/ssrn.4777074.
74. Klay D, Platenburg M, van Rijswijk R, Grutters JC, van Moorsel CHM. ABCA3 mutations in adult pulmonary fibrosis patients: a case series and review of literature. Curr Opin Pulm Med. 2020;26(3):293–301. https://doi.org/10.1097/MCP.0000000000000680.
75. Mulugeta S, Nureki S, Beers MF. Lost after translation: insights from pulmonary surfactant for understanding the role of alveolar epithelial dysfunction and cellular quality control in fibrotic lung disease. Am J Physiol Lung Cell Mol Physiol. 2015;309(6):L507–25. https://doi.org/10.1152/ajplung.00139.2015.
76. Nathan N, Giraud V, Picard C, Nunes H, Dastot-Le Moal F, Copin B, Galeron L, De Ligniville A, Kuziner N, Reynaud-Gaubert M, Valeyre D, Couderc LJ, Chinet T, Borie R, Crestani B, Simansour M, Nau V, Tissier S, Duquesnoy P, Mansour-Hendili L, Legendre M, Kannengiesser C, Coulomb-L'Hermine A, Gouya L, Amselem S, Clement A. Germline SFTPA1 mutation in familial idiopathic interstitial pneumonia and lung cancer. Hum Mol Genet. 2016;25(8):1457–67. https://doi.org/10.1093/hmg/ddw014.
77. Nogee LM, Dunbar AE 3rd, Wert SE, Askin F, Hamvas A, Whitsett JA. A mutation in the surfactant protein C gene associated with familial interstitial lung disease. N Engl J Med. 2001;344(8):573–9. https://doi.org/10.1056/NEJM200102223440805.
78. Takezaki A, Tsukumo SI, Setoguchi Y, Ledford JG, Goto H, Hosomichi K, Uehara H, Nishioka Y, Yasutomo K. A homozygous SFTPA1 mutation drives necroptosis of type II alveolar epithelial cells in patients with idiopathic pulmonary fibrosis. J Exp Med. 2019;216(12):2724–35. https://doi.org/10.1084/jem.20182351.

79. Wang Y, Kuan PJ, Xing C, Cronkhite JT, Torres F, Rosenblatt RL, DiMaio JM, Kinch LN, Grishin NV, Garcia CK. Genetic defects in surfactant protein A2 are associated with pulmonary fibrosis and lung cancer. Am J Hum Genet. 2009;84(1):52–9. https://doi.org/10.1016/j.ajhg.2008.11.010.
80. Alonso-Gonzalez A, Tosco-Herrera E, Molina-Molina M, Flores C. Idiopathic pulmonary fibrosis and the role of genetics in the era of precision medicine. Front Med (Lausanne). 2023;10:1152211. https://doi.org/10.3389/fmed.2023.1152211.
81. Revy P, Kannengiesser C, Bertuch AA. Genetics of human telomere biology disorders. Nat Rev Genet. 2023;24(2):86–108. https://doi.org/10.1038/s41576-022-00527-z.
82. Fernandes SG, Dsouza R, Khattar E. External environmental agents influence telomere length and telomerase activity by modulating internal cellular processes: implications in human aging. Environ Toxicol Pharmacol. 2021;85:103633. https://doi.org/10.1016/j.etap.2021.103633.
83. Adegunsoye A, Morisset J, Newton CA, Oldham JM, Vittinghoff E, Linderholm AL, Strek ME, Noth I, Garcia CK, Wolters PJ, Ley B. Leukocyte telomere length and mycophenolate therapy in chronic hypersensitivity pneumonitis. Eur Respir J. 2021;57:3. https://doi.org/10.1183/13993003.02872-2020.
84. Adegunsoye A, Newton CA, Oldham JM, Ley B, Lee CT, Linderholm AL, Chung JH, Garcia N, Zhang D, Vij R, Guzy R, Jablonski R, Bag R, Voogt RS, Ma SF, Sperling AI, Raghu G, Martinez FJ, Strek ME, Wolters PJ, Garcia CK, Pierce BL, Noth I. Telomere length associates with chronological age and mortality across racially diverse pulmonary fibrosis cohorts. Nat Commun. 2023;14(1):1489. https://doi.org/10.1038/s41467-023-37193-6.
85. Alder JK, Stanley SE, Wagner CL, Hamilton M, Hanumanthu VS, Armanios M. Exome sequencing identifies mutant TINF2 in a family with pulmonary fibrosis. Chest. 2015;147(5):1361–8. https://doi.org/10.1378/chest.14-1947.
86. Armanios MY, Chen JJ, Cogan JD, Alder JK, Ingersoll RG, Markin C, Lawson WE, Xie M, Vulto I, Phillips JA 3rd, Lansdorp PM, Greider CW, Loyd JE. Telomerase mutations in families with idiopathic pulmonary fibrosis. N Engl J Med. 2007;356(13):1317–26. https://doi.org/10.1056/NEJMoa066157.
87. Borie R, Renzoni E. Pulmonary fibrosis associated with telomere-related gene mutations: a complex inheritance. Respirology. 2021;26(12):1098–100. https://doi.org/10.1111/resp.14168.
88. Cogan JD, Kropski JA, Zhao M, Mitchell DB, Rives L, Markin C, Garnett ET, Montgomery KH, Mason WR, McKean DF, Powers J, Murphy E, Olson LM, Choi L, Cheng DS, Blue EM, Young LR, Lancaster LH, Steele MP, Brown KK, Schwarz MI, Fingerlin TE, Schwartz DA, Lawson WE, Loyd JE, Zhao Z, Phillips JA 3rd, Blackwell TS. Rare variants in RTEL1 are associated with familial interstitial pneumonia. Am J Respir Crit Care Med. 2015;191(6):646–55. https://doi.org/10.1164/rccm.201408-1510OC.
89. Kropski JA, Mitchell DB, Markin C, Polosukhin VV, Choi L, Johnson JE, Lawson WE, Phillips JA 3rd, Cogan JD, Blackwell TS, Loyd JE. A novel dyskerin (DKC1) mutation is associated with familial interstitial pneumonia. Chest. 2014;146(1):e1–7. https://doi.org/10.1378/chest.13-2224.
90. Ley B, Torgerson DG, Oldham JM, Adegunsoye A, Liu S, Li J, Elicker BM, Henry TS, Golden JA, Jones KD, Dressen A, Yaspan BL, Arron JR, Noth I, Hoffmann TJ, Wolters PJ. Rare protein-altering telomere-related gene variants in patients with chronic hypersensitivity pneumonitis. Am J Respir Crit Care Med. 2019;200(9):1154–63. https://doi.org/10.1164/rccm.201902-0360OC.
91. Mackintosh JA, Pietsch M, Lutzky V, Enever D, Bancroft S, Apte SH, Tan M, Yerkovich ST, Dickinson JL, Pickett HA, Selvadurai H, Grainge C, Goh NS, Hopkins P, Glaspole I, Reynolds PN, Wrobel J, Jaffe A, Corte TJ, Chambers DC. TELO-SCOPE study: a randomised, double-blind, placebo-controlled, phase 2 trial of danazol for short telomere related pulmonary fibrosis. BMJ Open Respir Res. 2021;8(1):e001127. https://doi.org/10.1136/bmjresp-2021-001127.

92. Newton CA, Oldham JM, Ley B, Anand V, Adegunsoye A, Liu G, Batra K, Torrealba J, Kozlitina J, Glazer C, Strek ME, Wolters PJ, Noth I, Garcia CK. Telomere length and genetic variant associations with interstitial lung disease progression and survival. Eur Respir J. 2019;53(4):1801641. https://doi.org/10.1183/13993003.01641-2018.
93. Stanley SE, Gable DL, Wagner CL, Carlile TM, Hanumanthu VS, Podlevsky JD, Khalil SE, DeZern AE, Rojas-Duran MF, Applegate CD, Alder JK, Parry EM, Gilbert WV, Armanios M. Loss-of-function mutations in the RNA biogenesis factor NAF1 predispose to pulmonary fibrosis-emphysema. Sci Transl Med. 2016;8(351):351ra107. https://doi.org/10.1126/scitranslmed.aaf7837.
94. Stuart BD, Choi J, Zaidi S, Xing C, Holohan B, Chen R, Choi M, Dharwadkar P, Torres F, Girod CE, Weissler J, Fitzgerald J, Kershaw C, Klesney-Tait J, Mageto Y, Shay JW, Ji W, Bilguvar K, Mane S, Lifton RP, Garcia CK. Exome sequencing links mutations in PARN and RTEL1 with familial pulmonary fibrosis and telomere shortening. Nat Genet. 2015;47(5):512–7. https://doi.org/10.1038/ng.3278.
95. Zhang D, Adegunsoye A, Oldham JM, Kozlitina J, Garcia N, Poonawalla M, Strykowski R, Linderholm AL, Ley B, Ma SF, Noth I, Strek ME, Wolters PJ, Garcia CK, Newton CA. Telomere length and immunosuppression in non-idiopathic pulmonary fibrosis interstitial lung disease. Eur Respir J. 2023;62(5):2300441. https://doi.org/10.1183/13993003.00441-2023.
96. Falfan-Valencia R, Camarena A, Pineda CL, Montano M, Juarez A, Buendia-Roldan I, Perez-Rubio G, Resendiz-Hernandez JM, Paramo I, Vega A, Granados J, Zuniga J, Selman M. Genetic susceptibility to multicase hypersensitivity pneumonitis is associated with the TNF-238 GG genotype of the promoter region and HLA-DRB1*04 bearing HLA haplotypes. Respir Med. 2014;108(1):211–7. https://doi.org/10.1016/j.rmed.2013.11.004.
97. Fanning GC, Welsh KI, Bunn C, Du Bois R, Black CM. HLA associations in three mutually exclusive autoantibody subgroups in UK systemic sclerosis patients. Br J Rheumatol. 1998;37(2):201–7. https://doi.org/10.1093/rheumatology/37.2.201.
98. Karlson EW, Chang SC, Cui J, Chibnik LB, Fraser PA, De Vivo I, Costenbader KH. Gene-environment interaction between HLA-DRB1 shared epitope and heavy cigarette smoking in predicting incident rheumatoid arthritis. Ann Rheum Dis. 2010;69(1):54–60. https://doi.org/10.1136/ard.2008.102962.
99. Ha YJ, Lee YJ, Kang EH. Lung involvements in rheumatic diseases: update on the epidemiology, pathogenesis, clinical features, and treatment. Biomed Res Int. 2018;2018:6930297. https://doi.org/10.1155/2018/6930297.
100. Barnes H, Hoy R. Occupational lung diseases: why an occupational history is important. Respir Med Today. 2022;7(2):8–14.
101. Johannson KA, Barnes H, Bellanger AP, Dalphin JC, Fernández Pérez ER, Flaherty KR, Huang YT, Jones KD, Kawano-Dourado L, Kennedy K, Millerick-May M, Miyazaki Y, Morisset J, Morell F, Raghu GR, Robbins C, Sack CS, Salisbury ML, Selman M, Vasakova M, Walsh SLF, Rose CS. Exposure assessment tools for hypersensitivity pneumonitis. An official American Thoracic Society workshop report. Ann Am Thorac Soc. 2020;17(12):1501–9. https://doi.org/10.1513/AnnalsATS.202008-942ST.
102. Raghu G, Remy-Jardin M, Ryerson CJ, Myers JL, Kreuter M, Vasakova M, Bargagli E, Chung JH, Collins BF, Bendstrup E, Chami HA, Chua AT, Corte TJ, Dalphin J-C, Danoff SK, Diaz-Mendoza J, Duggal A, Egashira R, Ewing T, Gulati M, Inoue Y, Jenkins AR, Johannson KA, Johkoh T, Tamae-Kakazu M, Kitaichi M, Knight SL, Koschel D, Lederer DJ, Mageto Y, Maier LA, Matiz C, Morell F, Nicholson AG, Patolia S, Pereira CA, Renzoni EA, Salisbury ML, Selman M, Walsh SLF, Wuyts WA, Wilson KC. Diagnosis of hypersensitivity pneumonitis in adults: an official ATS/JRS/ALAT clinical practice guideline. Am J Respir Crit Care Med. 2020;202(3):e36–69. https://doi.org/10.1164/rccm.202005-2032ST.
103. Millerick-May ML, Mulks MH, Gerlach J, Flaherty KR, Schmidt SL, Martinez FJ, LeVeque RM, Rosenman KD. Hypersensitivity pneumonitis and antigen identification – an alternate approach. Respir Med. 2016;112:97–105. https://doi.org/10.1016/j.rmed.2015.09.001.

104. Australian Government. National dust disease taskforce; 2021. Final Report. Canberra, ACT.
105. Aronson KI, Hayward BJ, Robbins L, Kaner RJ, Martinez FJ, Safford MM. 'It's difficult, it's life changing what happens to you' patient perspective on life with chronic hypersensitivity pneumonitis: a qualitative study. BMJ Open Respir Res. 2019;6(1):e000522.

# Chapter 7
# Influence of Race and Ethnicity on the Precision Diagnosis and Treatment of ILD

**Vincent Ferraro and Julie Morisset**

Within the field of precision medicine, it is essential to acknowledge the intersectionality of race and ethnicity, genetics, environmental factors, as well as healthcare access. Precision medicine, as previously explored in this textbook, is an evolving concept often defined as an approach to disease treatment and prevention that considers every individual's unique genes and environment and is aimed at offering personalized and effective healthcare interventions [1, 2]. By integrating all these crucial factors in our decision-making process, precision medicine represents a promising path for advancement of the management of interstitial lung disease (ILD), which is known as a complex and diverse group of diseases [3]. When exploring the impact of race and ethnicity on ILD, one must be mindful of the challenges regarding defining, interpreting, and comparing research related to these concepts.

## Defining Race, Ethnicity, and Its Importance in Medical Literature

Race, although often used as a proxy of human differences, has been shown to be a poor indicator of genetic diversity [4, 5]. Moreover, the continual overlap among different populations diminishes any significant genetic distinctions [6]. Caution must always be taken when addressing the influence of race and ethnicity on medical conditions. Medicine that categorizes individuals based on race, rather than a race-conscious approach, can perpetuate stereotypes and undermine the necessity

---

V. Ferraro (✉) · J. Morisset (✉)
Département de Médecine, Centre Hospitalier de L'Université de Montréal (CHUM), Montreal, QC, Canada
e-mail: vincent.ferraro@umontreal.ca; julie.morisset@umontreal.ca



B. F. Collins, S. B. Montesi (eds.), *Precision Medicine in Interstitial Lung Disease*, Respiratory Medicine, https://doi.org/10.1007/978-3-031-87183-2_7

for research to identify more accurate biomarkers to explain disparities between populations [4].

Defining race and ethnicity is complex as these are multifaceted societal concepts with no unanimous definitions in the medical literature. Historically, race has been based on social perceptions of physical traits such as skin color, hair texture, and facial features, whereas ethnicity refers to shared cultural characteristics such as language, religion, cuisine, or nationality [7, 8]. These concepts are often underused or misused in the medical literature and can perpetuate racial healthcare disparities [9, 10]. Their incorrect usage can conceal fundamental social determinants of health, thus preventing efforts to address these structural inequities. Furthermore, poorly captured race and ethnicity data can lead to the propagation of erroneous associations between race and disease incidence or outcome [11]. Research conducted with an inadequate understanding of these concepts can lead to the formulation of flawed guidelines [12]. A recent systematic review by Martinez et al. of the major epidemiology journals from 1995 to 2018 demonstrated that most authors did not express how race and ethnicity were measured, nor did they comprehensibly define these concepts. The terms most often used were: "Black, White" (Race), "Hispanic, non-Hispanic" (Ethnicity), or "Black, White, Hispanic" (Ethnoracial). These findings remained similar throughout the studied period. An example of a clinically embedded term that is often misused is "Caucasian," which is frequently used to describe individuals of European descent and thus White. In contrast, the term refers to the populations of the Caucasoid regions which include Europe but also Afghanistan, Pakistan, and subcontinental India [13]. With the goal of providing uniform and comparable data in the literature, the 2015 US National Institutes of Health (NIH) *Policy on Reporting Race and Ethnicity Data* issued updated definitions of five minimum racial and two ethnic categories based on the 1997 directives of the Office of Management and Budget (Table 7.1) [7, 14]. Ultimately, high-quality racial and ethnic data as well as a race-conscious approach, in the context of precision medicine, can help identify additional structural health barriers that overlap with race, in a way to reduce the risk of selection bias in research all while urging the need to identify more precise biomarkers to explain these health disparities [4, 15].

## Influence of Race and Ethnicity on Respiratory Health

To gain a more comprehensive understanding of the significant variations in respiratory health among various racial and ethnic groups, it is essential to consider not only genetic predispositions but also the role of environmental factors, socioeconomic determinants and healthcare access. Although genetic components are continuously being discovered for many respiratory diseases, environmental factors remain, in most cases, the primary driver of disease as few respiratory conditions arise exclusively based on genetic predisposition [16]. Respiratory health disparities are omnipresent due to significant differences among demographic groups in key

**Table 7.1** Race and ethnicity categories based on the US National Institutes of Health (NIH) policy on reporting race and ethnicity data and the 1997 Directives of the Office of Management and Budget [14]

| | |
|---|---|
| **Race category** | |
| White | Individual having origins in any of the original peoples of Europe, the Middle East, or North Africa. |
| Black or African American | Individual having origins in any of the Black racial groups of Africa |
| Asian | Individual having origins in any of the original peoples of the Far East, Southeast Asia, or the Indian subcontinent including, for example, Cambodia, China, India, Japan, Korea, Malaysia, Pakistan, the Philippine Islands, Thailand, and Vietnam |
| Native Hawaiian or other Pacific Islander | Individual having origins in any of the original peoples of Hawaii, Guam, Samoa, or other Pacific Islands |
| American Indian or Alaska Native | Individual having origins in any of the original peoples of North and South America (including Central America), and who maintains tribal affiliation or community attachment |
| **Ethnic category** | |
| Hispanic or Latino (Or not) | Individual of Cuban, Mexican, Puerto Rican, South or Central American, or other Spanish culture or origin, regardless of race |

risk factors such as air pollution exposure, tobacco use, or hazardous occupations [16, 17]. Inequality in healthcare leads to a greater rate of death from respiratory illnesses than from disease in any other organ [17, 18]. As the literature on the impact of race and ethnicity on ILD remains limited, the following section will explore the influence of these societal concepts on respiratory health in general as well as the most recent evidence in the field of ILD.

## Healthcare Access and Delivery in Racial and Ethnic Minorities

Minority racial and ethnic groups often face numerous barriers to accessing medical care but also experience poorer quality of care [19, 20]. These findings are of paramount importance, because once a respiratory conditions develop, variations in access to and quality of care can result in differences in disease evolution and mortality.

The availability of health insurance is an essential factor in the inequalities in healthcare access. According to the 2021 report by the United States Census Bureau, approximately 8.6% of Americans were uninsured with an important variation in coverage by race and ethnicity. While only 5.7% of White individuals were uninsured, 9.6% of Afro-Americans and 17.7% of Hispanic individuals did not have coverage. In addition, 18.8% of American Indian and Alaskan Native people were uninsured [21] (Fig. 7.1).

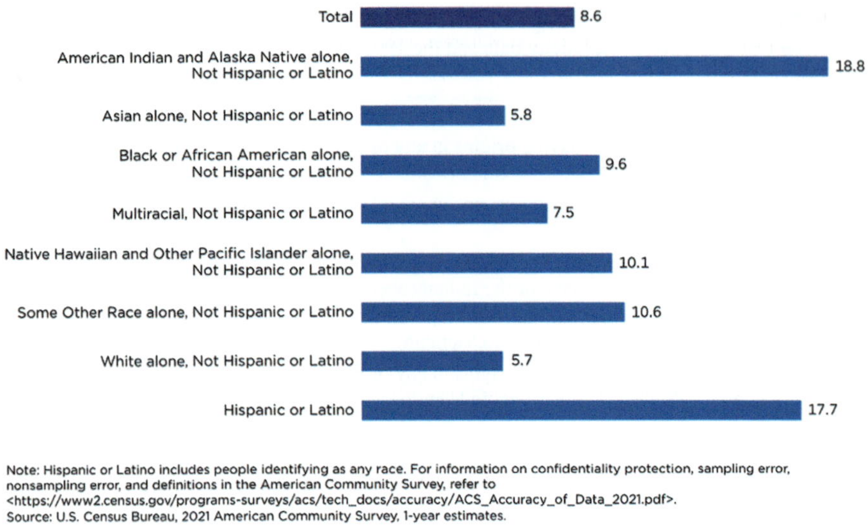


**Fig. 7.1** Percentage of people without health insurance coverage by race and Hispanic origin. (Reproduced from the U.S. Census Bureau, 2021 American Community Survey, 1-year estimates [21])

Furthermore, studies have shown that individuals with health insurance coverage are more likely to receive preventative care services, such as vaccinations and screening, which can help prevent respiratory illnesses and mitigate the impact of chronic respiratory conditions [22]. Coverage has the potential to prompt earlier diagnosis, treatment, and specialist care [23]. Among patients with asthma, individuals with public or no insurance were found to be more likely to have visited the emergency department more than twice over the past year when compared to individuals with private coverage. Uninsured individuals, despite having more severe disease, were less likely to receive guideline-recommended therapy and care from an asthma specialist [24]. Similar findings have been observed in COPD patients. Patients with high-deductible health coverage more commonly experienced delayed or foregone care, nonadherence to medication, and an increased frequency of emergency room visits or hospitalizations over the past year [25].

These disparities further exist in the field of thoracic oncology. A retrospective 2-year survival analysis of 1681 patients with lung cancer revealed that underinsured (those without insurance or on Medicaid) patients were 1.34 times more likely to die than those with commercial insurance, even after accounting for numerous potential confounding variables, including among others age, comorbidity index, and tobacco use. In addition, 41.4% of the insured patients had stage IV lung cancer compared to 56.7% of underinsured individuals. Notably, 25.1% of individuals with commercial coverage were current tobacco users compared to 40.7% of underinsured patients, highlighting the intricate and interconnected nature of respiratory health disparities [26].

Although the literature on the impact of health insurance on the diagnosis and treatment of ILD is scarce, similar findings regarding delayed care and suboptimal therapy are to be expected. A common obstacle to the timely diagnosis of ILD in resource-constrained settings and emerging countries is the limited access to CT scans and spirometry [27]. Beyond health insurance, race and ethnicity have been shown to be factors limiting access to diagnostic methods. Ross et al. conducted a retrospective observational study that spanned an 11-year period, involving more than 131 million patient encounters in the emergency room per year. The results indicated that White individuals were significantly more likely to undergo imaging than non-White patients, even after accounting for confounding variables such as age, sex, comorbidities, health insurance, and hospital settings [28].

Limited access to health care and inconsistent quality of care are of great concern in the context of ILD diagnosis and treatment as delayed referrals to tertiary centers are associated with increased mortality in IPF, independent of disease severity [27]. Early referral of patients with ILD is crucial to enable accurate diagnosis of the ILD subtype by conducting a thorough evaluation of contributing factors, including occupational or environmental exposures, medication, and underlying connective tissue disease [29]. This further permits the initiation of proper therapeutic interventions such as antifibrotics in the context of IPF or other progressive fibrosing phenotypes, which may slow progression but cannot reverse the damage already incurred [30–32].

Providing comprehensive health insurance coverage for all individuals would significantly reduce respiratory health disparities; however, it is important to recognize that numerous other racial and ethnic barriers to the accessibility and quality of health care persist and must not be overlooked. In this manner, inadequate health literacy, personal beliefs, language barriers, lack of transportation in underserved communities, and providers' limited cultural competency may all compromise patients' respiratory health by limiting access to care [16]. Individuals with limited education and income typically experience reduced access to health care but also a lower quality of care [33].

Patient-provider communication may also be a barrier to accessibility. Poor communication often leads to patient mistrust and hesitancy in accepting treatment. A lack of cultural proficiency, such as when health professionals fail to consider the patient's cultural background and therefore do not adapt their health promotion messages, can also play a significant role in healthcare disparities [15, 34]. The COVID-19 pandemic has helped expose these barriers to universal respiratory health. Individuals whose preferred language was not English were shown to be three times more likely to test positive [35]. Compared with their English-speaking counterparts, non-English-speaking individuals were more likely to be hospitalized within the first 45 days of diagnosis. Moreover, minority racial and ethnic populations, regardless of their area of deprivation index (ADI), were at increased risk of severe COVID-19 [36]. Identifying elements that can be more easily addressed such as communication may help reduce the burden on respiratory health [15].

## Race, Ethnicity, and Socioeconomic Determinants

Socioeconomic standing, which can be assessed through income, education, or occupational status, is among the strongest predictors of health disparities in nearly all societies [37, 38]. There is evidence that the impact of race and ethnicity on health outcomes attenuates considerably when socioeconomic position is controlled suggesting that the individual's standing is a greater predictor of health outcomes [39]. On the other hand, studies have shown that race matters beyond socioeconomic determinants when considering health disparities. In fact, these determinants are not equivalent across different racial groups. Blacks and Hispanics classically earn lower incomes for the same education levels and possess significantly less wealth at equivalent income levels [38, 40]. These racial and ethnic minorities, even at similar socioeconomic standing, undoubtedly face racism at the interpersonal and institutional levels consequently resulting in segregated neighborhoods, hazardous occupations, as well as stigma and stereotyping in the healthcare setting [38].

The impact of socioeconomic determinants on respiratory health becomes evident at an early age. Children from underprivileged backgrounds exhibit a higher likelihood of having asthma [41]. Minority racial and ethnic children have a greater prevalence of asthma than non-Hispanic White individuals and are at severely increased risk of mortality [42]. In addition, individuals from low-income households are more likely to have COPD, also characterized by more frequent exacerbations than are individuals from high-income households [43, 44]. People with lower education levels are also at greater risk of COPD exacerbation and are more likely to die from all causes [45].

In fact, individuals with limited education and income face higher rates of mortality and comorbidities, occupational hazards, and risk-taking behaviors [33]. As shown in the World Health Organization (WHO) conceptual framework, social determinants, education, occupation, and income are not only interconnected but also central to attaining good health [46] (Fig. 7.2).

A multicenter study of 70,496 individuals from four European countries (United Kingdom, France, Switzerland, and Portugal) examined the impact of socioeconomic disadvantage on lung function and years of lung function loss. Lifelong socioeconomic standing was assessed through paternal occupation, education level, and their own occupation. An underprivileged status was associated with a lower FEV1 and a loss of 4–5 years of healthy lung function by the age of 45 years when controlling for factors such as smoking, obesity, sedentary behavior, and cardiovascular or respiratory diseases [47].

The influence of socioeconomic determinants on ILD remains largely unexplored, especially in non-IPF diseases. Unfortunately, crucial data on these factors are often missing from ILD registries [48]. Low income has recently been shown to predict poor survival in IPF patients. In a study of 200 IPF patients from a French multicenter prospective cohort by Sésé et al., patients were divided into low- or high-income groups based on an estimated annual income of less than €18,170. After adjusting for age, sex, forced vital capacity (FVC), geographical origin, and

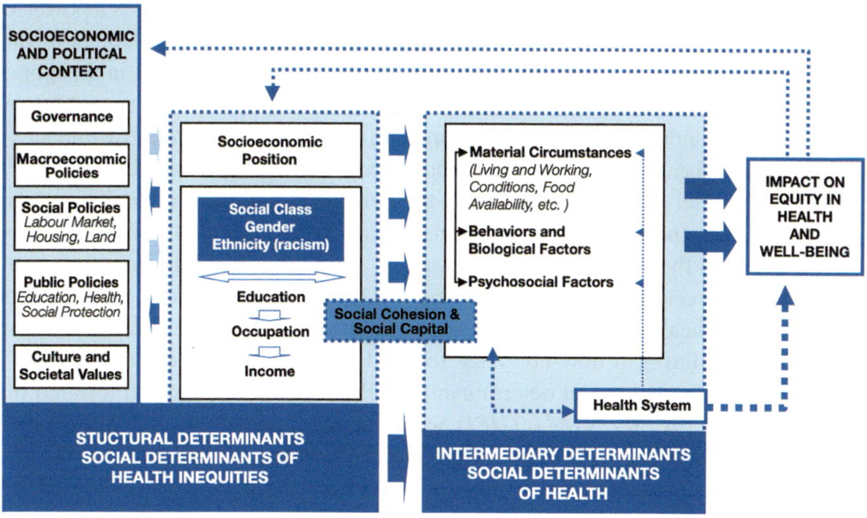


**Fig. 7.2** World Health Organization. Commission on Social Determinants of Health conceptual framework. (Reproduced from A conceptual framework for action on the social determinants of health. Social Determinants of Health Discussion Paper 2 [46])

occupational exposure, low income was associated with poorer progression-free survival and overall survival. In addition, there was a significant association between low-income and non-European origin [49].

A study using the *Nationwide Inpatient Sample*, a database of all hospitalizations from a nationally representative 20% sample of US hospitals, revealed that low socioeconomic status, uninsured, and Medicaid IPF patients were much less likely to receive lung transplants. Uninsured and Medicaid individuals were also less likely to undergo a VATS biopsy or be discharged to an inpatient pulmonary rehabilitation facility [50]. Notably, pulmonary rehabilitation may improve functional status and quality of life, and lung transplantation is one of the only life-prolonging interventions for severe progressive fibrosing ILD patients. Therefore, these disparities can have significant implications for IPF patient outcomes [51, 52].

Furthermore, through a multicenter international prospective cohort study of 4729 patients in 1 US and 8 Canadian ILD centers, Goobie et al. analyzed the impact of neighborhood-level disadvantages on fibrotic ILD. The *Area Deprivation Index* and the *Canadian Index of Multiple Deprivation* were used in the USA and Canada, respectively, to measure neighborhood-level disadvantage. Non-White individuals were more heavily represented in the disadvantaged group. In the USA, the greatest disadvantage was associated with a 1.51-fold increase in mortality, and IPF patients experienced a lower likelihood of lung transplantation, whereas no difference was observed in Canada. This is the first study to identify differences in fibrotic ILD outcomes between nonuniversal and universal healthcare systems, highlighting potentially avoidable disparities [53].

As shown in the study by Goobie et al., neighborhood disadvantage is a powerful predictor of outcomes in patients with fibrotic ILD [53]. The exact element of this complex socioeconomic indicator that contributes to poorer outcomes in this population remains uncertain as it has been evaluated as a composite measure. Most of the research conducted thus far has aimed to evaluate the cumulative impact of neighborhood health on fibrotic ILD outcomes, without distinguishing between physical or social factors present within the neighborhood. This methodology may fail to consider the distinct contributions of various aspects of the neighborhood environment to the severity of the disease and survival of individuals with fibrotic ILD. Thus, a recent retrospective study by DeDent et al. investigated the impact of neighborhood health on IPF severity using lung function at the initial assessment and mortality during follow-up. They focused on the role of the neighborhood's intrinsic physical and social determinants on IPF outcomes evaluated through the *California Healthy Places Index (HPI)*, which includes 25 indicators of health, such as education, economics, transportation, clean environment, housing, and healthcare access. In this study, each 10% increase in HPI was associated with a 1% increase in predicted FVC and DLCO. The strongest factors were the economics, education, healthcare access, and social domains. Moreover, a decrease in HPI was associated with an increase in mortality in patients with normal to mild FVC and DLCO impairment but not in those with moderate to severe impairment [54]. These findings suggest that in advanced stages of IPF, disease evolution becomes unchangeable, urging the need for early diagnosis, treatment, and modification of socioeconomic determinants to improve patient outcomes [55].

The *Area Deprivation Index*, a measure of socioeconomic disadvantage, ranges from 0 to 100, where 100 reflects the most underprivileged. While the US median resides at 50, the median in DeDent et al. was of 12, indicating a very privileged study population. A more drastic impact of neighborhood disadvantages, through socioeconomic disparities, on fibrotic ILD is to be expected [55]. Addressing socioeconomic inequalities is crucial for reducing the burden of ILD, particularly in low-resource settings.

## Impact of Race and Ethnicity on Environmental and Occupational Exposures

Environmental or occupational exposures often occur disproportionally in ethnic minorities and in those with lower socioeconomic status [17]. A study by Liu et al. quantified the disparities in air pollution exposure in the USA from 1990 to 2010. Despite the decline in air pollutants during that period, racial and ethnic exposure disparities remained in all US states, urban or rural areas and income levels. Minorities were found to be two times more likely than non-Hispanic Whites to reside in a census block group with the highest pollution levels. Exposures were more significant in low-income than in high-income households. The absolute exposure disparities were larger among minorities than among income levels, thus making the notion that racial and ethnic exposure can be attributed solely to income differences among these societal groups improbable [56]. In addition, exposure disparities among minorities have been shown to be greater in urban areas with higher levels of residential segregation [57].

The effect of air pollution on respiratory health can be influenced by factors such as race, ethnicity, and socioeconomic determinants. In fact, different types of air pollution inequalities exist such as the exclusion of certain groups from public policies regarding exposure mitigation (e.g., the decision to install a chemical infrastructure in a residential area) or the possibly adverse effects of air quality policies on lower-income households (e.g., the regressive impact of energy taxation). Individuals from disadvantaged neighborhoods may also experience unequal exposure and vulnerability to air pollution, as well as a lower pollution footprint than wealthier households [58].

Ferguson et al. refer to the respiratory inequalities induced by air pollution as a "triple jeopardy" scenario. Lower-income individuals who are exposed to more substantial environmental hazards such as air pollution also have an increase susceptibility to poorer outcomes from the exposure due to underlying health conditions, and as their condition progresses, they may be forced to spend more time in that detrimental environment [59].

These findings are most preoccupying as they may impact the development and progression of ILD. Environmental and occupational exposure have long been recognized as significant risk factors for ILD. Inhalation exposure plays a critical role in the pathophysiology of different ILDs such as pneumoconiosis or hypersensitivity pneumonitis. Air pollutants can trigger or contribute to the ongoing alveolar injury, compromised repair process, and fibrosis observed in ILD [60]. Even in IPF, ambient pollution has been associated with an increased risk of acute exacerbation in the 6 weeks following exposure [61]. A study from a French national multicenter prospective IPF cohort of 192 patients demonstrated that mortality was associated with increases in $PM_{2.5}$ and $PM_{10}$ levels [62].

Ambient air pollution exposure has been linked to qualitative and quantitative measurements of subclinical ILD, such as interstitial lung abnormalities (ILA) and high attenuation areas (HAA). The associations between the levels of pollutants and HAA varied by race and ethnicity. The strongest effect of pollution was found in non-Hispanic Whites [60]. We believe that these findings are more likely to be explained by unmeasured racial healthcare disparities that may mask the impact of pollution in minority subgroups, necessitating multifaceted interventions in these populations.

Hazardous occupations, such as construction, manufacturing, and transportation, are more frequently found in lower socioeconomic settings and are disproportionally held by racial and ethnic minorities [63]. Studies have revealed that when controlling for education and experience, Hispanic and African-American workers are more likely to be employed in dangerous occupations [64]. Even within the same occupation, workers from socially and economically disadvantaged populations are exposed to more hazardous tasks [64]. A tragic example of this is the *Hawks Nest*

*Tunnel* in the 1930s, where race-based job assignment (e.g., assigning African-Americans to the deeper, dustier parts of the tunnel compared to White workers who were more frequently working outside) contributed to a disproportionate incidence of pneumoconiosis (silicosis) and death among African-Americans compared to White workers [64, 65].

When assessing the influence of race and ethnicity on ILD risk factors, geographic variability in the prevalence of ILD subtypes may offer additional insights. In North America and Europe, IPF and sarcoidosis are the most prevalent ILDs, whereas the relative frequency of hypersensitivity pneumonitis (HP) is much greater in Asia, particularly in India and Pakistan [66]. The extensive use of evaporative air coolers in India was partly responsible for the high prevalence of HP. [67] Additionally, the frequency of connective tissue-associated ILD (CTD-ILD) varies greatly between countries. Differences in ILD prevalence are likely influenced by factors such as study design, data collection, and disease classification but may also result from underlying population characteristics [66].

## Genetic Predisposition in Racial and Ethnic Groups

As the literature rapidly progresses, associations between genetic susceptibility and environmental factors are being discovered. In the context of environmental exposure, individual genetic factors may influence the phenotypic expression of ILD [68]. Genetic approaches, including genome-wide association studies, have proven useful in discovering new pathways involved in the pathogenesis of ILD [69]. Known genetic susceptibilities to ILD include telomeropathies (short telomeres) caused by mutations in telomere-related genes (TRG), surfactant-related gene mutations, and MUC5B polymorphisms among others [70, 71]. Genetic predisposition in racial and ethnic groups may be due to both underlying genetic differences between these populations and the impact of associated exposures such as air pollution and environmental factors on genetic susceptibility.

In fact, as previously explored in this chapter, racial and ethnic minorities tend to experience higher levels of exposure to air pollution even when income is taken into account [56]. Recent studies have shown that air pollution exposure may serve as a trigger for several pathophysiological processes associated with IPF, including chronic inflammation, telomere shortening, oxidative stress, surfactant protein abnormalities, and endoplasmic reticulum stress [72]. Prolonged air pollutant exposure may increase the risk of IPF [70]. Furthermore, to better understand the influence of genetic mutations, polygenic risk scores (using 13 independent single nucleotide polymorphisms) have been proposed as the impact of single gene mutation is believed to be fairly small [70, 73]. A large prospective UK Biobank cohort study of 433 738 individuals demonstrated not only an association between air pollution and IPF in an exposure-response fashion but also a synergistic effect between air pollutant exposure and polygenic risk scores on the risk of IPF [72].

In regard to specific genetic predispositions among racial and ethnic minorities, a few genetic differences have been identified. The MUC5B polymorphism is a known risk factor for IPF as well as various progressive fibrosing ILD [70, 74]. This polymorphism, although frequent among individuals of European origin, is almost absent in individuals of African ancestry [75, 76]. When it comes to drug-induced ILD, Japanese patients are at increased risk compared to other ethnic groups which suggest that genetic differences may play a role [77, 78].

Current knowledge concerning the influence of genetics on ILD is hindered by the lack of racial and ethnic representation in most genetic studies conducted thus far. Polygenic risk scores are more precise for individuals of European ancestry than for those of other backgrounds [79, 80]. In a recent study by Adegunsoye et al., telomeres were shown to be a predictor of mortality in ILD patients among all racial groups. The shortest telomeres were shown to be in Asian and White men with ILD, among whom IPF was the most frequent diagnosis. Black individuals with ILD had the least short telomeres and the lowest IPF prevalence, which supports the causal role of telomeropathies in IPF [79]. Studies, which will be discussed further in this chapter, have shown that Black individuals develop ILD at a significantly younger age compared to White patients, which may suggest that telomeropathies play a lesser role in ILD development in this racial group [79, 81].

The inclusion of racial and ethnic minorities in genetic research and providing them with access to genetic services are crucial. This will improve genomic medicine as a whole and help reduce health disparities as these discoveries most often translate into clinical public health interventions [82, 83].

## Impact of Race and Ethnicity on Pulmonary Function Tests

Pulmonary function tests (PFT) play an important role in the diagnosis, treatment follow-up, and prognostication of ILD. The predicted values of PFT in the context of ILD may determine treatment eligibility, referral for lung transplant evaluation, health insurance coverage, and access to clinical trials [84]. Population-specific predicted values are based on historical studies of PFT differences between racial groups which often overlooked crucial factors such as environmental exposures, living conditions, or nutrition [84, 85]. Although part of standard practice, there is no biological basis supporting this approach. There is growing concern that incorporating racial and ethnic factors in PFT interpretation may foster a misconception of inherent distinctions between racial groups and disguise the consequences of underlying exposures and conditions [86]. This approach results in decreased lower limit of normal (LLN) predicted values of $FEV_1$ and FVC in Black individuals. For a given absolute value, Black patients may seem to have less impairment than White patients. Ultimately, Black individuals with ILD may not receive treatment until a more advanced stage of disease, and limited access to clinical trials could impact the relevance of the data that shape future clinical guidelines [84, 87, 88]. As of 2023, the American Thoracic Society (ATS) recommends using a race-neutral approach to

PFT to avoid inferring biological characteristics based on race. The Global Lung Function Initiative (GLI) eq. (GLI Global) is a recommended race-neutral reference [86].

A study conducted by Moffett et al. reviewed 14,080 PFT of individuals who self-identified as Black or Afro-American and compared the results with and without race adjustment. The removal of adjustment led to an increase in the number of patients with any pulmonary defect from 59.5% to 81.7% [89]. In addition, Adegunsoye et al. demonstrated that the use of race-neutral eqs. (GLI) increased the number of Black patients who fell under the FVC cutoff for ILD clinical trial participation, antifibrotic access, and lung transplant referral [84].

As demonstrated in these studies, race-neutral equations may positively impact the care received by racial and ethnic minorities. However, some patients, including White individuals, may become ineligible for treatment, clinical trials, or disability due to an upshift in function [84, 87]. Some authors believe that these changes will promote health equity among racial and ethnic groups [84]. Further research examining the impact of race-neutral equations on the management of ILD and its effect on clinically significant and long-term outcomes is needed to comprehensively understand the most effective method of PFT interpretation across various racial and ethnic subgroups.

## Impact of Race and Ethnicity on Research

The limited enrollment of racial and ethnic minorities in clinical trials and registries has hindered our understanding of the differences in ILD presentation and outcome among these populations [90]. Disparities in enrollment lead to biased medical knowledge and prevent these minorities from benefiting from trial participation [91]. As the field of ILD rapidly progresses and new medications become available, concerns arise that inequity may further occur due to low minority enrollment [88, 92].

Despite the National Institutes of Health Revitalization Act of 1993 and numerous institutional and governmental initiatives to increase representation in trials, the enrollment of minorities remains poor, although a modest improvement has been observed in a large study of all US clinical trials from 2000 to 2020 by Turner et al. Underrepresentation was most significant in Latinos and Asians [91]. While industry-funded trials featured the least diverse participant populations, US-government-funded studies exhibited the most diverse enrollment [91]. The greater enrollment of White patients in industry-funded clinical trials may be attributed to regulatory and financial incentives that promote homogeneity, thus minimizing cofounding variables and allowing more predictable treatment outcomes and a reduced risk of adverse events [91].

Many system- and individual-based barriers to clinical trials exist for racial and ethnic minorities. As previously explored, these minorities are more likely to be underinsured but also to receive care from under-resourced hospitals that lack the proper infrastructure to support trials. Minorities are also more likely to have comorbid conditions which may limit enrollment [93]. On an individual level, some minority patients may be unaware of the available trials or present with distrust in the process. On the other hand, a study of over 4500 racially diverse cancer patients revealed no significant differences in the refusal rate or "no desire to participate in research" among racial and ethnic groups [94]. Implicit biases, which may be conscious or unconscious, against minority groups may hinder the patient-physician relationship and ultimately affect the treatment course, as well as the likelihood of being offered participation in a clinical trial as a racial or ethnic minority (Fig. 7.3) [93].

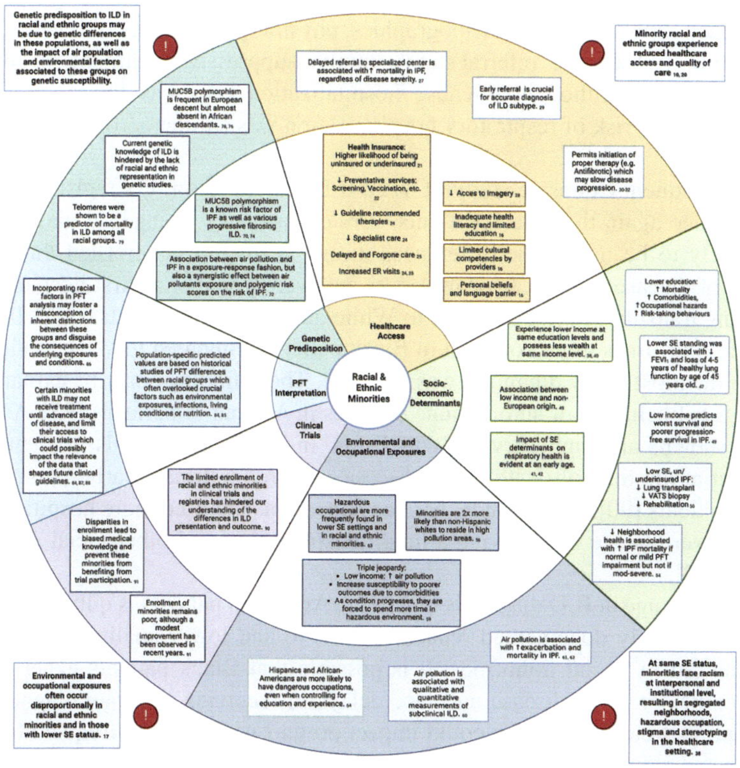


**Fig. 7.3** Overview of the impact of race and ethnicity on respiratory health and more precisely interstitial lung disease

## Influence of Specific Racial and Ethnic Groups on ILD Diagnosis and Treatment

### *African American Population*

Recent studies have revealed a distinctive phenotype in the presentation and progression of ILD among African American patients. In a large multicenter study conducted on 1640 ILD patients (excluding patients with sarcoidosis), 13% of whom were African Americans, Adegunsoye et al. reported that African-American patients exhibited an earlier age at diagnosis (58 years) compared to non-African-Americans (68 years), and a lower male prevalence compared to White, Hispanic, and Asian patients [81]. CTD-ILD was the most frequent form of ILD in Black patients (46.9% vs. 10.7% in White patients), while IPF comprised only 12.6% of the ILD compared to 44.4% in White patients [81].

Furthermore, survival was shown to be greater in Black individuals with ILD. The mean survival time and 10-year mortality were 8.6 years and 19%, respectively, compared to 7.1 years and 27% in non-Black patients. These differences persisted after accounting for baseline demographics, physiological indices of severity, GAP-ILD score, ILD subtype, referral status, immunosuppressive treatment, income, and insurance type. Although all-cause hospitalization risk was lower in African-Americans, the risk of respiratory hospitalization was similar across races and ethnicities [81].

A subsequent extensive study of 4792 ILD patients from US registries demonstrated once again that Black patients were consistently younger at diagnosis and less likely to be male. The differences in age at diagnosis persisted through the course of disease such as African Americans were younger at first hospitalization and lung transplantation compared to White and Hispanic patients. CTD-ILD was three to four times more common in Black patients compared to White patients, in whom the most likely diagnosis was IPF [90]. These findings may be explained by the higher likelihood of autoimmune diseases in African-Americans [95]. As previously shown, although survival was better in Black individuals, patients were younger at the time of death as the disease occurred a decade earlier than in non-Black patients [90]. In this study, African Americans incurred more hospitalizations and a lower chance of receiving a lung transplant than did other racial and ethnic groups [90].

The early age at ILD diagnosis in African American patients is quite concerning, given the widely documented reduced access to and lower quality of health care experienced by racial minorities. It is possible that Black patients experience an even earlier onset of disease and face delays in receiving accurate diagnosis and appropriate treatment, which could impact prognosis. The more frequent hospitalization and reduced number of lung transplant recipients may result from the numerous racial health disparities previously explored in this chapter.

The significant differences in ILD subtypes among Black patients may be due to variations in the several lung stressors that disproportionally affect African

Americans such as sporadic autoimmune conditions, air pollution, environmental antigens, and socioeconomic determinants [90]. Genetic differences may further contribute to the ILD disparities across racial and ethnic groups, and additional investigations through the inclusion of these populations in clinical trials and registries are needed.

In regard to ILD treatment, a study of more than 47,000 IPF patients in the USA, of whom 11% were Black patients, demonstrated that antifibrotics, the cornerstone treatment for IPF, were less frequently used in Black patients compared to Whites (6.2% vs. 11.4%), and other minorities such as Asians and Hispanics [30, 31, 96]. Similar results were observed in Black patients with diminished lung function, which is particularly worrisome. In contrast to White patients, for whom a significant difference in 3-year mortality was evident between those who received and those who did not receive antifibrotics, surprisingly, no such difference was observed among Blacks, Hispanics, and Asians [96]. We believe that the lack of a survival advantage associated with the administration of antifibrotics to racial and ethnic minorities with IPF may be attributed to an overshadowing impact of the substantial racial health disparities that these populations encounter and that have been extensively documented in the medical literature.

Furthermore, a cohort study of 19,504 lung transplant donors and recipients revealed that Black lung transplant recipients and recipients of Black donors experienced poorer posttransplant survival. Despite accounting for neighborhood socioeconomic status using the *Area Deprivation Index*, the association remained unchanged [97]. These alarming results raise numerous questions regarding whether unmeasured variables, such as racism at the institutional and personal level, quality of care, comorbidities, reduced access to health care, delayed diagnosis, and treatment faced by minorities, could contribute to the poorer survival rates observed.

## *Hispanic Population*

Few studies have explored the influence of Hispanic ethnicity on ILD presentation and evolution. Similar to non-Hispanic White individuals, Hispanic patients with ILD are predominantly male, and IPF is the most common ILD subtype among them. Notably, fibrotic HP is more prevalent among Hispanic patients than among other racial and ethnic subgroups, which may be partly attributed to the prevalent use of birds as pets in Hispanic culture [90, 98]. The survival rates in Hispanic patients with ILD are comparable to those in White individuals, and although hospitalizations are frequent in all ILD patients, regardless of race and ethnicity, Hispanic patients experience fewer episodes than Black patients and have similar rates to White patients [90].

## *Asian Population*

Although the Asian continent comprises approximately 60% of the world's population, epidemiologic data on the prevalence, subtypes, and progression of ILD are scarce. The inclusion of Asian patients in clinical trials conducted outside of East Asia is particularly limited. Despite prior research suggesting that East Asian IPF patients are at higher risk of acute exacerbation (AE), recent data from randomized controlled trials, such as the subgroup analysis in the INPULSIS trials, did not reveal differences in AE between Asian and White patients [99]. Furthermore, as large-scale genomic studies continue to be conducted, differences in genetic predisposition to clinical ILD are being discovered among racial and ethnic groups. For instance, studies have revealed an absence of association between MUC5B polymorphisms and IPF in Korean patients, in contrast to White or Hispanic populations [100].

# Conclusions

As we strive to provide personalized and effective healthcare interventions for individuals with ILD, it is essential to better recognize the significant intersectionality of race and ethnicity with socioeconomic determinants and with environmental and genetics factors. All of these aspects can influence the risk of ILD and its prognosis. To reduce racial healthcare disparities, more robust definitions and systematic usage of these crucial societal concepts are undoubtedly needed. The inclusion of racial and ethnic minorities in clinical trials is necessary to challenge stereotypes and erroneous associations as well as to identify possibly overlooked fundamental determinants of health arising from poorly captured racial and ethnic data. Embracing a race-conscious approach in the rapidly advancing fields of genomic and precision medicine will enable clinicians to better serve these populations and bridge the gap in ILD diagnosis and treatment.

**Acknowledgments** Figure 7.3 was created by the authors using BioRender.com.

During the preparation of this work, the authors corrected the language using the Curie software by the American Journal Expert (AJE) which uses machine-learning algorithms.

# References

1. Evans JP, Powell BC, Berg JS. Finding the rare pathogenic variants in a human genome. JAMA. 2017;317(18):1904–5. https://doi.org/10.1001/jama.2017.0432.
2. König IR, Fuchs O, Hansen G, von Mutius E, Kopp MV. What is precision medicine? Eur Respir J. 2017;50(4):1700391. https://doi.org/10.1183/13993003.00391-2017.
3. Maher TM, Nambiar AM, Wells AU. The role of precision medicine in interstitial lung disease. Eur Respir J. 2022;60(3):2102146. https://doi.org/10.1183/13993003.02146-2021.

4. Cerdeña JP, Plaisime MV, Tsai J. From race-based to race-conscious medicine: how anti-racist uprisings call us to act. Lancet. 2020;396(10257):1125–8. https://doi.org/10.1016/S0140-6736(20)32076-6.
5. Mersha TB, Abebe T. Self-reported race/ethnicity in the age of genomic research: its potential impact on understanding health disparities. Hum Genomics. 2015;9(1):1. https://doi.org/10.1186/s40246-014-0023-x.
6. Fuentes A, Ackermann RR, Athreya S, et al. AAPA statement on race and racism. Am J Phys Anthropol. 2019;169(3):400–2. https://doi.org/10.1002/ajpa.23882.
7. Lewis C, Cohen PR, Bahl D, Levine EM, Khaliq W. Race and ethnic categories: a brief review of global terms and nomenclature. Cureus. 2023;15(7):e41253. https://doi.org/10.7759/cureus.41253.
8. Haozous EA, Strickland CJ, Palacios JF, Solomon TGA. Blood politics, ethnic identity, and racial misclassification among American Indians and Alaska natives. J Environ Public Health. 2014;2014:1–9. https://doi.org/10.1155/2014/321604.
9. Flanagin A, Frey T, Christiansen SL. AMA manual of style committee. updated guidance on the reporting of race and ethnicity in medical and science journals. JAMA. 2021;326(7):621–7. https://doi.org/10.1001/jama.2021.13304.
10. Maduka RC, Broderick M, White EM, et al. The reporting of race and ethnicity in surgery literature. JAMA Surg. 2021;156(11):1036–41. https://doi.org/10.1001/jamasurg.2021.3752.
11. Hoang K, Gold J, Powell C, et al. Concordance between electronic health record-recorded race/ethnicity and parental report in hospitalized children. J Hosp Med. 2023;18(7):610–6. https://doi.org/10.1002/jhm.13140.
12. Christina A, Kaliya G, Adjoa M, et al. Misrepresenting race – The role of medical schools in propagating physician bias. N Engl J Med. 2021;384(9):872–8. https://doi.org/10.1056/NEJMms2025768.
13. Bhopal R, Donaldson L. White, European, Western, Caucasian, or what? Inappropriate labeling in research on race, ethnicity, and health. Am J Public Health. 1998;88(9):1303–7. https://doi.org/10.2105/AJPH.88.9.1303.
14. Evans L. NOT-OD-15-089: Racial and ethnic categories and definitions for NIH diversity programs and for other reporting purposes; 2015. Accessed April 11, 2024. https://grants.nih.gov/grants/guide/notice-files/NOT-OD-15-089.html#.
15. Kilbourne AM, Switzer G, Hyman K, Crowley-Matoka M, Fine MJ. Advancing health disparities research within the health care system: a conceptual framework. Am J Public Health. 2006;96(12):2113–21. https://doi.org/10.2105/AJPH.2005.077628.
16. Celedón JC, Roman J, Schraufnagel DE, Thomas A, Samet J. Respiratory health equality in the United States. The American Thoracic society perspective. Ann Am Thorac Soc. 2014;11(4):473–9. https://doi.org/10.1513/AnnalsATS.201402-059PS.
17. Schraufnagel DE, Blasi F, Kraft M, Gaga M, Finn PW, Rabe KF. An official American thoracic society/European respiratory society policy statement: disparities in respiratory health. Am J Respir Crit Care Med. 2013;188(7):865–71. https://doi.org/10.1164/rccm.201308-1509ST.
18. Hubbard R. The burden of lung disease. Thorax. 2006;61(7):557–8. https://doi.org/10.1136/thx.2006.066050.
19. Institute of Medicine (US) Committee on Understanding and Eliminating Racial and Ethnic Disparities in Health Care. Unequal Treatment: confronting racial and ethnic disparities in health care. (Smedley BD, Stith AY, Nelson AR, eds.). National Academies Press (US); 2003. Accessed April 15, 2024. http://www.ncbi.nlm.nih.gov/books/NBK220358/
20. Bulatao RA, Anderson NB, National Research Council (US) Panel on Race E. Health Care. In: Understanding racial and ethnic differences in health in late life: a research agenda. National Academies Press (US); 2004. https://www.ncbi.nlm.nih.gov/books/NBK24693/. . Accessed 15 Apr 2024
21. Branch B, Conway D. Health insurance coverage by race and Hispanic origin: 2021. Am Community Surv Briefs U S Census Bur. Published online; 2021.

22. Simon K, Soni A, Cawley J. The impact of health insurance on preventive care and health behaviors: evidence from the first two years of the ACA medicaid expansions. J Policy Anal Manage. 2017;36(2):390–417. https://doi.org/10.1002/pam.21972.
23. Lyon SM, Douglas IS, Cooke CR. Medicaid expansion under the affordable care act. Implications for insurance-related disparities in pulmonary, critical care, and sleep. Ann Am Thorac Soc. 2014;11(4):661–7. https://doi.org/10.1513/AnnalsATS.201402-072PS.
24. Hasegawa K, Stoll SJ, Ahn J, Kysia RF, Sullivan AF, Camargo CA. Association of insurance status with severity and management in ED patients with asthma exacerbation. West J Emerg Med Integrating Emerg Care Popul Health. 2016;17(1):22. https://doi.org/10.5811/westjem.2015.11.28715.
25. Gaffney A, White A, Hawks L, et al. High-deductible health plans and healthcare access, use, and financial strain in those with chronic obstructive pulmonary disease. Ann Am Thorac Soc. 2020;17(1):49–56. https://doi.org/10.1513/AnnalsATS.201905-400OC.
26. Mohamed MK, Herndon D, Schmidt M, Manning MA. The effect of under and uninsured status on survival in lung cancer while adjusting for other mortality risk factors. J Clin Oncol. 2020;38(15_suppl):e21734. https://doi.org/10.1200/JCO.2020.38.15_suppl.e21734.
27. Lamas DJ, Kawut SM, Bagiella E, Philip N, Arcasoy SM, Lederer DJ. Delayed access and survival in idiopathic pulmonary fibrosis. Am J Respir Crit Care Med. 2011;184(7):842–7. https://doi.org/10.1164/rccm.201104-0668OC.
28. Ross AB, Kalia V, Chan BY, Li G. The influence of patient race on the use of diagnostic imaging in United States emergency departments: data from the National Hospital Ambulatory Medical Care survey. BMC Health Serv Res. 2020;20:840. https://doi.org/10.1186/s12913-020-05698-1.
29. Mageto YN. Health care disparities in pulmonary fibrosis – time to move the needle forward. JAMA Netw Open. 2023;6(3):e232442. https://doi.org/10.1001/jamanetworkopen.2023.2442.
30. King TE, Bradford WZ, Socorro C-B, et al. A phase 3 trial of pirfenidone in patients with idiopathic pulmonary fibrosis. N Engl J Med. 2014;370(22):2083–92. https://doi.org/10.1056/NEJMoa1402582.
31. Luca R, du Bois Roland M, Ganesh R, et al. Efficacy and safety of nintedanib in idiopathic pulmonary fibrosis. N Engl J Med. 2014;370(22):2071–82. https://doi.org/10.1056/NEJMoa1402584.
32. Flaherty KR, Wells AU, Vincent C, et al. Nintedanib in progressive fibrosing interstitial lung diseases. N Engl J Med. 2019;381(18):1718–27. https://doi.org/10.1056/NEJMoa1908681.
33. Frieden TR. Centers for disease control and prevention (CDC). CDC health disparities and inequalities report – United States, 2013. Foreword. MMWR Suppl. 2013;62(3):1–2.
34. Freimuth VS, Quinn SC. The contributions of health communication to eliminating health disparities. Am J Public Health. 2004;94(12):2053–5.
35. Cohen-Cline H, Li HF, Gill M, et al. Major disparities in COVID-19 test positivity for patients with non-English preferred language even after accounting for race and social factors in the United States in 2020. BMC Public Health. 2021;21(1):2121. https://doi.org/10.1186/s12889-021-12171-z.
36. Ingraham NE, Purcell LN, Karam BS, et al. Racial and ethnic disparities in hospital admissions from COVID-19: determining the impact of neighborhood deprivation and primary language. J Gen Intern Med. 2021;36(11):3462–70. https://doi.org/10.1007/s11606-021-06790-w.
37. Marmot M, Friel S, Bell R, Houweling TAJ, Taylor S. Commission on social determinants of health. closing the gap in a generation: health equity through action on the social determinants of health. Lancet Lond Engl. 2008;372(9650):1661–9. https://doi.org/10.1016/S0140-6736(08)61690-6.
38. Williams DR, Priest N, Anderson N. Understanding associations between race, socioeconomic status and health: patterns and prospects. Social Med Reader. 2016;35(4):407–11. https://doi.org/10.1037/hea0000242.

39. Egede LE. Race, ethnicity, culture, and disparities in health care. J Gen Intern Med. 2006;21(6):667–9. https://doi.org/10.1111/j.1525-1497.2006.0512.x.
40. Williams DR, Mohammed SA, Leavell J, Collins C. Race, socioeconomic status, and health: complexities, ongoing challenges, and research opportunities. Ann N Y Acad Sci. 2010;1186:69–101. https://doi.org/10.1111/j.1749-6632.2009.05339.x.
41. Foronda CL, Kelley CN, Nadeau C, et al. Psychological and socioeconomic burdens faced by family caregivers of children with asthma: an integrative review. J Pediatr Health Care. 2020;34(4):366–76. https://doi.org/10.1016/j.pedhc.2020.02.003.
42. Forno E, Celedón JC. Health disparities in asthma. Am J Respir Crit Care Med. 2012;185(10):1033–5. https://doi.org/10.1164/rccm.201202-0350ED.
43. Osman S, Ziegler C, Gibson R, Mahmood R, Moraros J. The Association between risk factors and chronic obstructive pulmonary disease in Canada: a cross-sectional study using the 2014 Canadian community health survey. Int J Prev Med. 2017;8:86. https://doi.org/10.4103/ijpvm.IJPVM_330_17.
44. Kowalczyk A, Kosiek K, Godycki-Cwirko M, Zakowska I. Community determinants of COPD exacerbations in elderly patients in Lodz province, Poland: a retrospective observational Big Data cohort study. BMJ Open. 2022;12(10):e060247. https://doi.org/10.1136/bmjopen-2021-060247.
45. Lange P, Marott JL, Vestbo J, Ingebrigtsen TS, Nordestgaard BG. Socioeconomic Status and Prognosis of COPD in Denmark. COPD J Chronic Obstr Pulm Dis. 2014;11(4):431–7. https://doi.org/10.3109/15412555.2013.869580.
46. Solar O, Irwin A. A conceptual framework for action on the social determinants of health. *WHO*. Published online 2010:76.
47. Rocha V, Fraga S, Moreira C, et al. Life-course socioeconomic disadvantage and lung function: a multicohort study of 70 496 individuals. Eur Respir J. 2021;57(3):2001600. https://doi.org/10.1183/13993003.01600-2020.
48. Sesé L, Cavalin C, Bernaudin JF, Maesano IA, Nunes H. Patient registries in idiopathic pulmonary fibrosis: don't forget socioeconomic status. Am J Respir Crit Care Med. 2020;201(8):1014–5. https://doi.org/10.1164/rccm.201911-2275LE.
49. Sesé L, Caliez J, Annesi-Maesano I, et al. Low income and outcome in idiopathic pulmonary fibrosis: An association to uncover. Respir Med. 2021;183:106415. https://doi.org/10.1016/j.rmed.2021.106415.
50. Gaffney AW, Woolhander S, Himmelstein D, McCormick D. Disparities in pulmonary fibrosis care in the United States: an analysis from the Nationwide Inpatient Sample. BMC Health Serv Res. 2018;18(1):618. https://doi.org/10.1186/s12913-018-3407-0.
51. Huppmann P, Sczepanski B, Boensch M, et al. Effects of inpatient pulmonary rehabilitation in patients with interstitial lung disease. Eur Respir J. 2013;42(2):444–53. https://doi.org/10.1183/09031936.00081512.
52. Wong AW, Ryerson CJ, Guler SA. Progression of fibrosing interstitial lung disease. Respir Res. 2020;21(1):32. https://doi.org/10.1186/s12931-020-1296-3.
53. Goobie GC, Ryerson CJ, Johannson KA, et al. Neighborhood-level disadvantage impacts on patients with fibrotic interstitial lung disease. Am J Respir Crit Care Med. 2022;205(4):459–67. https://doi.org/10.1164/rccm.202109-2065OC.
54. DeDent AM, Collard HR, Thakur N. Neighborhood health and outcomes in idiopathic pulmonary fibrosis. Ann Am Thorac Soc. 2024;21:402. https://doi.org/10.1513/AnnalsATS.202304-323OC.
55. Goobie GC. Neighborhood disparities in interstitial lung disease: how do we capture the most vulnerable? Ann Am Thorac Soc. 2024;21(3):377–80. https://doi.org/10.1513/AnnalsATS.202311-959ED.
56. Liu J, Clark LP, Bechle MJ, et al. Disparities in air pollution exposure in the United States by race/ethnicity and income, 1990–2010. Environ Health Perspect. 2021;129(12):127005. https://doi.org/10.1289/EHP8584.

57. Woo B, Kravitz-Wirtz N, Sass V, Crowder K, Teixeira S, Takeuchi DT. Residential segregation and racial/ethnic disparities in ambient air pollution. Race Soc Probl. 2019;11(1):60–7. https://doi.org/10.1007/s12552-018-9254-0.
58. Laurent É. Air (ine)quality in the European Union. Curr Environ Health Rep. 2022;9(2):123–9. https://doi.org/10.1007/s40572-022-00348-6.
59. Ferguson L, Taylor J, Zhou K, et al. Systemic inequalities in indoor air pollution exposure in London, UK. Build Cities. 2021;2(1):425–48. https://doi.org/10.5334/bc.100.
60. Sack C, Vedal S, Sheppard L, et al. Air pollution and subclinical interstitial lung disease: the Multi-Ethnic Study of Atherosclerosis (MESA) air–lung study. Eur Respir J. 2017;50(6):1700559. https://doi.org/10.1183/13993003.00559-2017.
61. Johannson KA, Vittinghoff E, Lee K, et al. Acute exacerbation of idiopathic pulmonary fibrosis associated with air pollution exposure. Eur Respir J. 2014;43(4):1124–31. https://doi.org/10.1183/09031936.00122213.
62. Sesé L, Nunes H, Cottin V, et al. Role of atmospheric pollution on the natural history of idiopathic pulmonary fibrosis. Thorax. 2018;73(2):145–50. https://doi.org/10.1136/thoraxjnl-2017-209967.
63. Fujishiro K, Hajat A, Landsbergis PA, Meyer JD, Schreiner PJ, Kaufman JD. Explaining racial/ethnic differences in all-cause mortality in the Multi-Ethnic Study of Atherosclerosis (MESA): Substantive complexity and hazardous working conditions as mediating factors. SSM - Popul Health. 2017;3:497–505. https://doi.org/10.1016/j.ssmph.2017.05.010.
64. Okechukwu CA, Souza K, Davis KD, de Castro AB. Discrimination, harassment, abuse and bullying in the workplace: Contribution of workplace injustice to occupational health disparities. Am J Ind Med. 2014;57(5):573–86. https://doi.org/10.1002/ajim.22221.
65. Cherniack M. The Hawk's Nest Incident : America's worst industrial disaster. New Haven: Yale University Press; 1986.
66. Kaul B, Cottin V, Collard HR, Valenzuela C. Variability in global prevalence of interstitial lung disease. Front Med. 2021;8:751181. https://doi.org/10.3389/fmed.2021.751181.
67. Singh S, Collins BF, Sharma BB, et al. Interstitial lung disease in India. results of a prospective registry. Am J Respir Crit Care Med. 2017;195(6):801–13. https://doi.org/10.1164/rccm.201607-1484OC.
68. Johannson KA, Balmes JR, Collard HR. Air pollution exposure: a novel environmental risk factor for interstitial lung disease? Chest. 2015;147(4):1161–7. https://doi.org/10.1378/chest.14-1299.
69. Manichaikul A, Wang XQ, Sun L, et al. Genome-wide association study of subclinical interstitial lung disease in MESA. Respir Res. 2017;18(1):97. https://doi.org/10.1186/s12931-017-0581-2.
70. Stanel SC, Callum J, Rivera-Ortega P. Genetic and environmental factors in interstitial lung diseases: current and future perspectives on early diagnosis of high-risk cohorts. Front Med. 2023;10:10. https://doi.org/10.3389/fmed.2023.1232655.
71. Borie R, Kannengiesser C, Antoniou K, et al. European respiratory society statement on familial pulmonary fibrosis. Eur Respir J. 2023;61(3):2201383. https://doi.org/10.1183/13993003.01383-2022.
72. Cui F, Sun Y, Xie J, et al. Air pollutants, genetic susceptibility and risk of incident idiopathic pulmonary fibrosis. Eur Respir J. 2023;61(2):2200777. https://doi.org/10.1183/13993003.00777-2022.
73. Huang Y, Zhu M, Ji M, et al. Air pollution, genetic factors, and the risk of lung cancer: a prospective study in the UK Biobank. Am J Respir Crit Care Med. 2021;204(7):817–25. https://doi.org/10.1164/rccm.202011-4063OC.
74. Seibold MA, Wise AL, Speer MC, et al. A common MUC5B promoter polymorphism and pulmonary fibrosis. N Engl J Med. 2011;364(16):1503–12. https://doi.org/10.1056/NEJMoa1013660.
75. Shah Gupta R, Koteci A, Morgan A, George PM, Quint JK. Incidence and prevalence of interstitial lung diseases worldwide: a systematic literature review. BMJ Open Respir Res. 2023;10(1):e001291. https://doi.org/10.1136/bmjresp-2022-001291.

76. Auton A, Abecasis GR, Altshuler DM, et al. A global reference for human genetic variation. Nature. 2015;526(7571):68–74. https://doi.org/10.1038/nature15393.
77. Shidara K, Hoshi D, Inoue E, et al. Incidence of and risk factors for interstitial pneumonia in patients with rheumatoid arthritis in a large Japanese observational cohort, IORRA. Mod Rheumatol. 2010;20(3):280–6. https://doi.org/10.1007/s10165-010-0280-z.
78. Furukawa H, Oka S, Shimada K, Tsuchiya N, Tohma S. Genetics of interstitial lung disease: Vol de Nuit (Night Flight). Clin Med Insights Circ Respir Pulm Med. 2015;9s1:CCRPM.S23283. https://doi.org/10.4137/CCRPM.S23283.
79. Adegunsoye A, Newton CA, Oldham JM, et al. Telomere length associates with chronological age and mortality across racially diverse pulmonary fibrosis cohorts. Nat Commun. 2023;14:1489. https://doi.org/10.1038/s41467-023-37193-6.
80. Martin AR, Kanai M, Kamatani Y, Okada Y, Neale BM, Daly MJ. Clinical use of current polygenic risk scores may exacerbate health disparities. Nat Genet. 2019;51(4):584–91. https://doi.org/10.1038/s41588-019-0379-x.
81. Adegunsoye A, Oldham JM, Bellam SK, et al. African-American race and mortality in interstitial lung disease: a multicentre propensity-matched analysis. Eur Respir J. 2018;51(6):1800255. https://doi.org/10.1183/13993003.00255-2018.
82. Knerr S, Wayman D, Bonham VL. Inclusion of racial and ethnic minorities in genetic research: advance the spirit by changing the rules? J Law Med Ethics. 2011;39(3):502–12. https://doi.org/10.1111/j.1748-720X.2011.00617.x.
83. Saulsberry K, Terry SF. The need to build trust: a perspective on disparities in genetic testing. Genet Test Mol Biomark. 2013;17(9):647–8. https://doi.org/10.1089/gtmb.2013.1548.
84. Adegunsoye A, Bachman WM, Flaherty KR, Li Z, Gupta S. Use of race-specific equations in pulmonary function tests impedes potential eligibility for care and treatment of pulmonary fibrosis. Ann Am Thorac Soc. 2024;21:1156. https://doi.org/10.1513/AnnalsATS.202309-797OC.
85. Lujan HL, DiCarlo SE. Science reflects history as society influences science: brief history of “race,” “race correction,” and the spirometer. Adv Physiol Educ. 2018;42(2):163–5. https://doi.org/10.1152/advan.00196.2017.
86. Bhakta NR, Bime C, Kaminsky DA, et al. Race and ethnicity in pulmonary function test interpretation: an official American thoracic society statement. Am J Respir Crit Care Med. 2023;207(8):978–95. https://doi.org/10.1164/rccm.202302-0310ST.
87. Bhakta NR, Kaminsky DA, Bime C, et al. Addressing race in pulmonary function testing by aligning intent and evidence with practice and perception. Chest. 2022;161(1):288–97. https://doi.org/10.1016/j.chest.2021.08.053.
88. Adegunsoye A, Vela M, Saunders M. Racial disparities in pulmonary fibrosis and the impact on the black population. Arch Bronconeumol. 2022;58(8):590–2. https://doi.org/10.1016/j.arbres.2021.09.012.
89. Moffett A et al. The impact of race correction on the interpretation of pulmonary function testing among black patients. In: A7. A007 impact of race, ethnicity, and social determinants on individuals with lung diseases. American Thoracic Society International Conference Abstracts. American Thoracic Society; 2021 doi:https://doi.org/10.1164/ajrccm-conference.2021.203.1_MeetingAbstracts.A1030.
90. Adegunsoye A, Freiheit E, White EN, et al. Evaluation of pulmonary fibrosis outcomes by race and ethnicity in us adults. JAMA Netw Open. 2023;6(3):e232427. https://doi.org/10.1001/jamanetworkopen.2023.2427.
91. Turner BE, Steinberg JR, Weeks BT, Rodriguez F, Cullen MR. Race/ethnicity reporting and representation in US clinical trials: a cohort study. Lancet Reg Health—Am. 2022;11:11. https://doi.org/10.1016/j.lana.2022.100252.
92. Geller SE, Koch AR, Roesch P, Filut A, Hallgren E, Carnes M. The more things change, the more they stay the same: a study to evaluate compliance with inclusion and assessment of women and minorities in randomized controlled trials. Acad Med. 2018;93(4):630–5. https://doi.org/10.1097/ACM.0000000000002027.

93. Hamel LM, Penner LA, Albrecht TL, Heath E, Gwede CK, Eggly S. Barriers to clinical trial enrollment in racial and ethnic minority patients with cancer. Cancer Control J Moffitt Cancer Cent. 2016;23(4):327–37.
94. Langford AT, Resnicow K, Dimond EP, et al. Racial/ethnic differences in clinical trial enrollment, refusal rates, ineligibility, and reasons for decline among patients at sites in the National Cancer Institute's Community Cancer Centers Program. Cancer. 2014;120(6):877–84. https://doi.org/10.1002/cncr.28483.
95. Roberts MH, Erdei E. Comparative United States autoimmune disease rates for 2010–2016 by sex, geographic region, and race. Autoimmun Rev. 2020;19(1):102423. https://doi.org/10.1016/j.autrev.2019.102423.
96. Zhao J, Fares J, George G, et al. Racial and ethnic disparities in antifibrotic therapy in idiopathic pulmonary fibrosis. Respirology. 2023;28(11):1036–42. https://doi.org/10.1111/resp.14563.
97. Lehr CJ, Valapour M, Gunsalus PR, et al. Association of socioeconomic position with racial and ethnic disparities in survival after lung transplant. JAMA Netw Open. 2023;6(4):e238306. https://doi.org/10.1001/jamanetworkopen.2023.8306.
98. The use of birds as pets in Mexico | Journal of ethnobiology and ethnomedicine | Full Text; 2024. https://ethnobiomed.biomedcentral.com/articles/10.1186/s13002-017-0161-z. Accessed 10 June
99. Saito S, Lasky JA, Hagiwara K, Kondoh Y. Ethnic differences in idiopathic pulmonary fibrosis: the Japanese perspective. Respir Investig. 2018;56(5):375–83. https://doi.org/10.1016/j.resinv.2018.06.002.
100. Peljto AL, Selman M, Kim DS, et al. The MUC5B promoter polymorphism is associated with idiopathic pulmonary fibrosis in a Mexican cohort but is rare among Asian ancestries. Chest. 2015;147(2):460–4. https://doi.org/10.1378/chest.14-0867.

# Chapter 8
# In the Air: Exhaled Breath Analysis and Airway-Based Biomarkers in Interstitial Lung Diseases

**Mi Ho Jeong, Joong-Yub Kim, and Hyungsoon Im**

## Introduction

Interstitial lung diseases (ILDs) encompass a range of conditions marked by diffuse inflammation, fibrosis, or both within the pulmonary interstitium, frequently resulting in impaired gas exchange and physiological decline [1]. ILDs are classified by etiology, distinguishing between conditions with known causes, such as environmental exposure, drug toxicity, or connective tissue diseases, and those without a specific cause [2, 3]. Accurate diagnosis is crucial given the heterogeneity of the natural course, treatment response, and outcomes among ILDs. However, despite comprehensive history taking, imaging studies, and even surgical biopsies, diagnosis can remain challenging due to the lack of diagnostic specificity among available tests and the similarities observed across different ILDs [4]. Furthermore, limited options for assessing disease progression can make it difficult to determine when to initiate anti-inflammatory or anti-fibrotic treatment. Consequently, developing sensitive and specific biomarkers and technologies capable of distinguishing between diseases and monitoring the course and treatment response in patients with ILD is essential.

M. H. Jeong (✉)
Center for Systems Biology, Massachusetts General Hospital, Boston, MA, USA
e-mail: MJEONG2@mgh.harvard.edu

J.-Y. Kim
Division of Pulmonary and Critical Care Medicine, Department of Internal Medicine, Seoul National University Hospital, Seoul National University College of Medicine, Seoul, South Korea

H. Im (✉)
Center for Systems Biology, Massachusetts General Hospital, Boston, MA, USA

Department of Radiology, Massachusetts General Hospital, Boston, MA, USA
e-mail: im.hyungsoon@mgh.harvard.edu



B. F. Collins, S. B. Montesi (eds.), *Precision Medicine in Interstitial Lung Disease*, Respiratory Medicine, https://doi.org/10.1007/978-3-031-87183-2_8

In current clinical practice, diagnosis relies on radiological images, histological findings, and pulmonary function tests. However, these approaches often identify diseases at late stages when symptoms become evident. On the other hand, molecular diagnosis offers the potential for earlier detection, even before clinical manifestations arise [5]. While lung biopsies or less invasive bronchoalveolar lavage (BAL) analysis provide detailed molecular profiles, the high costs and potential risks limit their utility for early diagnosis and screening. Thus, exhaled breath condensate (EBC) analysis has emerged as a noninvasive alternative to address this clinical need [6]. EBC is collected noninvasively from the condensed vapor of a patient's breath [7]. EBC originates from an airway lining fluid, which covers the epithelium and contains various compounds from lung resident cells. Because of the proximity to the respiratory system, EBC is expected to contain biomolecules associated with lung diseases [8]. For instance, volatile organic compounds (VOCs) in EBC have been studied for ILD [9, 10]. Powered by machine learning, an electronic nose (eNose) system analyzes multiple VOCs in EBC to distinguish pneumoconiosis patients from healthy subjects by VOC pattern recognition [11]. A recent study using eNose technology with machine learning differentiated systemic sclerosis patients with and without ILD with an accuracy of 0.81 based on VOC profiles in exhaled breaths [12]. However, state-of-the-art eNose systems still have limitations in differential diagnosis and detection of other nonvolatile components in EBC.

This book chapter aims to provide an overview of the current understanding of EBC, including its composition, collection methods, biomolecules, and analytical techniques. We also discuss current technical challenges and the need for highly sensitive analysis technologies for EBCs to better understand the clinical potential of EBC biomarkers. Finally, we provide perspectives on future technology developments and clinical translation of EBC analysis.

## Characteristics of EBC

### *Source and Generation*

EBC comprises mainly water (>99%) containing a variety of volatile and nonvolatile molecules, liquid particles, and microbes vaporized from an airway lining fluid of the respiratory tract [13, 14]. The airspace is covered with an alveolar subphase fluid and surfactants, which contribute volatile components [15]. Surfactants, secreted from type II alveolar epithelial cells and Clara cells, consist of phospholipids (~80%), proteins (~10%), and cholesterols (~10%) [15]. Nonvolatile components are generally vaporized from an airway lining fluid that covers the respiratory tract. When airway lining fluid aerosolizes, nonvolatile components combine with water vapor and other volatile compounds to form EBC. These nonvolatile components, such as urea, are present in low concentrations in EBC, exhibiting an 8600-fold dilution compared to urea in the airway surface [16, 17].

Figure 8.1 depicts the generation of EBC from the respiratory system. The respiratory cycle creates turbulence in the airways, facilitating airway lining fluid aerosolization [6, 19]. Aerosols are predominantly generated in areas where turbulence occurs, influenced by surface tension and velocity of exhaled airflow [9]. These aerosols flow with exhaled air in highly diluted concentrations, ranging from 0.1 to 4 particles/cm$^3$ with diameters smaller than 0.3 μm [20–22]. It is still unclear which regions in the respiratory system could contribute to EBC components [17, 23]. Considering certain ILDs developing in specific parts of the lung, such as respiratory bronchiolitis-associated ILD and pulmonary alveolar microlithiasis, it is important to explore which diseases might be suitable for investigation through EBC analysis.

## EBC Collection

EBC collection methods have been established by the Task Force of the American Thoracic Society and European Respiratory Society [25]. There is no specific preference for condensing equipment for collecting EBC; individuals can choose between commercial and customized equipment depending on their purposes

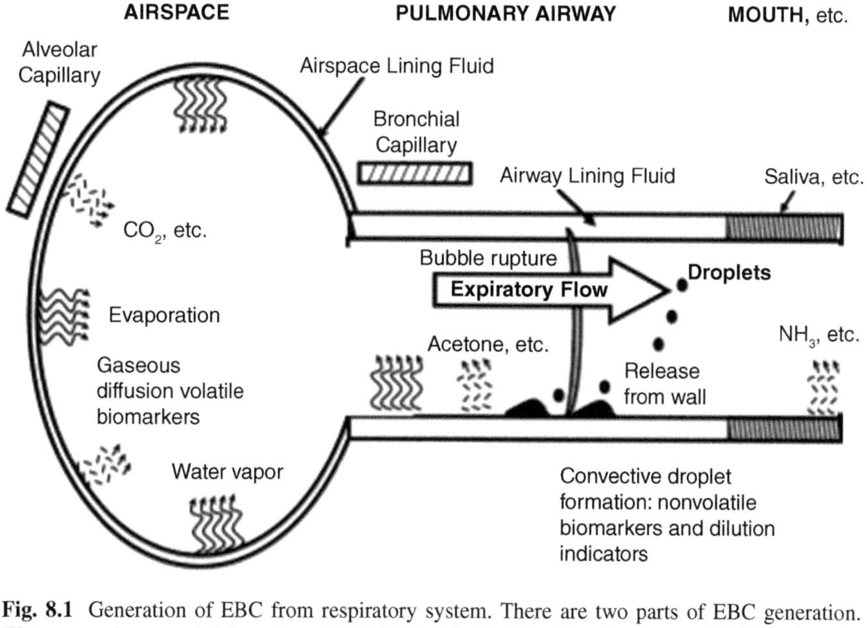


**Fig. 8.1** Generation of EBC from respiratory system. There are two parts of EBC generation. Water vapor is generated from the epithelial lining fluid of the alveolar space and diffuses into the airway. Airway lining fluid is aerosolized, especially when it encounters the turbulence. (Reprinted with permission of the American Thoracic Society. Copyright © 2024 American Thoracic Society. All rights reserved. Effros et al. [18])

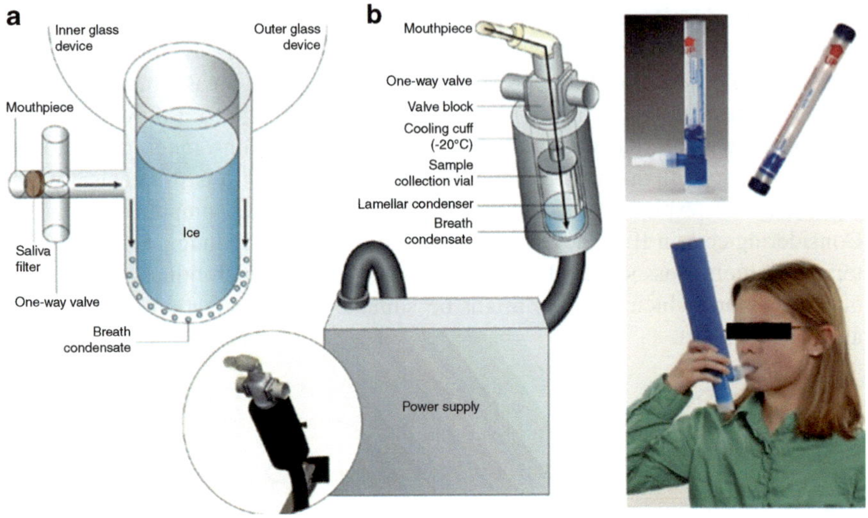


**Fig. 8.2** EBC collection systems. (**a**) Fundamental EBC collection device with inner and outer glass containers. (**b**) A commercial EBC collecting device (EcoScreen). (Reprinted with permission from Montuschi [24]. Copyright 2002 by Nature Reviews Drug Discovery. (**c**) A portable EBC condenser (RTube). Reprinted from Konstantinidi et al. [8]. Copyright 2015)

(Fig. 8.2). However, the principle to condensate the EBC is similar as cooling is critical for EBC collection. For instance, with ice cooling in the inner glass device, EBC can be condensed and collected between the inner and outer glass containers (Fig. 8.2a). For one of the commercial devices, the breath passes through from the mouthpiece to the cooling cuff zone for condensation and is collected in a collection vial (Fig. 8.2b). Collection tubes are made up of different materials, such as Teflon or polypropylene, and designed in various shapes [26–29]. Aerosolized particles in the tubes are cooled to allow condensation for collection. Typically, these methods require approximately 10 min to collect 1–3 mL of EBC samples. There are several portable EBC collecting tubes, such as Rtube, which is made with disposable polypropylene tubes with a syringe-type plunger (Fig. 8.2c). One study comparing commercial and customized collection methods found them interchangeable [30]. For more precise use of EBC for diagnosis and longitudinal monitoring, inter-subject and intra-subject reproducibility requires further validation. Therefore, detailed documentation of the method used for collection is highly recommended [25].

During EBC collection and handling, several precautions are recommended to minimize contamination with unintended components (e.g., nasal airway lining fluid, saliva, nitrogen oxides). Nasal airway lining fluid is a common contaminant that can enter the main airstream during inhalation and exhalation; therefore, the use of nose clips is recommended [25]. Salivary contamination also occurs occasionally. Saliva shares common components with the lower airways; thus, preventing contamination is essential [13, 31]. However, because amylase is also present in the lung, its presence does not conclusively indicate salivary contamination. Thus, using a saliva trap at the mouthpiece with a unidirectional filter is recommended to reduce risk of saliva contamination (Fig. 8.2a). Nitrogen oxides can be introduced from laboratory wares such as conical tubes and pipette tips [32]. When collecting EBC, it is recommended to use laboratory wares free of nitrogen oxides to avoid contamination [25].

Another important consideration is the varying volumes of collected samples. Ambient humidity and temperature at collection can affect the sample volumes [25]. Reported dilution factors for nonvolatile components vary widely, ranging from 8,300 to 48,400 between subjects [16]. Thus, normalization with internal components, such as urea [13, 16], total protein concentration [33], or conductance [23], have been suggested. Analysis of highly diluted EBC can be technically challenging. Thus, ambient temperature and humidity control should be considered for consistent test results.

## EBC Components as ILD Biomarkers

Various components detected in EBC hold the potential to aid in the diagnosis and therapeutic monitoring of ILD. Several types of EBC markers have been identified and proposed as potential biomarkers for ILDs.

### *RNA/DNA*

EBC contains components derived not only from the human respiratory system but also from microorganisms such as bacteria, viruses, and fungi in the lungs. This approach provides opportunities to differentiate other pulmonary infections presenting with patterns similar to ILDs by identifying unique nucleic acids in EBCs associated with common pathogens. For instance, a recent study showed that SARS-CoV-2 RNA detection in EBC demonstrated 93.5% accuracy by reverse transcriptase polymerase chain reaction (RT-PCR) with four gene targets. The accuracy was higher than nasopharyngeal swabs with fewer false negatives [34].

Lung cancer and ILD share common risk factors, such as smoking, and lung cancer is approximately three to seven times more common in people with ILD. Given that nearly 10% of patients with ILD die from lung cancer, early detection of lung cancer in ILD is critical [35]. Consequently, mutations associated with lung cancer, such as EGFR T790M, were detectable in EBC using UltraSEEK technology based on mass spectrometry. It showed relatively good sensitivity (90%) and specificity (100%) compared to plasma analysis with 70% sensitivity and 100% specificity [36]. Furthermore, telomere mutations (e.g., TERT, TERC) or single-nucleotide polymorphisms (e.g., SP-B, TOLLIP), which have been observed more frequently in patients with ILD, could serve as potential biomarkers in EBC [37–40].

## *Protein*

Researchers have conducted proteomic analyses to identify proteins present in EBC [41, 42] and used enzyme-linked immunosorbent assay (ELISA) to detect cytokines in EBCs [43]. Tandem mass tags quantitative mass spectrometry was used in recent studies [41, 42] to analyze EBC markers for chronic obstructive pulmonary disease (COPD) and pulmonary embolism. A study by Gade et al. reported that the protein concentration in EBC was around 0.5 μg/mL [41], requiring approximately 7 mL of EBC to meet the minimum protein amount of 3–4 μg for analysis. In analyzing 77 EBC samples, on average, they detected 81 proteins in each of the EBC samples with high variability and absence between samples. They identified 11 proteins (C3, IGHG1, KRT6, GAPDH, PIP, DSP, ACTG1, DGS1, SERPINB12, CALML5, UBA52) that were commonly present in 77 EBC samples.

ELISA allows direct use of EBC samples without pre-concentration or lysis. For instance, one study used ELISA to demonstrate that periostin, a crucial protein involved in fibrogenesis, was elevated in the EBCs of patients with idiopathic pulmonary fibrosis (IPF) compared to healthy controls, effectively distinguishing the two groups with an area under the curve of 0.88 [44]. Another study evaluated VEGF-A concentration in EBC after treatment with Pirfenidone, one of the approved anti-fibrotic medications for IPF [43]. The change in EBC VEGF-A concentration measured with ELISA was correlated with the change in 6-min walking distance, implying that it could be a promising biomarker for monitoring therapeutic efficacy.

The specific proteins present in EBC for ILD patients remain poorly understood. For example, several other cytokines, such as TNF-α and IL-15, that are known to modulate immune responses in IPF were not detected in the aforementioned study on VEGF-A. Further investigation is needed to determine whether this is related to the limited sensitivity of ELISA. This also highlights the need and opportunities for highly sensitive proteomic analysis to identify potential candidate protein biomarkers and validate their clinical potential.

## *Lipid*

Lipids are more abundantly present in EBC at relatively higher concentrations than proteins, because phospholipid accounts for 80% of the surfactant in an airway lining fluid. In a study by Montesi et al., lipidomic analysis showed that docosatetraenoyl (22:4) lysophosphatidic acid (LPA) was ~27 times more frequently detected in EBC from IPF patients compared to a control group [45]. Intriguingly, LPA species in blood did not show a significant difference between IPF patients and control groups. This highlights the potential utility of 22:4 LPA as an EBC biomarker for IPF diagnosis. Another study successfully detected *Mycobacterium tuberculosis* (Mtb)-specific lipids in EBC by immunoassays [46]. By analyzing EBC samples from pulmonary tuberculosis patients and evaluating the levels of Mtb-specific lipids with antibodies, researchers were able to monitor the therapeutic effects of antibiotics. Lipidomics is indispensable for understanding the lipid composition in EBC. After identifying biomarker candidates from untargeted lipidomics, a simple and robust targeted method could be applied to detect specific biomarkers with higher detection sensitivity.

## *Metabolite*

Metabolomics involves the profiling of metabolites in EBC. This is generally conducted with nuclear magnetic resonance (NMR) spectroscopy and mass spectrometry to quantify the metabolites. In cystic fibrosis, the metabolites in EBC were detected with liquid chromatography coupled with mass spectrometry [47]. They developed a machine learning model to distinguish pre-acute pulmonary exacerbations and stable cystic fibrosis patients from normal subjects, which showed an accuracy of 87.7 and 85.7%, respectively. Additionally, EBC metabolites were also detected with NMR. NMR requires minimal sample preparation and enables untargeted metabolomics [48]. In a study involving asthma-COPD overlap (ACO) patients, a machine learning model based on eight dysregulated metabolites showed a good area under the curve (AUC) value of 0.852 in distinguishing ACO from asthma or COPD [48]. In another study, 58 metabolites displayed different patterns in IPF patients compared to control subjects when analyzed using liquid chromatography coupled with mass spectrometry [49]. Similar to other molecular analyses, further refinement of target metabolites and clinical validation is necessary for practicality in future studies.

Mass spectrometry, which has sub-femtomole sensitivity with high resolving power and accurate mass measurement, has been widely used in proteomics, lipidomics, and metabolomics [50]. However, mass spectrometry has been primarily applied for marker screening due to long analysis time and high operational costs. Thus, for clinical adaption, accessibility and assay costs should also be considered. For example, laser-based spectroscopy, such as mid-infrared laser sources, show high sensitivity and convenience at reasonable prices [51, 52]. One study demonstrated rapid (< 1 hour assay time), accurate (AUC: 0.849), and sensitive detection of SARS-COV-2 infection from exhaled breath using laser spectroscopic technology [53].

## *Extracellular Vesicles*

Extracellular vesicles (EVs) are emerging biomarkers as they carry biomolecules reflective of their originating parental cells. In previous studies, EVs were isolated from EBC by size-exclusion chromatography [54], immunoisolation [55], and ultracentrifugation [56]. These studies consistently identified the presence of EVs in EBC by observing their spherical shape and sizes through electron micrography [54, 56]. Lucchetti et al. analyzed small EVs from asthma patients and showed that EV protein concentrations were significantly higher than those of COPD patients and healthy subjects [56]. The presence of EBC EVs was further confirmed by detecting protein markers enriched in EVs (e.g., CD63) [54, 56]. Additionally, several EV miRNAs in EBC showed different levels in asthma patients compared with healthy subjects [55]. Notably, miR-556-5p significantly decreased in asthma patients, but further studies are required to understand the reverse correlation between miR-556-5p expression and asthma. Given that EVs can encapsulate various biomolecules such as nucleotides, proteins, and lipids, EBC EVs could be promising biomarkers for ILD. The current bottleneck is the insufficient sensitivity of EV analysis technology to analyze these EV biomarkers in EBC precisely. Thus, further improving the sensitivity of EV detection is crucial for EBC EV biomarker studies.

## *Oxidative Stress Biomarkers*

Environmental pollutants, redox cycling drugs, radiation, and other factors can generate reactive oxygen species, leading to lung tissue damage [57, 58]. However, they lack specificity for distinguishing ILD from other respiratory diseases.

Nitrogen oxides have garnered interest in EBC due to their potential to provide insights into the balance between lung nitrogen and oxygen redox [59]. Total nitrogen oxide concentrations did not significantly differ between ILD patients and healthy patients [60]. However, the fraction of exhaled nitric oxide levels was lower in systemic sclerosis patients compared to the control group [61].

Hydrogen peroxide ($H_2O_2$) is a major source of reactive oxygen species. $H_2O_2$ in EBC originates from the airway wall as a gas phase [28]. The level of EBC $H_2O_2$ increased in IPF patients [62]. However, another study did not observe a correlation between EBC $H_2O_2$ and lung function, whereas EBC $H_2O_2$ showed a good correlation with nitrogen oxides and 8-isoprostane [60].

8-isoprostane is an end product of lipid peroxidation from arachidonic acid. Higher levels of 8-isoprostane were measured by ELISA in pulmonary fibrosis patients compared to healthy subjects, because reactive oxygen can induce nonenzymatic oxidation of arachidonic acid to 8-isoprostane [60, 62].

**Table 8.1** Summary for conventional analytical methods to detect various molecules in EBCs

| Target molecules | Method | Types | Notes |
|---|---|---|---|
| Nucleic acid | PCR-based methods | Targeted | Fast, high sensitivity and specificity |
| | UltraSEEK | Targeted | For marker screening, expensive |
| | Sequencing | Nontargeted | Marker screening, expensive |
| Protein | Mass spectrometry-based proteomics | Nontargeted, targeted | For marker screening, complicated, expensive |
| | ELISA | Targeted | Fast, cheap, low sensitivity |
| Lipid | Mass spectrometry-based lipidomics | Nontargeted, targeted | For marker screening, complicated, expensive |
| | ELISA | Targeted | Fast, cheap, low sensitivity, low variety |
| Metabolites | Mass spectrometry-based metabolomics | Nontargeted, targeted | For marker screening, complicated, expensive |
| | Nuclear magnetic resonance | Nontargeted, targeted | Low sensitivity, high reproducible, low specificity (compared to mass spectrometry) |
| Extracellular vesicles | PCR-based methods | Targeted | Fast, high sensitivity and specificity |

## EBC Analysis Technologies

### *Conventional Analytical Methods*

Table 8.1 summarizes conventional analytical methods used in EBC marker analysis. Most multi-analyze methods, such as chromatography and mass spectrometry, have been instrumental in omics studies, especially in proteomics and metabolomics research [41, 42, 47]. Advanced nucleic acid sequencing techniques also have enabled the quantification and qualification of RNA and DNA in EBC [63, 64]. Some studies have developed their own computational models using the omics data of patients' EBC to predict the diseases, achieving high accuracies of over 85% [47, 48]. However, contamination can lead to varying outcomes [9]. Therefore, putative markers identified through multi-analyte data should be validated with other conventional targeted detection methods.

Conventional assays, such as immunoassay, photometry, fluorometry, and pH meter, have been utilized in EBC studies. These methods are typically employed to detect specific target molecules identified from biomarker screening. As EBC is a highly diluted matrix, the concentrations of the compounds of interest are often below the assay's detection limit. Therefore, understanding the target concentration ranges for each analytical method and target molecules is advisable.

## Next Generation of Analytical Technologies

A major challenge associated with EBC analysis is detecting biomarkers in a highly diluted specimen. This requires high sensitivity, ideally down to single-molecular detection sensitivity. For nucleic acid targets, droplet digital PCR could be a promising candidate for identifying target genes in EBC. However, detecting short miRNA or fragmented genes still requires a sophisticated primer design to improve its specificity. More importantly, target genes for differential diagnosis should be identified first. Increasing the level of multiplexing for multiple DNA/RNA targets is also essential, considering the heterogeneity of ILDs. Recent studies demonstrated RNA extracted from EBC could be analyzed with a sequencing method. HiSeq® platform showed better sensitivity and consistency in miRNA detection compared to MiSeq® platform [65]. Hence, high-throughput next-generation sequencing could be a promising tool to study nucleic acids in EBC.

For proteins, ultrasensitive single-molecular arrays (SIMOA) could be a good candidate for well-established cytokine and chemokine panels [66]. SIMOA enables the digital detection of protein targets in the fg/mL concentration. Adapting other novel technologies for point-of-care cytokine profiling developed for other diseases should be considered [67]. These single-molecular detection platforms could deepen our understanding of protein biomarkers in the EBC of patients with different physiological conditions and help establish normal ranges. Conventional ELISA assays have limited detection sensitivity and may only be suitable for target molecules over pg/mL concentrations. The limited sensitivity of conventional ELISA resulted in key cytokines remaining undetected in EBC [43]. It was reported that many cytokines are expected to be in the sub-pg/mL concentrations in EBC (Table 8.2). Thus, developing and applying highly sensitive protein detection

**Table 8.2** Concentration of EBC components

| Analyte | Values | References |
|---|---|---|
| Hydrogen peroxide (μmol/L) | 0–0.9 | Dodig and Cepelak [9] |
| pH (mean ± SD) | 7.70 ± 0.49 / 7.85 ± 0.02 | |
| 8-isoprostane (ng/mL) (mean ± SD) | 6.2 ± 0.4 / 4.7 ± 1.8 | |
| Malondialdehyde (nmol/L) (IQR) | 15.6 (4–25) | |
| IL-6 (ng/L) (mean ± SD) | 2.7 ± 0.6 | |
| Nitrite (μmol/L) (IQR) | 2.9 (1.6–5.3) | |
| IL-1 (pg/mL) (IQR) | 0.2 (0.08–1.10) | Aliberti et al. [68] |
| IL-1α (pg/mL) (IQR) | 0.11 (0.05–0.22) | |
| IL-1β (pg/mL) (IQR) | 0.00 (0.00–0.95) | |
| IL-2 (pg/mL) (IQR) | 0.80 (0.00–1.24) | |
| IL-6 (pg/mL) (IQR) | 0.00 (0.00–0.10) | |
| IL-8 (pg/mL) (IQR) | 0.36 (0.00–0.47) | |
| IFNγ (pg/mL) (IQR) | 0.00 (0.00–0.16) | |
| TNFα (pg/mL) (IQR) | 0.00 (0.00–0.76) | |

*IQR* interquartile range, *SD* standard deviation, *IL* interleukin

technologies with sub-pg/mL sensitivity could be suggested for EBC protein biomarkers.

For extracellular vesicles, there are ongoing efforts to develop single EV analysis technologies. These allow for multiparametric analysis of biophysical and biochemical analysis at a single EV level [69, 70]. This could eventually enable us to identify and discriminate EVs based on their cellular origins. If available, this will be a powerful tool to quantitatively analyze EV biomarkers in EBC. The multiplexed single EV analysis requires sophisticated signal amplification strategies while minimizing sample losses. This is particularly challenging for EVs due to their small sizes, which are under a micrometer. Therefore, it is important to keep the sample processing simple while achieving sufficient sensitivity to detect multiple biomarkers [71]. A combination of different amplification strategies with novel detection approaches (e.g., proximity ligation, CRISPR technologies) could be considered [72].

For machine learning-based multi-analyze approaches, such as electronic-nose systems for VOC analysis [11], it is crucial to validate the algorithm with various patient populations in large cohorts from multiple institutions. A machine learning algorithm trained on a local population is vulnerable to over-fitting [73]. Many current machine learning methods have black-box issues in which the exact parameters that the algorithms generate for classification are unknown, which hinders the clinical translation of many AI algorithms [74]. Developing explainable AI algorithms, large, various cohort validation, or both, will be required for more robust and acceptable analysis in the clinical communities.

## *Other Considerations*

Analysis of serially collected samples: Considering the heterogeneity of ILDs and variations between patients, it is important to collect and analyze serially collected samples from the same patient groups. This requires joint efforts from clinicians, engineers, and biostatisticians to recruit high-risk group patients and frequently monitor their status while collecting serial samples. Collecting paired samples (e.g., surgical tissue, BAL fluids, blood samples) will produce an invaluable repository to understand better the correlation of biomolecules between specimens and further support using EBC as a source of surrogate biomarkers.

Cross-Validation: Validation of biomarkers in EBC studies is rarely demonstrated [75]. The quantities or concentrations of biomarkers can vary significantly depending on the methods, research groups, and sample handling. It is pivotal to confirm the reproducibility of differentially expressed markers in EBC within and between different laboratories [76].

Normalization Factor: Collected EBC sample volumes could vary by several conditions. A normalization factor could be considered to compensate for the experimental conditions [9]. Some studies used urea concentration, total proteins, and EBC conductivity for normalization [13, 33, 77]. However, a universally accepted normalization factor has yet to be established [78]. Future research endeavors should focus not only on identifying biomarkers but also on discovering and validating suitable normalization factors.

## Conclusion

EBC shows significant promise as a noninvasive biomarker source for ILD, but addressing key challenges is essential for its successful implementation in clinical practice. Advancements in detection technologies hold promise for discovering and validating robust ILD biomarkers, potentially improving disease management. Standardizing EBC collection and analytic methods is a crucial first step in this process.

**Acknowledgments** This work was partly supported by the National Institute of Health grant (R01GM138778) and the US Army Medical Research Acquisition Activity through the Congressionally Directed Medical Research Programs (HT94252410040). M.H.J. was supported by the National Institute of Health grant (T32CA079443).

## References

1. Aronson KI, Danoff SK, Russell AM, Ryerson CJ, Suzuki A, Wijsenbeek MS, Bajwah S, Bianchi P, Corte TJ, Lee JS, Lindell KO, Maher TM, Martinez FJ, Meek PM, Raghu G, Rouland G, Rudell R, Safford MM, Sheth JS, Swigris JJ. Patient-centered outcomes research in interstitial lung disease: an official american thoracic society research statement. Am J Respir Crit Care Med. 2021;204:e3–e23.
2. Fischer A, Antoniou KM, Brown KK, Cadranel J, Corte TJ, du Bois RM, Lee JS, Leslie KO, Lynch DA, Matteson EL, Mosca M, Noth I, Richeldi L, Strek ME, Swigris JJ, Wells AU, West SG, Collard HR, Cottin V, et al. An official European respiratory society/American thoracic society research statement: interstitial pneumonia with autoimmune features. Eur Respir J. 2015;46:976–87.
3. Park SW, Baek AR, Lee HL, Jeong SW, Yang SH, Kim YH, Chung MP, Korean ILDSG. Korean guidelines for diagnosis and management of interstitial lung diseases: part 1. Introduction Tuberc Respir Dis (Seoul). 2019;82:269–76.
4. Wallis A, Spinks K. The diagnosis and management of interstitial lung diseases. BMJ. 2015;350:h2072.
5. Stainer A, Faverio P, Busnelli S, Catalano M, Della Zoppa M, Marruchella A, Pesci A, Luppi F. Molecular biomarkers in idiopathic pulmonary fibrosis: state of the art and future directions. Int J Mol Sci. 2021;22:6255.
6. Horváth I, Lázár Z, Gyulai N, Kollai M, Losonczy G. Exhaled biomarkers in lung cancer. Eur Respir J. 2009;34:261–75.
7. Liang Y, Yeligar SM, Brown LA. Exhaled breath condensate: a promising source for biomarkers of lung disease. ScientificWorldJournal. 2012;2012:217518.
8. Konstantinidi EM, Lappas AS, Tzortzi AS, Behrakis PK. Exhaled breath condensate: technical and diagnostic aspects. ScientificWorldJournal. 2015;2015:435160.
9. Dodig S, Cepelak I. Exhaled breath condensate – from an analytical point of view. Biochem Med (Zagreb). 2013;23:281–95.

10. Hashoul D, Haick H. Sensors for detecting pulmonary diseases from exhaled breath. Eur Respir Rev. 2019;28:190011.
11. Yang HY, Peng HY, Chang CJ, Chen PC. Diagnostic accuracy of breath tests for pneumoconiosis using an electronic nose. J Breath Res. 2017;12:016001.
12. Marges ER, van der Sar IG, Vries-Bouwstra JK, Huizinga TWJ, van Daele PLA, Wijsenbeek MS, Moor CC, Geelhoed JJM. Detection of systemic sclerosis-associated interstitial lung disease by exhaled breath analysis using electronic nose technology. Am J Respir Crit Care Med. 2024;210:512.
13. Effros RM, Hoagland KW, Bosbous M, Castillo D, Foss B, Dunning M, Gare M, Lin W, Sun F. Dilution of respiratory solutes in exhaled condensates. Am J Respir Crit Care Med. 2002;165:663–9.
14. Montuschi P. Analysis of exhaled breath condensate in respiratory medicine: methodological aspects and potential clinical applications. Ther Adv Respir Dis. 2007;1:5–23.
15. Ng AW, Bidani A, Heming TA. Innate host defense of the lung: effects of lung-lining fluid pH. Lung. 2004;182:297–317.
16. Dwyer TM. Sampling airway surface liquid: non-volatiles in the exhaled breath condensate. Lung. 2004;182:241–50.
17. Hunt J. Exhaled breath condensate: an evolving tool for noninvasive evaluation of lung disease. J Allergy Clin Immunol. 2002;110:28–34.
18. Effros RM, Casaburi R, Porszasz J, Morales EM, Rehan V. Exhaled breath condensates: analyzing the expiratory plumn. Am J Respir Crit Care Med. 2012;185:803–4.
19. American TS, European RS. ATS/ERS recommendations for standardized procedures for the online and offline measurement of exhaled lower respiratory nitric oxide and nasal nitric oxide, 2005. Am J Respir Crit Care Med. 2005;171:912–30.
20. Fairchild CI, Stampfer JF. Particle concentration in exhaled breath. Am Ind Hyg Assoc J. 1987;48:948–9.
21. Fritter D, Knobler CM, Beysens DA. Experiments and simulation of the growth of droplets on a surface (breath figures). Phys Rev A. 1991;43:2858–69.
22. Papineni RS, Rosenthal FS. The size distribution of droplets in the exhaled breath of healthy human subjects. J Aerosol Med. 1997;10:105–16.
23. Effros RM, Biller J, Foss B, Hoagland K, Dunning MB, Castillo D, Bosbous M, Sun F, Shaker R. A simple method for estimating respiratory solute dilution in exhaled breath condensates. Am J Respir Crit Care Med. 2003;168:1500–5.
24. Montuschi P. Indirect monitoring of lung inflammation. Nat Rev Drug Discov. 2002;1:238.
25. Horváth I, Hunt J, Barnes PJ, et al. Exhaled breath condensate: methodological recommendations and unresolved questions. Eur Respir J. 2005;26:523–48.
26. Horváth I, Donnelly LE, Kiss A, Kharitonov SA, Lim S, Chung KF, Barnes PJ. Combined use of exhaled hydrogen peroxide and nitric oxide in monitoring asthma. Am J Respir Crit Care Med. 1998;158:1042–6.
27. Kietzmann D, Kahl R, Müller M, Burchardi H, Kettler D. Hydrogen peroxide in expired breath condensate of patients with acute respiratory failure and with ARDS. Intensive Care Med. 1993;19:78–81.
28. Schleiss MB, Holz O, Behnke M, Richter K, Magnussen H, Jörres RA. The concentration of hydrogen peroxide in exhaled air depends on expiratory flow rate. Eur Respir J. 2000;16:1115–8.
29. Sznajder JI, Fraiman A, Hall JB, Sanders W, Schmidt G, Crawford G, Nahum A, Factor P, Wood LD. Increased hydrogen peroxide in the expired breath of patients with acute hypoxemic respiratory failure. Chest. 1989;96:606–12.
30. Corradi M, Rubinstein I, Andreoli R, Manini P, Caglieri A, Poli D, Alinovi R, Mutti A. Aldehydes in exhaled breath condensate of patients with chronic obstructive pulmonary disease. Am J Respir Crit Care Med. 2003;167:1380–6.
31. Huszár E, Vass G, Vizi E, Csoma Z, Barát E, Molnár Világos G, Herjavecz I, Horváth I. Adenosine in exhaled breath condensate in healthy volunteers and in patients with asthma. Eur Respir J. 2002;20:1393–8.

32. Ishibashi T, Himeno M, Imaizumi N, Maejima K, Nakano S, Uchida K, Yoshida J, Nishio M. NO(x) contamination in laboratory ware and effect of countermeasures. Nitric Oxide. 2000;4:516–25.
33. Gessner C, Kuhn H, Seyfarth HJ, Pankau H, Winkler J, Schauer J, Wirtz H. Factors influencing breath condensate volume. Pneumologie. 2001;55:414–9.
34. Ryan DJ, Toomey S, Madden SF, Casey M, Breathnach OS, Morris PG, Grogan L, Branagan P, Costello RW, De Barra E, Hurley K, Gunaratnam C, McElvaney NG, et al. Use of exhaled breath condensate (EBC) in the diagnosis of SARS-COV-2 (COVID-19). Thorax. 2021;76:86–8.
35. Naccache JM, Gibiot Q, Monnet I, Antoine M, Wislez M, Chouaid C, Cadranel J. Lung cancer and interstitial lung disease: a literature review. J Thorac Dis. 2018;10:3829–44.
36. Smyth RJ, Toomey SM, Sartori A, O'Hanrahan E, Cuffe SD, Breathnach OS, Morgan RK, Hennessy BT. Brief report on the detection of the EGFR T790M mutation in exhaled breath condensate from lung cancer patients. J Thorac Oncol. 2018;13:1213–6.
37. Alder JK, Hanumanthu VS, Strong MA, DeZern AE, Stanley SE, Takemoto CM, Danilova L, Applegate CD, Bolton SG, Mohr DW, Brodsky RA, Casella JF, Greider CW, Jackson JB, Armanios M. Diagnostic utility of telomere length testing in a hospital-based setting. Proc Natl Acad Sci USA. 2018;115:E2358–65.
38. Courtwright AM, El-Chemaly S. Telomeres in interstitial lung disease: the short and the long of it. Ann Am Thorac Soc. 2019;16:175–81.
39. Kubbara A, Amundson WH, Herman A, Lee AM, Bishop JR, Kim HJ. Genetic variations in idiopathic pulmonary fibrosis and patient response to pirfenidone. Heliyon. 2023;9:e18573.
40. Stanel SC, Callum J, Rivera-Ortega P. Genetic and environmental factors in interstitial lung diseases: current and future perspectives on early diagnosis of high-risk cohorts. Front Med (Lausanne). 2023;10:1232655.
41. Gade IL, Riddersholm SJ, Stilling-Vinther T, Brøndum RF, Bennike TB, Honoré B. A clinical proteomics study of exhaled breath condensate and biomarkers for pulmonary embolism. J Breath Res. 2023;18
42. Sun C, Zhou T, Xie G, Fu S, Gao L, Liao J, Wu Y, Wang G. Proteomics of exhaled breath condensate in stable COPD and non-COPD controls using tandem mass tags (TMTs) quantitative mass spectrometry: A pilot study. J Proteome. 2019;206:103392.
43. Jaskiewicz K, Mycroft K, Maskey-Warzechowska M, Paralusz K, Siemiez N, Nejman-Gryz P, Barnas M, Krenke R, Gorska K. Exhaled biomarkers in idiopathic pulmonary fibrosis-a six-month follow-up study in patients treated with pirfenidone. J Clin Med. 2020;9:2523.
44. Carpagnano GE, Soccio P, Scioscia G, Palladino GP, Foschino Barbaro MP, Lacedonia D. The potential role of airways periostin in the clinical practice of patients affected by idiopathic pulmonary fibrosis. Rejuvenation Res. 2021;24:302–6.
45. Montesi SB, Mathai SK, Brenner LN, Gorshkova IA, Berdyshev EV, Tager AM, Shea BS. Docosatetraenoyl LPA is elevated in exhaled breath condensate in idiopathic pulmonary fibrosis. BMC Pulm Med. 2014;14:5.
46. Mosquera-Restrepo SF, Zuberogoïtia S, Gouxette L, Layre E, Gilleron M, Stella A, Rengel D, Burlet-Schiltz O, Caro AC, Garcia LF, Segura C, Peláez Jaramillo CA, Rojas M, Nigou J. A mycobacterium tuberculosis fingerprint in human breath allows tuberculosis detection. Nat Commun. 2022;13:7751.
47. Zang X, Monge ME, Gaul DA, McCarty NA, Stecenko A, Fernández FM. Early detection of cystic fibrosis acute pulmonary exacerbations by exhaled breath condensate metabolomics. J Proteome Res. 2020;19:144–52.
48. Ghosh N, Choudhury P, Joshi M, Bhattacharyya P, Roychowdhury S, Banerjee R, Chaudhury K. Global metabolome profiling of exhaled breath condensates in male smokers with asthma COPD overlap and prediction of the disease. Sci Rep. 2021;11:16664.
49. Rindlisbacher B, Strebel C, Guler S, Kollár A, Geiser T, Martin Fiedler G, Benedikt Leichtle A, Bovet C, Funke-Chambour M. Exhaled breath condensate as a potential biomarker tool for idiopathic pulmonary fibrosis-a pilot study. J Breath Res. 2017;12:016003.

50. Nagornov KO, Gorshkov MV, Kozhinov AN, Tsybin YO. High-resolution Fourier transform ion cyclotron resonance mass spectrometry with increased throughput for biomolecular analysis. Anal Chem. 2014;86:9020–8.
51. Henderson B, Khodabakhsh A, Metsälä M, Ventrillard I, Schmidt FM, Romanini D, Ritchie GAD, Te Lintel HS, Briot R, Risby T, Marczin N, Harren FJM, Cristescu SM. Laser spectroscopy for breath analysis: towards clinical implementation. Appl Phys B Lasers Opt. 2018;124:161.
52. Kiss H, Örlős Z, Gellért Á, Megyesfalvi Z, Mikáczó A, Sárközi A, Vaskó A, Miklós Z, Horváth I. Exhaled biomarkers for point-of-care diagnosis: recent advances and new challenges in breathomics. Micromachines (Basel). 2023;14:391.
53. Liang Q, Chan YC, Toscano J, Bjorkman KK, Leinwand LA, Parker R, Nozik ES, Nesbitt DJ, Ye J. Breath analysis by ultra-sensitive broadband laser spectroscopy detects SARS-CoV-2 infection. J Breath Res. 2023;17:036001.
54. Dobhal G, Datta A, Ayupova D, Teesdale-Spittle P, Goreham RV. Isolation, characterization and detection of breath-derived extracellular vesicles. Sci Rep. 2020;10:17381.
55. Sinha A, Yadav AK, Chakraborty S, Kabra SK, Lodha R, Kumar M, Kulshreshtha A, Sethi T, Pandey R, Malik G, Laddha S, Mukhopadhyay A, Dash D, Ghosh B, Agrawal A. Exosome-enclosed microRNAs in exhaled breath hold potential for biomarker discovery in patients with pulmonary diseases. J Allergy Clin Immunol. 2013;132:219–22.
56. Lucchetti D, Santini G, Perelli L, Ricciardi-Tenore C, Colella F, Mores N, Macis G, Bush A, Sgambato A, Montuschi P. Detection and characterization of extracellular vesicles in exhaled breath condensate and sputum of COPD and severe asthma patients. Eur Respir J. 2021;58:2003024.
57. Bast A, Weseler AR, Haenen GR, den Hartog GJ. Oxidative stress and antioxidants in interstitial lung disease. Curr Opin Pulm Med. 2010;16:516–20.
58. van der Vliet A, Janssen-Heininger YMW, Anathy V. Oxidative stress in chronic lung disease: from mitochondrial dysfunction to dysregulated redox signaling. Mol Asp Med. 2018;63:59–69.
59. American TSW. ATS workshop proceedings: exhaled nitric oxide and nitric oxide oxidative metabolism in exhaled breath condensate: executive summary. Am J Respir Crit Care Med. 2006;173:811–3.
60. Chow S, Thomas PS, Malouf M, Yates DH. Exhaled breath condensate (EBC) biomarkers in pulmonary fibrosis. J Breath Res. 2012;6:016004.
61. Guillen-Del Castillo A, Sánchez-Vidaurre S, Simeón-Aznar CP, Cruz MJ, Fonollosa-Pla V, Muñoz X. Prognostic role of exhaled breath condensate pH and fraction exhaled nitric oxide in systemic sclerosis related interstitial lung disease. Arch Bronconeumol. 2017;53:120–7.
62. Psathakis K, Mermigkis D, Papatheodorou G, Loukides S, Panagou P, Polychronopoulos V, Siafakas NM, Bouros D. Exhaled markers of oxidative stress in idiopathic pulmonary fibrosis. Eur J Clin Investig. 2006;36:362–7.
63. Cherchi R, Cusano R, Orrù S, Ferrari PA, Massidda M, Fotia G, De Matteis S, Cocco P. Next generation sequencing for miRNA detection on the exhaled breath condensate: a pilot study. Epigenet Insights. 2023a;16:25168657231160985.
64. Youssef O, Knuuttila A, Piirilä P, Böhling T, Sarhadi V, Knuutila S. Presence of cancer-associated mutations in exhaled breath condensates of healthy individuals by next generation sequencing. Oncotarget. 2017;8:18166–76.
65. Cherchi R, Cusano R, Orrù S, Ferrari PA, Massidda M, Fotia G, De Matteis S, Cocco P. Next generation sequencing for miRNA detection on the exhaled breath condensate: a pilot study. Epigenet Insights. 2023b;16:25168657231160985.
66. Wu D, Milutinovic MD, Walt DR. Single molecule array (Simoa) assay with optimal antibody pairs for cytokine detection in human serum samples. Analyst. 2015;140:6277–82.
67. Chin LK, Yang JY, Chousterman B, Jung S, Kim DG, Kim DH, Lee S, Castro CM, Weissleder R, Park SG, Im H. Dual-enhanced plasmonic biosensing for point-of-care sepsis detection. ACS Nano. 2023;17:3610–9.

68. Aliberti S, Morlacchi LC, Faverio P, Fernandez-Botran R, Cosentini R, Mantero M, Peyrani P, Ramirez J, Bordon J, Blasi F. Serum and exhaled breath condensate inflammatory cytokines in community-acquired pneumonia: a prospective cohort study. Pneumonia (Nathan). 2016;8:8. https://doi.org/10.1186/s41479-016-0009-7. PMID: 28702287.
69. Ferguson S, Yang KS, Zelga P, Liss AS, Carlson JCT, Del Castillo CF, Weissleder R. Single-EV analysis (sEVA) of mutated proteins allows detection of stage 1 pancreatic cancer. Sci Adv. 2022;8:eabm3453.
70. Jeong MH, Son T, Tae YK, Park CH, Lee HS, Chung MJ, Park JY, Castro CM, Weissleder R, Jo JH, Bang S, Im H. Plasmon-enhanced single extracellular vesicle analysis for cholangiocarcinoma diagnosis. Adv Sci (Weinh). 2023;10:e2205148.
71. Petga MAD, Taylor C, Macpherson A, et al. A simple scalable extracellular vesicle isolation method using polyethylenimine polymers for use in cellular delivery. Extracellular Vesicle. 2024;3:100033.
72. Hong JS, Son T, Castro CM, Im H. CRISPR/Cas13a-based MicroRNA detection in tumor-derived extracellular vesicles, vol. 10. Advanced Science; 2023. p. e2301766.
73. Leming MJ, Bron EE, Bruffaerts R, Ou Y, Iglesias JE, Gollub RL, Im H. Challenges of implementing computer-aided diagnostic models for neuroimages in a clinical setting. NPJ Digit Med. 2023;6:129.
74. Yang G, Ye Q, Xia J. Unbox the black-box for the medical explainable AI via multi-modal and multi-centre data fusion: A mini-review, two showcases and beyond. Inf. Fusion. 2022;77:29.
75. Hayton C, Terrington D, Wilson AM, Chaudhuri N, Leonard C, Fowler SJ. Breath biomarkers in idiopathic pulmonary fibrosis: a systematic review. Respir Res. 2019;20:7.
76. Jeong MH, Han Y, Oh IS, Kim DM, Son DW, Jung MS, Yang H, Lee K, Shin JY, Kim HR, Chung KH. Pre-validation of a Calu-3 epithelium cytotoxicity assay for predicting acute inhalation toxicity of chemicals. Toxicol In Vitro. 2021;75:105136.
77. Effros RM, Dunning MB, Biller J, Shaker R. The promise and perils of exhaled breath condensates. Am J Physiol Lung Cell Mol Physiol. 2004;287:L1073–80.
78. Caffarelli C, Calcinai E, Rinaldi L, Povesi Dascola C, Terracciano L, Corradi M. Hydrogen peroxide in exhaled breath condensate in asthmatic children during acute exacerbation and after treatment. Respiration. 2012;84:291–8.

# Chapter 9
# Animal and Translational Models for Precision Medicine in ILD

**Jeremy Katzen and Rachel Knipe**

## Introduction

Animal and translational models can be invaluable tools in understanding disease pathogenesis, in part because they facilitate the determination of causal relationships. They permit critical modulation experiments such as gain or loss of function that answer fundamental questions about pathogenesis and the potential of therapeutic strategies. Genetic findings in patients with ILD detailed in this book have been leveraged to develop animal and translational models that link genetic associations with mechanistic biology. These preclinical studies are currently experiencing a growth phase. As new technologies develop, and novel genetic mutations are discovered, the ability to use these models to inform precision medicine strategies will continue to expand.

The most common animals used to model ILD in preclinical studies are mice. Mice have several advantages over larger animals, including lower costs for purchasing and housing, the ease of genetic manipulation, and the abundance of species-specific reagents [1]. However, it has been noted that the cellular composition of mouse airways differs from humans, and this has led to some investment in

J. Katzen
Division of Pulmonary, Allergy, and Critical Care Medicine, University of Pennsylvania Perelman School of Medicine and Penn-CHOP Lung Biology Institute, Philadelphia, PA, USA
e-mail: Jeremy.Katzen@pennmedicine.upenn.edu

R. Knipe (✉)
Division of Pulmonary and Critical Care Medicine and Center for Immunology and Inflammatory Diseases, Massachusetts General Hospital and Harvard Medical School, Boston, MA, USA
e-mail: rknipe@mgh.harvard.edu



B. F. Collins, S. B. Montesi (eds.), *Precision Medicine in Interstitial Lung Disease*, Respiratory Medicine, https://doi.org/10.1007/978-3-031-87183-2_9

larger animal models such as pigs and ferrets, especially for the study of airway diseases such as cystic fibrosis [2].

Within mouse models of ILD, the most used and best characterized model is delivery of a single intratracheal injection of bleomycin, which leads to the development of pulmonary fibrotic changes after several weeks of inflammation [3]. This model has some advantages, including reproducibility, predictability, and low cost; however, it fails to recapitulate some key findings in human fibrotic lung diseases, such as persistence of pulmonary fibrosis and progression of disease over time. In addition, there is considerably more inflammation in the bleomycin model than is seen in the prototypic human fibrotic lung disease, idiopathic pulmonary fibrosis (IPF).

Thus, in recent years, there has been increased use of mouse models that induce persistent fibrosis (aged mice, repetitive bleomycin injury and genetic models). It has been shown that repeated doses of intratracheal bleomycin, even in young mice, induce a progressive, persistent fibrosis in the lungs that more closely resembles that seen in IPF [4, 5].

Moving beyond the exogenous lung injury and fibrotic response from bleomycin, seminal papers have been published, which will be reviewed in this chapter, introducing human mutations identified in familial ILD cohorts into mice. These models can be characterized based on the biologic impact of the genetic mutation on a cellular level, and the lung phenotypes of these models range from an increased susceptibility to bleomycin-induced fibrosis to the development of a spontaneous persistent fibrotic phenotype without bleomycin stimulation. In addition, emerging murine models of connective tissue disease-associated ILDs, occupational exposure related ILDs, and rare diffuse parenchymal lung diseases further show a precision approach to modeling ILD for discovery biology and therapeutic testing.

Precision medicine has also been incorporated into translational models using inducible pluripotent stem cells (iPSC) from patients with pulmonary fibrosis, with demonstration of the abnormal cell phenotypes seen in disease. These emerging models marry stem cell biology with disease-specific cell biology using primary human cells which are at the forefront of precision medicine. Demonstrating genetic modulation in human cell phenotypes *in vitro* will be the first step toward personalized medicine in the field of interstitial lung diseases.

## Genetic and Molecular Precision Models

### *Disrupted Cellular Proteostasis: Pulmonary Surfactant Mutations and MUC5B Gain of Function*

Mutations in alveolar type 2 (AT2) cell-restricted pulmonary surfactant genes were among the first identified genetic driver mutations of adult pulmonary fibrosis and pediatric ILD. Since the first clinical surfactant protein C (*SFTPC*) mutation was identified in a child and her mother by Nogee and colleagues in 2001 [6], over 60 clinical mutations in *SFTPC* and surfactant protein A (*SFTPA1*; *SFTPA2*) have been identified in familial and sporadic cases of adult and pediatric ILD [7]. These mutations provide proof of concept for AT2 cell dysfunction as an upstream driver of disease and offer insight into the upstream cellular dysfunction that can initiate ILD pathogenesis.

When modeled *in vitro*, the majority of *SFTPC* mutations occur in the COOH-terminal (BRICHOS) domain and produce a misfolded and aggregation-prone pro-protein that challenges AT2 cell proteostasis activating the unfolded protein response (UPR) [7]. Similarly, *SFTPA1/2* mutations when modeled in vitro also activate AT2 cell UPR signaling [8]. Given that interrogation of AT2 cells from sporadic IPF explant lung tissue have also identified molecular signals of challenged proteostasis and UPR activation [9, 10], this particular AT2 cell dysfunction appears to be an upstream cellular endotype. However, not all clinical *SFTPC* mutations activate the UPR. The most common *SFTPC* mutation identified in the clinic ($SFTPC^{I73T}$) causes pro-protein mistrafficking and accumulates in the late endosomal pathway resulting in impaired autophagy and mitophagy with subsequent mitochondrial dysfunction [11]. AT2s from IPF also have impaired mitochondrial bioenergetics and cellular metabolism, suggesting this may be a second endotype of upstream AT2 cell dysfunction in ILD [12]. These mutations have thus become the basis for more complex preclinical models to interrogate how these upstream AT2 cell endotypes result in organ dysfunction.

While mutations in pulmonary surfactant genes represent a rare and severe form of genetic ILD, the identification of the gain-of-function *MUC5B* promoter variant rs35705950 in 2011 provided a dominant genetic risk factor for sporadic IPF [13]. Initial work modeling overexpression of *Muc5b* in mice defined a loss of mucociliary clearance from exaggerated mucin production as the pathophysiological consequence of the overexpression, with increased susceptibility to bleomycin-induced lung fibrosis [14]. However, subsequent studies have revealed a loss of cellular proteostasis and increased UPR signaling in the MUC5B-producing distal airway cells, which can be modeled *in vivo* [15].

## Preclinical Models

### BRICHOS Surfactant Protein C Mutations

The first murine SFTPC mutation model was based upon the first ILD-associated clinical *SFTPC* mutation, the delta-Exon4 mutation identified in 2001 [6]. Expression of this highly aggregation-prone mutant protein caused UPR activation and an arrest of lung development without viable mice. Subsequent modeling of inducible expression of less proteotoxic mutations in the adult mouse lung (C121G, C185G, L188Q) generated models demonstrating that AT2 cell UPR in the adult mouse lung could generate spontaneous lung fibrosis (C121G, C185G) or increased susceptibility to bleomycin-induced fibrosis (L188Q) [16–19]. Refinement of these models has become a tool to understand the consequences of AT2 cell UPR as an upstream driver of lung fibrosis.

#### Surfactant Protein A Mutations

Surfactant protein A (SP-A) has two isoforms, which are encoded by adjacent genes (*SFTPA1* and *SFTPA2*). *In vitro* modeling of SP-A mutations in alveolar epithelial cells lines demonstrated UPR and production of TGF-β [8]. The first murine model of a clinical *SFTPA1* resulted in AT2 cell UPR- and JNK-mediated necroptosis [20]. These mice developed spontaneous lung fibrosis that was accelerated by infection with influenza virus and responded to JNK inhibition.

#### *Muc5b* Overexpression

Based on the gain-of-function *MUC5B* promoter variant associated with IPF risk, murine models of *Muc5b* overexpression have been developed to understand the consequence of MUC5B on the distal lung epithelia in fibrosis [14, 15]. With increased MUC5B in the distal lung epithelial cells, there is disrupted proteostasis and UPR signaling. While these overexpression mice do not develop spontaneous lung fibrosis, they have increased susceptibility to exogenous fibrotic stimulants.

#### *Grp78* Knockout

While not a clinical mutation, perhaps the best link between disrupted AT2 proteostasis and lung fibrosis comes from a model of genetic knockout of the protein chaperone BIP encoded by the *Grp78* gene (glucose regulated protein 78) [21]. GRP78 interacts with endoplasmic reticulum stress sensors to repress UPR. Mice with induced knockout of this chaperone developed profound AT2 UPR and spontaneous lung fibrosis.

### *Organellar Dysfunction: Hermansky-Pudlak Syndrome and Surfactant Protein Mistrafficking Mutations*

Rare genetic drivers of pulmonary fibrosis have mechanistically linked cell-specific organellar dysfunctions to organ fibrosis. Modeling these mutations has provided important insights into the interplay between organelles and specifically the role of impaired mitochondrial function in the pathogenesis of IPF. Perhaps no better genetic ILD has linked organellar dysfunction with lung pathology than Hermansky-Pudlak syndrome (HPS), a rare autosomal recessive disorder caused by mutations in lysosome-related organelles (LRO) complex genes (*BLOC1–3*, *AP3*). Patients with HPS subtypes 1,2,4 develop early pulmonary fibrosis with UIP features [32]. The LRO mutations cause dysfunction in the lamellar bodies (LBs), the LROs in AT2 that are involved in surfactant homeostasis. These mutations cause a disruption in autophagy and mitophagy, thus mechanistically linking AT2 mitochondrial dysfunction to pulmonary fibrosis. While most of the aforementioned clinical *SFTPC* mutations disrupt AT2 proteostasis, mutations in the linker domain of the gene cause a mistrafficking of the proprotein, which blocks autophagy and mitophagy and also produces mitochondrial dysfunction [11]. Finally, mutations in *ABCA3*, an ATP-dependent transporter of phosphatidylcholine and cholesterol into LBs, further link organellar dysfunction and pulmonary fibrosis. Modeling these mutations has demonstrated the interdependence of organelle maintenance, specifically LB and mitochondria, in AT2 function, and how disruption leads to organ fibrosis.

## Preclinical Models

### Hermansky-Pudlak Syndrome (HPS)

Precision models for HPS include both human cell-based *in vitro* models and murine *in vivo* models. Human cell-based models have included genetically modified embryonic stem cells expressing HPS genes [33], and patient-specific-induced pluripotent stem cell-derived AT2 cells [34, 35]. Both these cell-based model approaches generated AT2s with disrupted LB form and function. They further demonstrated AT2 mitochondrial dysfunction, a hallmark of pulmonary fibrosis, and AT2 elaboration of profibrotic mediators. In vivo models of HPS-1 and HPS-2 have AT2 LB dysfunction and demonstrate increased sensitivity to bleomycin fibrosis, whereas the HPS1/2 double-mutant mice develop spontaneous fibrosis with aging [36]. Beyond providing proof of concept for AT2 dysfunction as an upstream initiator of fibrosis, these models have been used to identify key AT2-immune cell and AT2-fibroblast signaling in the disease pathogenesis.

### Mistrafficking Surfactant Protein C Mutations

Similar to HPS, modeling of the mistrafficking $SFTPC^{I73T}$ mutation has included both human cell-based models and in vivo murine models [37, 38]. The overlapping AT2 biology between these two model systems centers on the impact of the mistrafficked pro-protein on LB maturation and the subsequent disruption of AT2 macroautophagy and mitophagy. In both model systems, AT2s develop mitochondrial dysfunction through impaired mitophagy. These models demonstrate the proximal role of AT2 mitochondrial function in pulmonary fibrosis pathogenesis, and the in vivo model has been used to model the multicellular orchestration of lung fibrosis and test novel therapeutic approaches [39].

ABCA3 Mutations

Mutations in *ABCA3*, an ATP-dependent transporter of phosphatidylcholine and cholesterol into LBs, link LB dysfunction to fibrotic lung disease. While homozygous null *ABCA3* mutations result in absent LB and neonatal respiratory failure in humans and mice models [40], a number of clinical *ABCA3* mutations have been associated with pulmonary fibrosis [7]. Similar to *SFTPC*, clinical *ABCA3* mutations can result in AT2 UPR as well as LB dysfunction, with iPSC modeling showing activation of fibrogenic programs in mutation-expressing AT2 cells [41], and mice expressing a clinical mutation demonstrating susceptible to bleomycin-induced lung fibrosis [42].

## *DNA Damage and Cellular Senescense: Telomere-Associated Mutations*

Telomeres are structures that cap the ends of chromosomes, protecting the chromosome tips from DNA damage which can activate DNA damage pathways and induce disease [22]. Several genetic mutations have been found in familial cohorts with ILD, including loss-of-function mutations in genes related to telomere biology including telomerase activity (TERT, TERC), telomere stability (RTEL1), and other telomere functions (PARN). The consequence of these mutations is shortened telomere length. Supporting the broader relevance of these genetic cases, peripheral blood telomeres are shorter in sporadic PF patients than unaffected controls, and shortened telomere length is associated with disease progression [23]. Some patients have been identified to have short telomere syndrome, with a triad of ILD, bone marrow failure, and liver cirrhosis. Dyskeratosis congenita is the prototypic telomere biology disorder, with a classic triad of abnormal skin pigmentation, nail dystrophy, and oral leukoplakia in addition to bone marrow failure and ILD.

The cellular consequence of shortened telomeres activating DNA damage pathways is the adoption of senescence program with release of fibrotic remodeling-associated senescence-associated secretory proteins (SASPs) and stem cell failure. While the clinical measurement of telomere length in patients is through peripheral white blood cells, the structural lung cell affected by shortened telomere length is hypothesized to be the AT2 cell. This hypothesis is based on the identification of shortened AT2 telomere length in regions of fibrotic lung [24] and preclinical modeling.

### Preclinical Models

Telomerase Mutations

While initial modeling of lung telomerase deficiency in mice showed variable results after challenge with intratracheal bleomycin [25, 26], these models were limited by the basal longer telomere length in mouse cells compared to human.

More recent studies have generated mouse models in which they introduced mutations in telomerase-related genes specifically in epithelial cells, such as Trf1 deletion in AT2 cells, which induced severe telomere dysfunction specifically in the lungs and induced pulmonary fibrosis without a second hit external injury stimulus [27, 28]. In a proof-of-principle study, augmented telomerase expression using an adenoviral vector model showed therapeutic effects in a mouse model of pulmonary fibrosis due to low-dose bleomycin insult and short telomeres [29]. In this model, AAV9-Tert-treated mice showed improved lung function and lower inflammation and fibrosis at 1–3 weeks after viral treatment and improvement of fibrosis at 8 weeks after treatment. Telomeres were longer and epithelial cells had increased proliferation and lower DNA damage, apoptosis, and senescence after AAV-Tert treatment.

Sin3A Mutation

Modeling the process of alveolar epithelial cell senescence even in the absence of a genetic mutation linked to human disease can provide insights into disease pathogenesis. It has been shown that selective induction of cellular senescence in AT2 cells in a mouse through conditional loss of Sin3a, which regulates chromatin structure, in adult mice leads to spontaneous, progressive pulmonary fibrosis [30]. In this model, disease progression occurs over weeks in the absence of a second hit injury and progresses from the periphery of the lung to involve the more central regions, similar to how clinical disease progresses in patients.

Dyskeratosis Congenita iPSC-Derived AT2 Cells

Dyskeratosis congenita is a rare genetic disorder characterized by deficiencies in telomere maintenance leading to critically short telomeres and early onset of aging-related disease such as pulmonary fibrosis. Recently, human-induced pluripotent stem cells have been used to derive AT2 cells which can model how short telomeres impact AT2 cells. In these elegant studies, cultured mutant iAT2 cells develop characteristics of short telomeres, including uncapped ends, and shortened lengths, and result in epithelial cell dysfunction such as growth defects and senescence [31].

## *Exposure-Related ILD*

Given that most ILDs do not present until later in life, it is generally felt that ILD is the result of a multihit phenomenon, with one of the hits being genetic susceptibility and the other being environmental in origin. Through clinical studies, it has been recognized that increased inhalation of substances, often through occupational exposures, can result in the development of ILD [43]. Given that there are millions of workers across the globe exposed to high levels of inhaled substances, the burden of disease is likely underestimated. Inhalation of both inorganic and organic dusts/antigens has been associated with a variety of interstitial lung diseases most often pneumoconiosis and hypersensitivity pneumonitis. There are less understood associations between inhalational exposures and other ILDs including sarcoidosis and idiopathic pulmonary fibrosis [44].

## Preclinical Models

### Inhaled Silica

ILD can be caused by chronic inhalation of crystalline silica. This is often linked to occupational exposures, for instance, manufacturing and processing of artificial stone to produce kitchen and bathroom countertops. Silicosis is thought to result from inhalational exposure in humans; thus, intratracheal instillation has been developed as a model in mice for silicosis [45]. There have been increasing studies in the last several years showing intratracheal silica induces fibrosis in mice persistent at least 56 days after instillation, with increased extracellular matrix proteins collagen 1 and fibronectin in the lung tissue [46]. In this study, intervention with an adipokine apelin reduced fibrosis through inhibition of TGF-β-induced fibroblast activation.

### Inhaled Asbestos

Prior to changes in occupational regulations in the USA, exposure to asbestos through construction and shipbuilding was associated with asbestos-related lung disease, including pulmonary fibrosis. Animals challenged with even a single intratracheal administration of asbestos have been shown to develop lung injury and fibrosis [47]. Inhaled asbestos has been shown to lead to a persistent fibrosis in the lungs, with increased macrophage numbers between weeks 1 and 4 and fibrosis persistent through at least week 24, and has therefore been proposed as an animal model of persistent ILD with more potential relevance to human disease than a single injection of bleomycin, which has been shown to resolve over time [48, 49].

### Carbon Nanoparticles

Sarcoidosis is an ILD characterized by noncaseating granulomas presumed to be a response to an inhaled exposure. There have been reported links between carbon nanoparticles and pulmonary granulomas; thus, a mouse model has been developed induced by oropharyngeal administration of multiwell carbon nanotubes (MWCNT). Unlike other models of sarcoid published over the years, this model induces persistent granulomatous disease in the lungs for up to 90 days after exposure, also modeling a key characteristic of human disease [50].

## *Connective Tissue Disease-Associated ILD*

There are several systemic connective tissue diseases which have increased risk for the development of ILD. Those with the highest risk of ILD include rheumatoid arthritis (RA), systemic sclerosis (SSc), and myositis. There have been various attempts to model these diseases in animals to better understand disease mechanism and pathogenesis, and while they all model some aspects of disease, none fully recapitulate all aspects of disease such that they have led to precision medicine therapeutics.

Rheumatoid arthritis is a multisystem autoimmune disease characterized by erosive joint inflammation and destruction and fibrosis in the lungs. The pattern of progressive ILD in the lungs of patients with RA can have a very similar distribution to IPF, with traction bronchiectasis and honeycomb cystic changes. Thus, it has been hypothesized that models of IPF would similarly model RA, although it is not known at which point pathogenesis converges to generate a common pattern of end-stage lung pulmonary fibrosis.

Scleroderma is a multisystem autoimmune disease characterized by fibrosis of multiple organs in particular skin and lungs. Lung fibrosis has now become the leading cause of mortality in patients with scleroderma. There are several animal models which have been developed with the goal of recapitulating the systemic inflammation and fibrosis present in patients with scleroderma.

Both myositis- and amyopathic dermatomyositis-associated ILD have been associated with a rapidly progressive ILD often refractory to immunosuppression, leading to respiratory failure. Amyopathic dermatomyositis has been associated with autoantibodies against MDA5, which has been seen in patients with rapidly progressive ILD. While an animal model inducing MDA5 autoantibodies does not develop the rapidly progressive ILD seen in patients, the spontaneous fibrotic lung changes in this model connect the amyopathic dermatomyositis autoantibody to lung pathology.

### Preclinical Models

#### Systemic Delivery of Bleomycin

Systemic bleomycin has been one of the main models of SSc-ILD, initially with delivery of a low dose of bleomycin subcutaneously by injection daily for 3–4 weeks, which has been shown to induce skin and lung fibrosis [51]. More recently, systemic delivery of bleomycin has been achieved through the use of an implantable osmotic minipump, which delivers continuous infusion of bleomycin subcutaneously for 7 days, which has also been shown to induce skin and lung fibrosis [52].

#### Subcutaneous Injections of Hypochlorous Acid

Repeated injections of hypochlorous acid (HOCl), a member of a group of reactive oxygen species (ROS) believed to play a role in the inflammation and fibrosis seen in scleroderma, also induce skin and lung fibrosis [53, 54]. Interestingly, SC injections of HOCl led to the production of serum anti-DNA topoisomerase-1 autoantibodies (Anti-Topo-1), increased immune infiltration and pro-fibrotic cytokine expression, and perivascular inflammatory cell infiltration and microvessel wall thickening, all seen in SSc-ILD patients clinically.

#### Subcutaneous Injections of Topoisomerase-1

Given that the presence of anti-topoisomerase-1 (Scl-70) autoantibodies is associated with an increased risk of developing ILD, a model has been published injecting mice with repeated doses of recombinant topoisomerase-1 protein in combination with Complete Freund's Adjuvant (CFA) subcutaneously for four doses every 2 weeks, which has been shown to induce skin and lung fibrosis in mice [55, 56]. This model has also been shown to induce the production of anti-topoisomerase 1 autoantibodies, suggesting even more strongly a causal link between the development of these autoantibodies and the development of skin and lung fibrosis in SSc.

#### Tight Skin 1 Model (Fibrillin-1 Mutations)

There are several transgenic mice which have been used to model scleroderma skin fibrosis, including a mouse with duplication of the fibrillin-1 gene leading to the development of a tight skin mouse 1 (Tsk1/+). These mice have thickened fibrotic skin but lack the inflammation seen in scleroderma [57–59].

#### Tight Skin 2 Model (Col3a1 Mutations)

Another transgenic mouse, the tight skin 2 (Tsk2/+) mouse, has a mutation in Col3a1, leading to accumulation of collagen in the skin. Interestingly, these mice also develop anti-Scl70 autoantibodies, which are associated with increased risk of ILD among patients with SSc [60, 61].

#### SKG Model

Mice develop arthritic joint inflammation and progressive lung fibrosis in response to an immunological stimulation with zymogen. In this model, anti-fibrotic treatment with nintedinab has been shown to reduce pulmonary fibrosis [62].

#### Subcutaneous Injection of MDA5

Despite lack of clarify in the causal relationship between autoantibodies and ILD, mice have been challenged with weekly injections of subcutaneous MDA5 protein in conjunction with Freund's adjuvant and have been shown to develop autoantibodies against MDA5. When the mice are additionally challenged with a lung injury induced by poly (I:C), to mimic a viral infection, the mice develop lung injury and fibrosis [63].

## *Rare Diffuse Paranchymal Lung Diseases*

### Cystic Lung Disease Preclinical Models

#### Lymphangioleiomyomatosis (LAM)

The identification that mutations causing inactivation of the tumor suppressor gene tuberous sclerosis complex 1 (TSC1) or TSC2 are a cause of LAM led to initial murine models of the disease. Mice were injected with TSC2-null cells and developed the characteristic LAM cystic lesions in the lung [64]. Through leveraging this model, the impact of mTOR inhibition with rapamycin was shown to be efficacious and is now a standard therapy for LAM. In addition to iPSC patient-cell-based modeling [65], recent murine modeling of lung-specific Tsc2 knockout [64] has led to multiple LAM-specific preclinical platforms.

#### Brit-Hogg-Dube Syndrome (BHD)

Leveraging the known genetic basis of BHD, germline loss-of-function mutations in folliculin gene (FLCN), multiple murine models of *Flcn* loss of function have been developed [66]. Most of these models result in renal lesions. However, AT2-specific knockout of *Flcn* in adult mice resulted in enlarged alveolar airspaces [67]. This model demonstrated impaired AMPK activation and apoptosis in lung epithelial cells lacking folliculin, implicating these pathways in disease pathogenesis. A subsequent model of *Flcn* knockout in the lung mesenchyme during fetal lung development resulted in cystic lung development, with aberrant mTORC1 and AMPK signaling [68].

#### Pulmonary Langerhans Cell Histiocytosis (PLCH)

PCLH is a rare often smoking-related cystic lung disease, characterized by nodular opacities that progress to pulmonary cysts. Based on the identification that roughly half of PLCH patients harbor somatic BRAF-V600E mutations in myeloid lineage cells that activate MAPK pathway, a BRAF-V600E-mutant mouse model was developed [69]. Phenocopying the human disease, BRAF-V600E-mutant mice exposed to cigarette smoke developed inflammatory lesions with accumulation of dendritic cells in the lungs and cystic lung lesions.

### Other Rare Lung Disease Preclinical Models

Pulmonary Alveolar Microlithiasis (PAM)

PAM is a rare alveolar and parenchymal lung disease defined by progressive accumulation of calcium phosphate microliths. The genetic basis of the disease is autosomal recessive inactivating mutations in *SLC34A2*, which encodes a sodium-dependent phosphate cotransporter (Npt2b) expressed by AT2 cells. Modeling epithelial loss of *Npt2b* in mice lungs resulted in recapitulation of the human lung phenotype, and the model was used to demonstrate that a low-phosphate diet prevents microlith formation and reduces lung injury [70].

Pulmonary Alveolar Proteinosis (PAP)

The molecular basis of PAP involves disruption of alveolar epithelial-macrophage signaling causing a loss of pulmonary surfactant homeostasis and the accumulation of proteinaceous fluid in the alveolar space [71]. The congenital and idiopathic/acquired forms of PAP involve loss of granulocyte–macrophage colony-stimulating factor (GM-CSF) signaling through receptor mutations (congenital) and autoantibodies against GM-CSF (idiopathic/acquired). PAP has been modeled in mice through leveraging this biology where preclinical models of GM-CSF deficiency develop PAP [72, 73]. This provided the basis for GM-CSF replacement as a therapeutic approach to human disease [74, 75].

## *Multicellular Human Tissue Models*

Animal models provide all the components of an *in vivo* lung environment, such as complex cellular composition, air-liquid interface, mechanical influences, and circulating soluble mediators. However, results from animal studies benefit from validation with human tissue systems to increase the translational potential of the findings. Single cell-type culture systems are simple to use but lack the critical cell-cell interactions needed to fully understand complex diseases. Therefore, there has been growing interest in the use of multicellular human tissue systems. Tissue and cells can be used from either healthy or diseased subjects and then can be stimulated with pro-fibrotic mediators, to augment fibrotic processes, or they can be treated with potential inhibitors of pro-fibrotic mediators, to reduce fibrotic processes. In this way, the impact of various therapeutic strategies can be tested on human tissue, as a preclinical test prior to testing in early phase clinical trials.

**Preclinical Models**

Precision-Cut Lung Slices (PCLS)

PCLS have been obtained from normal human lung specimens, grown in *ex vivo* culture conditions, and then treated with a fibrotic cocktail of soluble mediators (LPA, Tgfβ, TNFα, PDGF-AB), which has been shown to induce early fibrosis-like changes in the tissue slices [76]. These slices are especially useful for studying cell-cell interactions and cell-matrix interactions, as these are preserved to some degree in the *ex vivo* culture condition. Valuable readouts have included production of extracellular matrix proteins, such as collagen, elastin and fibronectin, and tissue contraction. Less valuable readouts include vascular function, given the lack of flow and shear stress in the classic PCLS *ex vivo* model.

3D Multicellular Systems

Cells have also been added in series to *ex vivo* microfluidic flow systems, such as a "Lung on a chip" model, which attempts to recapitulate the alveolar-capillary subunit, by seeding alveolar epithelial cells and capillary cells on opposite sides of a porous membrane [77]. These biomimetic microsystems allow for modeling of cell-cell interactions, cyclic mechanical strain impact, and tissue-tissue interfaces. There are many readouts possible in these systems, including microscopy, collection of soluble mediators in the flow media, and collection of cells after perturbation for gene and protein analysis. In addition to expansion of the capabilities of standard cell culture models, they provide nonanimal alternative models for drug screening and toxicology applications.

## Conclusion

There are a number of disease-relevant, preclinical animal models for various interstitial lung diseases, particularly fibrotic lung diseases. As science and precision medicine advance, there will likely be additional development and ongoing integration of multicellular human tissue models. As genetic and molecular precision models (both animal and human tissue) are refined, there will hopefully be more precision options to guide ILD diagnosis and treatment in clinical practice.

## References


1. Fröhlich E. Animals in respiratory research. Int J Mol Sci. 2024;25
2. Basil MC, Alysandratos KD, Kotton DN, Morrisey EE. Lung repair and regeneration: Advanced models and insights into human disease. Cell Stem Cell. 2024;31:439–54.
3. Moore B, et al. Animal models of fibrotic lung disease. Am J Respir Cell Mol Biol. 2013;49:167–79.
4. Degryse AL, et al. Repetitive intratracheal bleomycin models several features of idiopathic pulmonary fibrosis. Am J Physiol Lung Cell Mol Physiol. 2010;299:L442–52.
5. Redente EF, et al. Persistent, progressive pulmonary fibrosis and epithelial remodeling in mice. Am J Respir Cell Mol Biol. 2021;64:669–76.
6. Nogee LM, et al. A mutation in the surfactant protein C gene associated with familial interstitial lung disease. N Engl J Med. 2001;344:573–9.
7. Mulugeta S, Nureki S, Beers MF. Lost after translation: insights from pulmonary surfactant for understanding the role of alveolar epithelial dysfunction and cellular quality control in fibrotic lung disease. Am J Physiol Lung Cell Mol Physiol. 2015;309:L507–25.
8. Maitra M, Cano CA, Garcia CK. Mutant surfactant A2 proteins associated with familial pulmonary fibrosis and lung cancer induce TGF-β1 secretion. Proc Natl Acad Sci USA. 2012;109:21064–9.
9. Korfei M, et al. Epithelial endoplasmic reticulum stress and apoptosis in sporadic idiopathic pulmonary fibrosis. Am J Respir Crit Care Med. 2008;178:838–46.
10. Lawson WE, et al. Endoplasmic reticulum stress in alveolar epithelial cells is prominent in IPF: association with altered surfactant protein processing and herpesvirus infection. Am J Physiol Lung Cell Mol Physiol. 2008;294:L1119–26.
11. Hawkins A, et al. A non-BRICHOS SFTPC mutant (SP-CI73T) linked to interstitial lung disease promotes a late block in macroautophagy disrupting cellular proteostasis and mitophagy. Am J Physiol Lung Cell Mol Physiol. 2015;308:L33–47.
12. Bueno M, et al. PINK1 deficiency impairs mitochondrial homeostasis and promotes lung fibrosis. J Clin Invest. 2015;125:521–38.
13. Seibold MA, et al. A common MUC5B promoter polymorphism and pulmonary fibrosis. N Engl J Med. 2011;364:1503–12.
14. Hancock LA, et al. Muc5b overexpression causes mucociliary dysfunction and enhances lung fibrosis in mice. Nat Commun. 2018;9:5363.
15. Dobrinskikh E, et al. Epithelial endoplasmic reticulum stress enhances the risk of Muc5b-associated lung fibrosis. Am J Respir Cell Mol Biol. 2023;68:62–74.
16. Lawson WE, et al. Endoplasmic reticulum stress enhances fibrotic remodeling in the lungs. Proc Natl Acad Sci USA. 2011;108:10562–7.
17. Katzen J, et al. An SFTPC BRICHOS mutant links epithelial ER stress and spontaneous lung fibrosis. JCI Insight. 2019;4
18. Katzen J, et al. Disruption of proteostasis causes IRE1 mediated reprogramming of alveolar epithelial cells. Proc Natl Acad Sci USA. 2022;119:e2123187119.
19. Rodriguez L, et al. Chronic expression of a clinical SFTPC mutation causes murine lung fibrosis with idiopathic pulmonary fibrosis features. Am J Respir Cell Mol Biol. 2023;68:358–65.
20. Takezaki A, et al. A homozygous SFTPA1 mutation drives necroptosis of type II alveolar epithelial cells in patients with idiopathic pulmonary fibrosis. J Exp Med. 2019;216:2724–35.
21. Borok Z, et al. Grp78 loss in epithelial progenitors reveals an age-linked role for endoplasmic reticulum stress in pulmonary fibrosis. Am J Respir Crit Care Med. 2020;201:198–211.
22. Blackburn EH, Epel ES, Lin J. Human telomere biology: a contributory and interactive factor in aging, disease risks, and protection. Science. 2015;350:1193–8.
23. Alder JK, et al. Short telomeres are a risk factor for idiopathic pulmonary fibrosis. Proc Natl Acad Sci USA. 2008;105:13051–6.
24. Snetselaar R, et al. Short telomere length in IPF lung associates with fibrotic lesions and predicts survival. PLoS One. 2017;12:e0189467.

25. Liu T, et al. Telomerase activity is required for bleomycin-induced pulmonary fibrosis in mice. J Clin Invest. 2007;117:3800–9.
26. Degryse AL, et al. Telomerase deficiency does not alter bleomycin-induced fibrosis in mice. Exp Lung Res. 2012;38:124–34.
27. Povedano JM, Martinez P, Flores JM, Mulero F, Blasco MA. Mice with pulmonary fibrosis driven by telomere dysfunction. Cell Rep. 2015;12:286–99.
28. Naikawadi RP, et al. Telomere dysfunction in alveolar epithelial cells causes lung remodeling and fibrosis. JCI Insight. 2016;1:e86704.
29. Povedano JM, et al. Therapeutic effects of telomerase in mice with pulmonary fibrosis induced by damage to the lungs and short telomeres. elife. 2018;7
30. Yao C, et al. Senescence of alveolar type 2 cells drives progressive pulmonary fibrosis. Am J Respir Crit Care Med. 2021;203:707–17.
31. Fernandez RJ, et al. GSK3 inhibition rescues growth and telomere dysfunction in dyskeratosis congenita iPSC-derived type II alveolar epithelial cells. elife. 2022;11
32. Vicary GW, Vergne Y, Santiago-Cornier A, Young LR, Roman J. Pulmonary fibrosis in hermansky-pudlak syndrome. Ann Am Thorac Soc. 2016;13:1839–46.
33. Strikoudis A, et al. Modeling of fibrotic lung disease using 3D organoids derived from human pluripotent stem cells. Cell Rep. 2019;27:3709–23.
34. Korogi Y, et al. In vitro disease modeling of hermansky-pudlak syndrome type 2 using human induced pluripotent stem cell-derived alveolar organoids. Stem Cell Rep. 2019;13:235.
35. Suezawa T, et al. Modeling of lung phenotype of Hermansky-Pudlak syndrome type I using patient-specific iPSCs. Respir Res. 2021;22:284.
36. Young LR, et al. Epithelial-macrophage interactions determine pulmonary fibrosis susceptibility in Hermansky-Pudlak syndrome. JCI Insight. 2016;1:e88947.
37. Alysandratos KD, et al. Patient-specific iPSCs carrying an SFTPC mutation reveal the intrinsic alveolar epithelial dysfunction at the inception of interstitial lung disease. Cell Rep. 2021;36:109636.
38. Nureki SI, et al. Expression of mutant Sftpc in murine alveolar epithelia drives spontaneous lung fibrosis. J Clin Invest. 2018;128:4008–24.
39. Rodriguez LR, et al. PGF2α signaling drives fibrotic remodeling and fibroblast population dynamics in mice. JCI Insight. 2023;8
40. Cheong N, et al. ABCA3 is critical for lamellar body biogenesis in vivo. J Biol Chem. 2007;282:23811–7.
41. Sun YL, et al. Human pluripotent stem cell modeling of alveolar type 2 cell dysfunction caused by ABCA3 mutations. J Clin Invest. 2024;134
42. Tomer Y, et al. The common ABCA3(E292V) variant disrupts AT2 cell quality control and increases susceptibility to lung injury and aberrant remodeling. Am J Physiol Lung Cell Mol Physiol. 2021;321:L291–l307.
43. Spagnolo P, et al. Occupational interstitial lung diseases. J Intern Med. 2023;294:798–815.
44. Gandhi SA, et al. The impact of occupational exposures on the risk of idiopathic pulmonary fibrosis: a systematic review and meta-analysis. Ann Am Thorac Soc. 2024;21:486–98.
45. Lam M, Mansell A, Tate MD. Preclinical mouse model of silicosis. Methods Mol Biol. 2023;2691:111–20.
46. Shen J, et al. Apelin Prevents and alleviates crystalline silica-induced pulmonary fibrosis via inhibiting transforming growth factor beta 1-triggered fibroblast activation. Int J Biol Sci. 2023;19:4004–19.
47. Guo L, et al. PM2.5 exposure induces lung injury and fibrosis by regulating ferroptosis via TGF-beta signaling. Dis Markers. 2022;2022:7098463.
48. Lemaire I, Beaudoin H, Masse S, Grondin C. Alveolar macrophage stimulation of lung fibroblast growth in asbestos-induced pulmonary fibrosis. Am J Pathol. 1986;122:205–11.
49. Lemaire I, Nadeau D, Dunnigan J, Masse S. An assessment of the fibrogenic potential of very short 4T30 chrysotile by intratracheal instillation in rats. Environ Res. 1985;36:314–26.
50. Huizar I, et al. Novel murine model of chronic granulomatous lung inflammation elicited by carbon nanotubes. Am J Respir Cell Mol Biol. 2011;45:858–66.

51. Yamamoto T, et al. Animal model of sclerotic skin. I: local injections of bleomycin induce sclerotic skin mimicking scleroderma. J Invest Dermatol. 1999;112:456–62.
52. Ravanetti F, et al. Modeling pulmonary fibrosis through bleomycin delivered by osmotic minipump: a new histomorphometric method of evaluation. Am J Physiol Lung Cell Mol Physiol. 2020;318:L376–85.
53. Meng M, et al. The fibrosis and immunological features of hypochlorous acid induced mouse model of systemic sclerosis. Front Immunol. 2019;10:1861.
54. Servettaz A, et al. Selective oxidation of DNA topoisomerase 1 induces systemic sclerosis in the mouse. J Immunol. 2009;182:5855–64.
55. Gronberg C, et al. Combined inhibition of IL-1, IL-33 and IL-36 signalling by targeting IL1RAP ameliorates skin and lung fibrosis in preclinical models of systemic sclerosis. Ann Rheum Dis. 2024;83:1156–68.
56. Yoshizaki A, et al. Immunization with DNA topoisomerase I and Freund's complete adjuvant induces skin and lung fibrosis and autoimmunity via interleukin-6 signaling. Arthritis Rheum. 2011;63:3575–85.
57. Saito E, et al. CD19-dependent B lymphocyte signaling thresholds influence skin fibrosis and autoimmunity in the tight-skin mouse. J Clin Invest. 2002;109:1453–62.
58. Shibata S, et al. Immunochemical and molecular characterization of anti-RNA polymerase I autoantibodies produced by tight skin mouse. J Clin Invest. 1993;92:984–92.
59. Hatakeyama A, Kasturi KN, Wolf I, Phelps RG, Bona CA. Correlation between the concentration of serum anti-topoisomerase I autoantibodies and histological and biochemical alterations in the skin of tight skin mice. Cell Immunol. 1996;167:135–40.
60. Christner PJ, Peters J, Hawkins D, Siracusa LD, Jimenez SA. The tight skin 2 mouse. An animal model of scleroderma displaying cutaneous fibrosis and mononuclear cell infiltration. Arthritis Rheum. 1995;38:1791–8.
61. Gentiletti J, et al. Demonstration of autoimmunity in the tight skin-2 mouse: a model for scleroderma. J Immunol. 2005;175:2418–26.
62. Redente EF, et al. Nintedanib reduces pulmonary fibrosis in a model of rheumatoid arthritis-associated interstitial lung disease. Am J Physiol Lung Cell Mol Physiol. 2018;314:L998–L1009.
63. Ichimura Y, et al. Autoimmunity against melanoma differentiation-associated gene 5 induces interstitial lung disease mimicking dermatomyositis in mice. Proc Natl Acad Sci USA. 2024;121:e2313070121.
64. Goncharova EA, et al. Prevention of alveolar destruction and airspace enlargement in a mouse model of pulmonary lymphangioleiomyomatosis (LAM). Sci Transl Med. 2012;4:154ra134.
65. Julian LM, et al. Human pluripotent stem cell-derived TSC2-haploinsufficient smooth muscle cells recapitulate features of lymphangioleiomyomatosis. Cancer Res. 2017;77:5491–502.
66. Kennedy JC, Khabibullin D, Boku Y, Shi W, Henske EP. New developments in the pathogenesis of pulmonary cysts in birt-hogg-dubé syndrome. Semin Respir Crit Care Med. 2020;41:247–55.
67. Goncharova EA, et al. Folliculin controls lung alveolar enlargement and epithelial cell survival through E-cadherin, LKB1, and AMPK. Cell Rep. 2014;7:412–23.
68. Chu L, et al. Mesenchymal folliculin is required for alveolar development: implications for cystic lung disease in Birt-Hogg-Dubé syndrome. Thorax. 2020;75:486–93.
69. Liu H, et al. MAPK mutations and cigarette smoke promote the pathogenesis of pulmonary Langerhans cell histiocytosis. JCI Insight. 2020;5
70. Saito A, et al. Modeling pulmonary alveolar microlithiasis by epithelial deletion of the Npt2b sodium phosphate cotransporter reveals putative biomarkers and strategies for treatment. Sci Transl Med. 2015;7:313ra181.
71. Trapnell BC, Whitsett JA, Nakata K. Pulmonary alveolar proteinosis. N Engl J Med. 2003;349:2527–39.
72. Dranoff G, et al. Involvement of granulocyte-macrophage colony-stimulating factor in pulmonary homeostasis. Science. 1994;264:713–6.

73. Stanley E, et al. Granulocyte/macrophage colony-stimulating factor-deficient mice show no major perturbation of hematopoiesis but develop a characteristic pulmonary pathology. Proc Natl Acad Sci USA. 1994;91:5592–6.
74. Reed JA, et al. Aerosolized GM-CSF ameliorates pulmonary alveolar proteinosis in GM-CSF-deficient mice. Am J Phys. 1999;276:L556–63.
75. Seymour JF, et al. Therapeutic efficacy of granulocyte-macrophage colony-stimulating factor in patients with idiopathic acquired alveolar proteinosis. Am J Respir Crit Care Med. 2001;163:524–31.
76. Alsafadi HN, et al. An ex vivo model to induce early fibrosis-like changes in human precision-cut lung slices. Am J Physiol Lung Cell Mol Physiol. 2017;312:L896–1902.
77. Huh D, et al. Reconstituting organ-level lung functions on a chip. Science. 2010;328:1662–8.

# Chapter 10
# Big Data: Pearls and Pitfalls for Precision Medicine in Interstitial Lung Disease

**Bhavika Kaul, Harold R. Collard, and Laura A. Petersen**

## Introduction

Interstitial lung diseases (ILD) first emerged as a distinct clinical entity in the mid-twentieth century when seminal work by Hamman and Rich in the 1940s described what we now recognize as acute interstitial pneumonia. Since then, our understanding of disease pathogenesis, natural history, and optimal treatments have evolved primarily through literature generated from a network of tertiary care referral centers. Although important in advancing knowledge and facilitating development of breakthrough therapies, this research methodology relies on individual patient recruitment, which has constrained efficiency. Furthermore, patients recruited from tertiary care referral centers may represent a select subset of patients with different socioeconomic and demographic features compared to ILD patients in the broader population, introducing bias into data sets. With the digitization of health records ushering in an era of "big data," the landscape of clinical research and care delivery have changed. In light of this opportunity, multiple agencies including the National Academy of Medicine and the US Food and Drug Administration have advocated for the restructuring of current healthcare systems to incorporate clinical research into a practice-based model of evidence generation called the "learning health care system," which relies on the aggregation of data generated from routine clinical encounters to further patient care and research [1, 2].

B. Kaul (✉) · L. A. Petersen
Baylor College of Medicine, Houston, TX, USA

Center for Innovations in Quality, Effectiveness and Safety, Department of Veterans Affairs, Houston, TX, USA
e-mail: Bhavika.Kaul@va.gov; Laura.Petersen@va.gov

H. R. Collard
University of California San Francisco, San Francisco, CA, USA
e-mail: Harold.Collard@ucsf.edu



B. F. Collins, S. B. Montesi (eds.), *Precision Medicine in Interstitial Lung Disease*, Respiratory Medicine, https://doi.org/10.1007/978-3-031-87183-2_10

Big data and the learning healthcare system model present a unique opportunity to study disease at population levels and optimize "precision medicine" in ILD. The National Institute of Health defines precision medicine as "an innovative approach that takes into account individual differences in patients' genes, environment and lifestyles," thus facilitating tailoring of treatment to individuals rather than population means [3]. Stated another way, **precision medicine is about connecting the *right patient to the right care at the right time***. In this chapter, we will first discuss the history of big data in health care and define current data sources, describe the epochs of ILD research, outline unique challenges and pitfalls including diversity and privacy concerns, and conclude with a shared priority agenda to further precision medicine in ILD.

## Understanding Big Data

### *History of Digitization of Healthcare Data*

The foundation of big data in health care was built against a broader backdrop of digital revolutions in the late twentieth and early twenty-first centuries. To encourage more rapid digitization of the healthcare sector, the 2009 Health Information Technology for Economic and Clinical Health Act provided significant incentives to healthcare systems to adopt electronic health records (EHR). Simultaneous advances in genomics and medical imaging led to rapid expansion of available biomedical data. The convergence with increasing computing power and advanced analytic techniques created new opportunities for data science in health care.

Against this backdrop, President Obama launched the Precision Medicine Initiative in 2015, a program designed to transform how we improve health and treat disease. The overall aim was to generate the scientific evidence needed to move the concept of precision medicine into clinical practice by empowering patients, researchers, and healthcare teams to work toward the development of individualized treatments while considering variability in genes, environment, and lifestyle. The three cornerstones of the initiative included (1) sequencing data from the human genome, (2) improving technologies for biomedical analysis (including longitudinal EHR data), and (3) developing new computational tools. The near-term goals focused on precision medicine in cancer by expanding cancer genomics research to develop tailored treatments. The longer-term goal through the *All of Us Research Program* focused on gathering genetic data, biological samples, diet, and lifestyle information, linked to electronic health records to pioneer a new model of scientific inquiry. Particularly for ILD, this infrastructure opens avenues for large-scale analysis in rare diseases and sets the stage for a more data-driven personalized approach to medicine including understanding the genetic basis of ILD subtypes, exploring environmental contributors of disease, developing targeted pharmacogenomics informed therapeutics, and ensuring that they reach patients. This new research paradigm relies on several key data sources that can be utilized to advance precision medicine in ILD.

## *Data Sources*

The key big data sources that are being leveraged to advance precision medicine in ILD are illustrated in Fig. 10.1.

1. Health Insurance Claims Data: Health insurance claims data originally generated for billing purposes provide valuable information about patient demographics, diagnosis, procedures, and healthcare utilization. Medicare Claims and MarketScan Research Databases have been used to study ILD disease epidemiology, disparities in care, uptake of novel therapeutics, and evaluate cost-effectiveness [4–8]. However, claims data primarily consist of structured data elements such as patient demographics, medication prescriptions, diagnosis, and procedure codes. Structured data elements are standardized predefined data fields that are typically collected via templated forms or drop-down menus making them easier to query using traditional data mining and statistical techniques. However, structured data in claims dataset lack the clinical detail and granularity of unstructured data elements such as free-text, narrative responses (e.g., clinical notes), pulmonary function test interpretation, or multimedia (e.g., imaging,

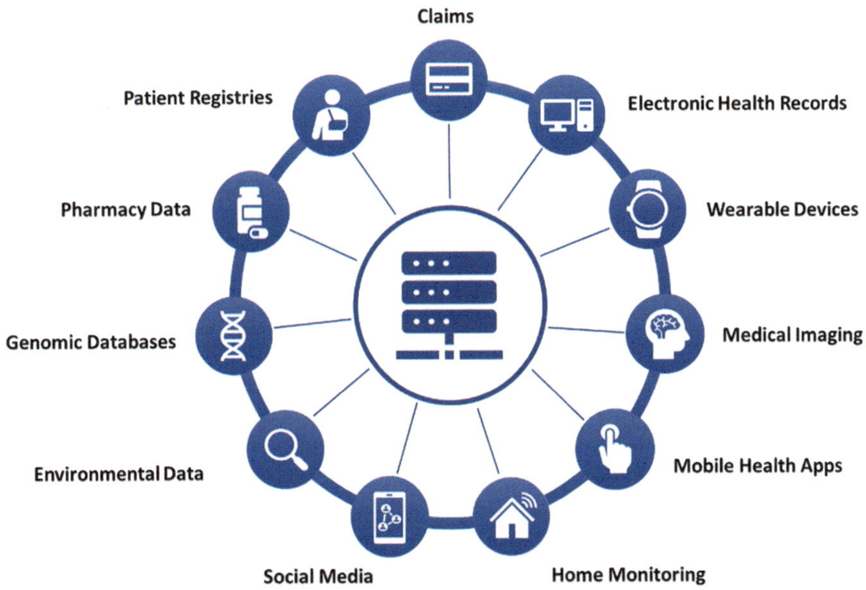


**Fig. 10.1** Big data sources

pathology slides) that provide richer context-specific information about patients' coexisting conditions, therapies, and outcomes.

2. Electronic Health Records (EHR): EHRs such as Epic Systems, Cerner, and Department of Veterans Affairs CPRS represent more comprehensive data sources and contain a mix of both structured data elements found in traditional claims data sets and unstructured data elements captured from patient-physician encounters. EHR data can be used to develop computable disease phenotypes and study longitudinal disease trajectories including differential impact of treatment responses. However, analyzing this data requires more advanced statistical methods such as natural language processing (NLP) to extract key features from clinical notes and machine learning for complex pattern recognition for sub-phenotype development.
3. Multi-omics Biospecimen Repositories: Over the last decade, national and international repositories have collated genomic, proteomic, and metabolomic data for mechanistic studies of disease biology, biomarker discovery, and development of personalized treatment approaches. The UK Biobank contains genetic and health data from over 500,000 participants, the Database of Genotypes and Phenotypes (dbGaP) archives studies investigating genotype-phenotype interaction, and the Metabolomics Workbench serves as a repository for metabolomic metadata. These national and international repositories are particularly valuable for rare disease research as they aggregate specimens from multiple sites to enhance sample sizes. Integration of these sources with clinical data can lead to development of more accurate risk prediction tools and therapeutics targeted to individual patients' molecular profiles as has been pioneered by precision oncology.
4. Wearable Devices, Mobile Apps, and Home-Based Monitoring: Ubiquitous wearable devices such as Apple Watch, Fitbit, and Aura Rings collect continuous, real-time health data outside of clinical settings including physiological parameters such as heart rate, blood oxygen saturation, respiratory rate, physical activity levels, and sleep patterns. The aggregate data can identify early signs of disease progression or exacerbations and facilitate more timely intervention. These devices can also set medication reminders, track adherence, and measure the impact of treatment on daily functioning to complement structured clinical data from healthcare settings.
5. Environmental Data: The Environmental Protection Agency (EPA) Air Quality System, National Oceanic and Atmospheric Administration Climate Data, and Occupational Safety and Health Administration Exposure Data can play a crucial role in advancing precision medicine for ILD yet have been underutilized to date. These databases offer comprehensive information about air pollution, climate patterns, and occupational clusters and provide valuable insights into how environmental factors (the "exposome") interact with individual susceptibilities to influence ILD onset, progression, and treatment response. For example, combining air quality data with clinical and genomic data can improve our understanding of how susceptibility to particulate matter leads to inflammation in ILD subtypes. Similarly, occupational exposure data can inform development of per-

sonalized risk assessments and targeted screening programs for high-risk populations.

## Epochs of Data Science in Interstitial Lung Disease

The increasingly sophisticated research questions that can be answered by big data have led to rapid advancements in ILD research over the last decade. Broadly, ILD research can be categorized into three epochs: Epoch 1, defined by epidemiological and observational research studies in the early part of the twenty-first century; Epoch 2, our current era of high-dimensional multimodal data integration; and Epoch 3, a future state that moves precision medicine from the theoretical research domain into practical real-time decision support and clinical implementation. Below we outline the data sources required to support each epoch and the research questions that have been answered.

### *Epoch 1: Foundational Epidemiological and Observational Research (2000–2019)*

The start of the twenty-first century was marked by a significant shift in how medical data was collected, stored, and analyzed, setting the stage for the first epoch of big data research for precision medicine in ILD. The era was characterized by a transition from paper-based records to digital systems, a crucial first step in aggregating and analyzing clinical data at a scale. These efforts resulted in the establishment of collaborative registries such as the Pulmonary Fibrosis Foundation Patient Registry, which supported retrospective epidemiological analyses and longitudinal outcome studies. Early biobanking efforts within these multi-institutional registries paved the way for early mechanistic studies. Complementing these efforts, investigators began leveraging claims data (e.g., CMS Medicare) to better understand population-level epidemiology and answer health services-oriented research questions.

Studies during this time characterized major ILD subtypes based on overlapping clinical features, estimated population incidence and prevalence, identified risk factors associated with disease development and progression, assessed treatment response, and examined care utilization patterns and economic impact. Through these early studies, we learned the following:

1. Changes in clinical and physiological variables predict outcomes in patients with idiopathic pulmonary fibrosis (IPF) supporting the subsequent uptake of physiological parameters as the primary endpoint of IPF clinical trials [9–11].
2. Immunosuppression does not alter survival in IPF and in fact is detrimental to patients. These findings were initially described in observational studies from

IPF registries and subsequently confirmed through clinical trials that utilized registries for patient identification and recruitment [12, 13].
3. Prognostication models such as the gender-age-physiology (GAP) index can leverage commonly measured clinical and physiological variables to predict ILD mortality [14, 15].
4. Genetics play an important role in fibrosis pathogenesis. Telomere length emerged as a prognostic biomarker with short leukocyte telomere length associated with worse survival in IPF [16]. Telomere-related genes were found to contribute to diagnostically heterogenous ILD phenotypes but were notably uniformly progressive [17].
5. Claims data demonstrated that the incidence and prevalence of ILD at a population level are higher than what has been described in registries and novel risk factors, including environmental exposures such as air pollution which are associated with increased risk for exacerbation [6, 7, 18–20]. These findings justified further research examining the impact of the "exposome" in ILD [21–25].

Although Epoch 1 represents the nascent stage of precision medicine, these initial studies set the foundation for our current epoch of big data in ILD in which we have begun to integrate multiple data modalities to develop a more comprehensive understanding of disease biology, sub-phenotypes, and optimal treatment responses.

## *Epoch 2: High-Dimensional, Multi-omics Integration (Present)*

Limitations of computation power and challenges with data stewardship restricted the sophistication of studies in Epoch 1. However, the digital infrastructure laid the foundation for high-dimensional, multi-omics research that characterize our current epoch. New technologies, particularly cloud-based computing platforms (e.g., Amazon Web Services, Google Cloud, Azure), have supported the rapid scale-up of storage capacity and computation power required to analyze large volumes of clinical, imaging, and molecular data. The multimodal data paired with new machine learning methods has enabled researchers to begin answering more complex questions about disease biology by identifying biomarkers of disease progression and treatment response. Biomarker studies to date have focused broadly on three areas: genetics, proteomics, and imaging.

1. Genetics: Genetics research in ILD has now moved beyond testing for telomere length in peripheral blood testing that defined Epoch 1 to genome-wide association studies (GWAS). Through GWAS, we have learned that in addition to rare genetic variants, common genetic variants contribute to IPF risk, and genetic risk assessment can be linked to clinically relevant outcomes [26–28]. More recent studies have examined polygenic risk scores for idiopathic pulmonary fibrosis and the association between medications (e.g., immunosuppression), genetic profile, and clinical outcomes [27, 29, 30]. The PANTHER study con-

firmed the harmful effects of immunosuppression in IPF [13]. However, a posthoc analysis of the clinical trial data noted a potential beneficial effect of NAC in a subgroup of individuals carrying a specific TOLLIP genetic variant which is present in 25% of patients with IPF. This sentinel observation of potential pharmacogenetic interaction between NAC and TOLLIP polymorphism has led to the first pharmacogenomic trial in IPF–PRECISIONS, which will use molecularly focused techniques to identify patients with IPF most likely to benefit from treatment [31].
2. Proteomics: In addition to genomic biomarkers, distinct proteomic markers of survival and progressive fibrosing ILD phenotypes have also been identified [32]. These signature profiles have the potential to improve prognostication at index diagnosis and avoid the need for antecedent progression when defining progressive fibrosing phenotypes [33]. Such molecular signatures can also support clinical trial enrichment for patients most at risk for adverse outcomes.
3. Radiomics: Deep learning models of high-resolution CT scans have been developed for disease quantification, automation of pattern recognition, and predictive modeling of disease behavior and treatment response. These tools have demonstrated efficacy in accurately quantifying extent of fibrosis and are now being incorporated into ILD clinical trials as secondary endpoints, potentially offering greater sensitivity in detecting treatment response. Imaging biomarkers have also shown efficacy in differentiating between usual interstitial pneumonia and other ILD patterns and in predicting IPF mortality with better accuracy than clinical prediction models [34–39]. Recent studies have demonstrated that baseline CT features can predict progressive disease phenotypes [39, 40]. Although still in its early phases, predicting progression and treatment response at index CT could match patients with appropriate therapies and identify high-risk patients who may benefit from more proactive care engagement, treatment, and referral to lung transplantation. Compared to genomics and proteomics, radiomics also offers the simplest pathway to clinical integration as imaging is already a part of standard clinical workflows.

Notably, the study of genetic, proteomic, and imaging biomarkers in ILD has largely progressed along parallel but separate tracks. There is a growing recognition that integrating genetic, proteomic, radiomic, and clinical data can uncover novel disease subtypes and develop more comprehensive patient profiles to guide individualized treatment. The volume of data processing required for multi-omics subphenotyping will also require new analytical methods that utilize unsupervised machine learning.

Despite these advancements in genetics, proteomics, and radiomics, we remain in the nascent stages of understanding the exposome and its interaction with the biological mechanisms that contribute to disease development. Progress in Epoch 2 will require more disciplined studies of environmental exposures captured through EPA data, lifestyle surveys, and occupational databases in addition to continued evolution of computational methods to facilitate multiomics data integration.

## *Epoch 3: Real-Time Decision Support and Clinical Implementation (Future)*

The third epoch of ILD research represents an ambitious future state that builds upon the multimodal data integration and biomarker discover currently underway. This epoch moves beyond theoretical research into practical, real-time clinical implementation, characterized by sophisticated decision support tools, individualized treatment approaches, and continuous disease monitoring. The path to clinical integration is not without significant challenges. Implementation science has shown that translating research into clinical practice take an average of 17 years [41]. This delay is often due to combination of factors including resistance to change, lack of awareness of emerging evidence, insufficient infrastructure to support new practices, regulatory hurdles, and concerns about cost-effectiveness. In the context of ILD and precision medicine, these challenges are further amplified by the complexity of data and interventions involved and the concentration of subspecialty expertise at a few tertiary care referral centers. For example, integration of omics-based discoveries such as polygenic risk scores or pharmacogenetic testing into clinical decision-making requires not only new tools and technologies but also a fundamental shift in how ILD physicians approach diagnosis and treatment planning.

To have the foresight to address these challenges and translate the promise of precision medicine in ILD into clinical reality, two key areas will require thoughtful change: development of clinical decision support tools with the end user in mind and education and training of clinicians. The development of user-friendly clinical decision support systems is crucial for the practical applications of precision medicine in ILD. These systems must be able to capture and synthesize complex, multimodal data (clinical, imaging, molecular, environmental) in real time, provide clear and actionable insights at the point of care, and integrate seamlessly into existing clinical workflows without significantly increasing administrative burden. Additionally, they must offer transparent reasoning for recommendations to build trust and have a clear pathway to iterative improvement as new evidence emerges over time. Potential clinical decision support tools include automated detection and quantification of disease patterns on imaging to improve monitoring, early warnings for acute exacerbations or clinical decompensation leveraging continuous monitoring data (e.g., wearable devices), personalized treatment recommendations based on molecular profiles, and predicted drug responses.

Implementation of real-time clinical decisions support tools requires a workforce equipped to interpret and act upon the volume of data and complexity of personalized treatment recommendations generated by advanced analytic platforms. Training end users in engaging with such platforms requires creating continuing education programs for practicing clinicians that can adapt to rapidly evolving precision medicine approaches and building competency in explaining precision medicine results to patients and families. Lastly, as precision medicine tools are implemented in clinical practice, it is crucial to establish systems to monitor and evaluate of the impact of interventions on patient outcomes and healthcare efficiency.

As precision medicine in ILD advances and moves into clinical spaces in Epoch 3, there is a risk that precision medicine will exacerbate existing health disparities. Addressing health equity at the forefront requires ensuring diverse representation in omics studies, developing policies and incentives to ensure equitable access to testing (e.g., whole genome sequencing), and creating strategies for implementing these advanced care approaches in both resource-rich academic medical centers, which will likely have the infrastructure and computational power to support new tools, and resource-constrained community-based practices. This is important, because a lack of diversity in source data can lead to biased findings, perpetuating inequities or exacerbating disparities. Ultimately, the success of this epoch will be measured not just by scientific breakthroughs in precision medicine but by the tangible improvements in patient outcomes and efficient healthcare delivery for patients with ILD. It will require close collaboration between researchers, clinicians, patients, health system leaders, and policy-makers to create an ecosystem that can fully leverage the power of data to drive tangible improvements in patient care.

## Methodological Challenges

There are several key methodological challenges (Fig. 10.2) spanning the life cycle of data use that need to be addressed as we progress in Epoch 2 and subsequently move into Epoch 3 of ILD research.

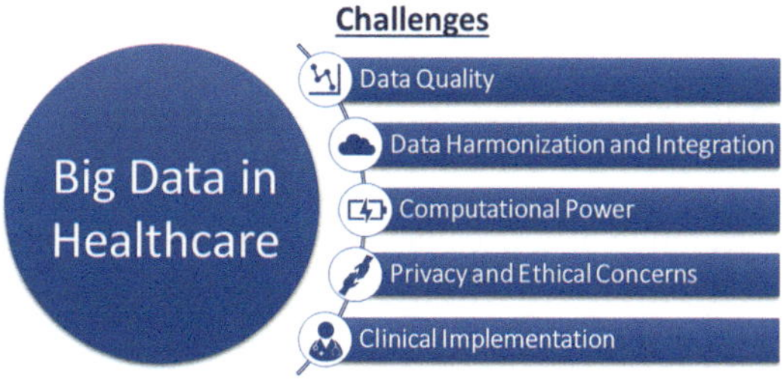
Challenges
Big Data in Healthcare
Data Quality
Data Harmonization and Integration
Computational Power
Privacy and Ethical Concerns
Clinical Implementation

**Fig. 10.2** Challenges of big data research

## *Data Quality*

Data quality issues, particularly those related to completeness and accuracy, are key challenges that have hindered the full realization of big data potential in health care. For example, administrative claims have inherent challenges as they are generally restricted to the structured data elements developed for billing purposes. The reliance on international classification of disease (ICD) codes for disease identification in claims databases has been limiting as ICD codes may be inaccurate or overly broad due to coding practices aimed at maximizing reimbursement rather than capturing precise clinical phenotypes. Electronic health records are more nuanced and have the potential to overcome the limitations of administrative claims databases as they contain both structured data elements and unstructured data. However, unstructured narrative information included in EHR is more difficult to systematically analyze. Particularly for ILD, many clinically relevant details such as specific radiologic patterns or nuanced description of symptom progression are captured in narrative data. Emerging tools such as natural language processing have the potential to overcome these methodological limitations.

Data missingness is another limitation impacting data quality, especially for patients seen outside integrated healthcare system. This type of missingness may not be random. Patients with more severe disease are likely to have frequent healthcare encounters and thus more complete data compared to patients at earlier stages of disease. Being cognizant of the patterns of missingness and how they introduce bias is important to generalizability of research that utilize these data resources.

Despite these challenges, the volume of data can help overcome limitations in data quality. For example, question related to healthcare utilization (e.g., proportion of patients with IPF prescribed antifibrotics) are less prone to data quality issues, whereas predictive modeling with missing or inaccurate data elements is more likely to lead to biased results. A thoughtful approach to defining use case questions during the early phases of big data and precision medicine research can advance our understanding, while efforts at improving data quality are underway.

## *Data Harmonization and Integration*

Integrating data from heterogenous sources and data formats remains a challenge. Imaging data is stored in Digital Imaging and Communications in Medicine (DICOM) files, and "omics" data formats vary, complicating integration efforts. Inconsistent terminology across data sets, particularly for ILD subtypes, must also be addressed as patient identification and case adjudication methods differ between data sets (e.g., ICD-code derived vs. individually case validated) [42]. To address these challenges, three key solutions have been proposed to support integration and harmonization: (1) standardization of data into a common data model, (2) federated

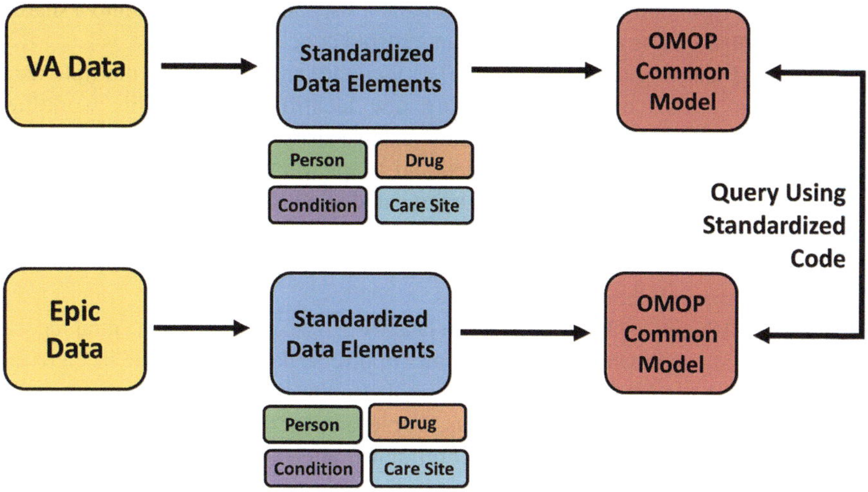


**Fig. 10.3** Common Data Models standardize healthcare data from diverse sources into common formats that can be queried using standardized codes. Abbreviations: *VA* veterans health, *OMOP* observational medical outcomes partnership

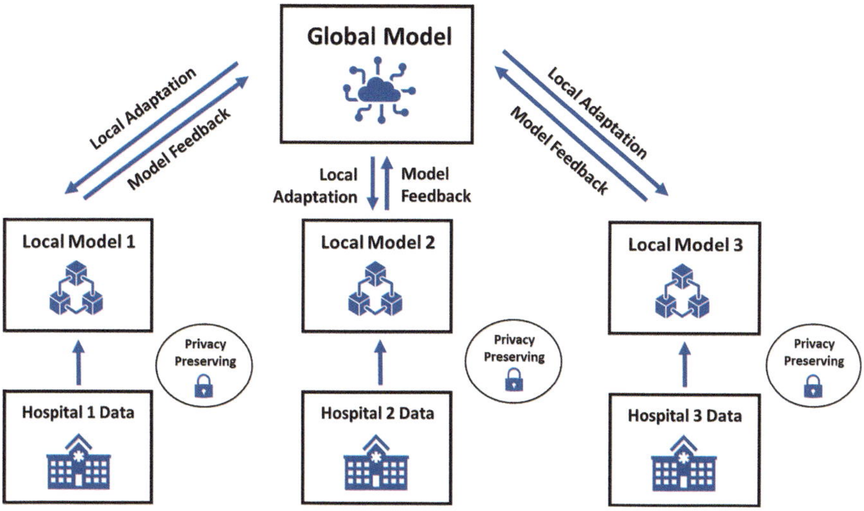


**Fig. 10.4** Federated learning models allow different clients (e.g., hospital systems) to collaboratively train algorithms and models while ensuring their data remains decentralized

learning solutions, and (3) creation of shared data lakes. The Observational Medical Outcomes Partnership (OMOP) Common Data Model is a widely adopted framework that standardizes healthcare data from diverse sources into a common format to facilitate data integration and analysis (Fig. 10.3). The OMOP common data model defines a standard data dictionary that allows researchers to combine and analyze data from multiple EHRs, claims databases, and clinical trials into a shared data model that can be queried using standardized code.

Federated learning solutions (Fig. 10.4) facilitate analysis across multiple data sets without centralizing or exchanging raw identifiable data. This workflow addresses privacy concerns and maintains data security and compliance. In federated learning, global models are trained and adapted locally on each dataset, and only model parameters are shared and aggregated allowing collaboration while preserving data privacy and ownership. Federated learning solutions are ideal for testing radiomics tools across diverse data sets to ensure that models perform well across different population demographics.

Lastly, collaborative platforms and data lakes (Fig. 10.5) can serve as central repositories for storing and managing large volumes of diverse data. Appropriate incentivization to contribute to these data lakes will facilitate collaboration to generate high-dimensional, multi-omics data sets. For example, the Open Source Imaging Consortium (OSIC) is a collaborative effort aimed at creating a shared repository of imaging and outcome data for ILD research. The OSIC platform provides access to a centralized imaging repository for researchers at academic medical centers who contribute to the platform, incentivizing users to contribute shared data, and enabling researchers to develop novel imaging biomarkers with multi-institutional validation cohorts.

Addressing the issues of harmonization upfront and creating incentives for implementation of common data models, federated learning, and collaborative platforms can overcome some of the current barriers to data integration and has been successfully pioneered by the field of precision oncology.

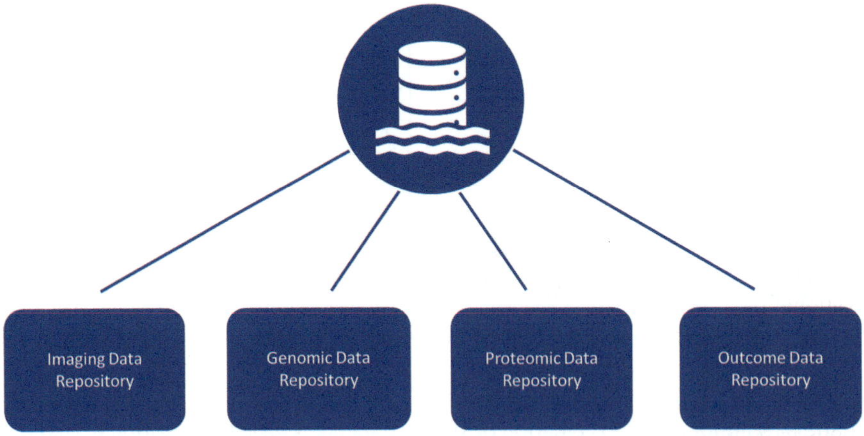


**Fig. 10.5** Data lakes are a way to hold different data types within storage platforms that have high scalability and durability potential

## Computational Power

The computational power required to integrate the volume and complexity of data can impede translation into actionable clinical insights. Processing vast amounts of data requires storage capabilities, infrastructure, and scalable algorithms. Imaging is a cornerstone of ILD research and high-resolution CT scans can range from 100 MB to 1GB of data each depending on resolution, number of series, and bit depth. When taken collectively at scale, these CT scans can generate petabytes of data that overwhelm traditional computing infrastructure. Current workstations used by clinical radiologists use multi-core processors to handle basic viewing capabilities with dedicated graphic processing units improving speed. However, advanced image processing including lung segmentation, texture analysis, or quantitative CT measurements that use deep learning algorithms require high-performance computing clusters or cloud-based solutions. To meet these challenges, institutions on the forefront of big data research are increasingly partnering with platforms like Amazon Web Services, Google Cloud, or Microsoft Azure to improve computing and processing. Yet, implementation of such infrastructure is expensive and requires expertise and resources that are often limited to well-funded large academic medical centers or the federal government. Balancing computational demands with the practical constraints of time and costs remains a critical challenge. To address these challenges more efficiently, a concerted effort to develop more efficient and scalable solutions, optimize data storage and retrieval systems, and create collaborative platforms that allow for sharing of computations resources across institutions is needed. Ultimately, this will require a multidisciplinary approach that brings together experts in computer science, bioinformatics, radiology, pulmonary medicine, and healthcare system leaders.

## Privacy and Ethical Concerns

Protecting patient privacy and ensuring data security is a priority when accessing sensitive health information. Privacy concerns with big data involve a few core issues—the inadvertent release of identifiable patient data, data ownership, patient autonomy, and ethical concerns related to incidental findings identified when repurposing observational data. Historically, research studies involving human subjects have required individual patient consent. In the era of big data, most studies require waiver of consent due to the volume of information being analyzed. There is an inherent tension between individual risk and the potential knowledge benefit to society. Several solutions have been proposed to address the privacy and ethical concerns related to the former. First, robust de-identification can minimize risk of sharing identifiable person information. Second, federated learning approaches described above can allow for algorithm development across multiple decentralized data sets without exchanging identifiable information. Lastly, clear policies for handing incidental findings, including criteria for when and how to disclose this information to patients or healthcare providers, can help navigate the ethical complexities and safeguard patients while still allowing for knowledge generation that is beneficial to the broader society.

## *Clinical Implementation*

Ultimately, delivering precision medicine requires translating data insights generated from research into clinical practice. However, while significant attention is given to data collection, analysis, and model development, the clinical integration of these tools is often overlooked in current practice. This results in a significant gap between the promise of big data analytics and practical impact on patient care. The field of precision medicine in ILD is still in its nascent stages. Tools (e.g., pharmacogenomics or radiomics solutions) still need to be evaluated as delivery interventions with attention to the resources required to integrate applications into pulmonary practice and the nimbleness of updating interventions as new data or techniques emerge. For example, introducing new decisions support tools can disrupt established routines and generate extra administrative burden for busy clinicians. "Black box" algorithms can impede uptake, especially when algorithmic output contradicts clinical intuition or established clinical practices or guidelines.

To overcome these challenges, a multifaceted approach is needed that involves clinicians both early and throughout development process. Frameworks such as human-centered design have been suggested to ensure that insights are clinically relevant and that end users are engaged from the outset. Additionally, ensuring that complex models that are used in decision support are transparent is crucial to effective clinical integration. This can be done by conducting robust prospective clinical validation in real-world studies, establishing feedback loops to refine models, and educating clinicians on how to interpret and interface with new models, including safeguards for when clinical acumen differs from algorithmic output. Initial pilot testing with iterative redesign can support a phased approach to successful clinical integration. By addressing the challenges of clinical implementation early, the field can more effectively translate promises of precision medicine in ILD into meaningful improvements in patient care.

## *Health Equity: Who Is Left Out of Big Data?*

Realizing the promise of the "All of Us" research program requires understanding limitations of our source cohorts. Current data sets have critical gaps that can exacerbate existing health disparities. Historically underrepresented populations, including racial and ethnic minorities, rural communities, and the socioeconomically disadvantaged, are frequently underrepresented in large-scale genomic studies, clinical trials, registries, and electronic heath record databases. These data sets tend to favor European ancestry, urban, and socioeconomically advantaged populations. Lack of diversity in source data can lead to biased algorithms and concentrate resources for genomic-informed targeted therapeutics to only a few demographics thus perpetuating inequities or exacerbating current disparities. Additionally, the implementation of precision medicine approaches both in research and clinical care requires resources and infrastructure, which are currently concentrated at major academic medical centers that favor a large urban patient population. Consequently, the benefits of data-driven precision medicine in ILD may disproportionately accrue at these centers and widen our current health outcome gaps. Addressing these potential pitfalls requires intentional efforts to diversify research cohorts, include marginalized populations, validate tools across populations, and ensure equitable access at time of implementation in both academic- and community-based settings.

## Conclusions and Future Directions

The advent of big data has transformed ILD research and will be the foundation for precision medicine, helping the field deliver the right care to the right patient at the right time. We are currently in the early phases of this new era of ILD research. Integrating diverse data sources—including electronic health records, claims data, multi-omics biospecimen repositories, wearable devices, and environmental databases—will continue to significantly expand our understanding of ILD pathogenesis, progression, and treatment response. This approach has already led to identification of novel genomic, proteomic, and radiomic biomarkers; the development of more accurate prognostic models; and potential for tailored therapeutic targets.

Looking ahead, several key priorities have emerged for advancing precision medicine in ILD: improving data harmonization and integration, developing advanced analytic tools that can efficiently analyze large volumes of data, expanding exposome research, therapeutic development, and subsequent translation of research findings into clinical care. To actualize this potential, researchers, clinicians, patients, and policy-makers in the ILD community need to make a consorted effort to invest in the data infrastructure, interdisciplinary collaborations, diverse patient inclusion, human-centered, and comprehensive training programs to ensure that patients and providers can engage with emerging tools at the point-of-care delivery. By addressing these priorities, we can rapidly move from Epoch 2 to Epoch 3 and usher in a new era of precision medicine in ILD, ensuring that we are able to deliver the right care to the right patient at the right time for these complex diseases.

**Acknowledgments** The authors would like to thank Noelle Nguyen who helped with development of some of the graphics used in this book chapter.

## References


1. McGinnis JM, Fineberg HV, Dzau VJ. Advancing the learning health system. N Engl J Med. 2021;385(1):1–5.
2. Olsen L, Aisner D, McGinnis JM, editors. The learning healthcare system: workshop summary. Washington; 2007.
3. The Promise of Precision Medicine. November 16, 2023 [cited 2024 September 10]; Available from: https://www.nih.gov/about-nih/what-we-do/nih-turning-discovery-into-health/promise-precision-medicine
4. Dempsey TM, et al. Adoption of the anti-fibrotic medications Pirfenidone and Nintedanib for patients with idiopathic pulmonary fibrosis. Ann Am Thorac Soc. 2021;18:1121.
5. Dempsey TM, et al. Clinical effectiveness of Antifibrotic medications for idiopathic pulmonary fibrosis. Am J Respir Crit Care Med. 2019;200(2):168–74.
6. Raghu G, et al. Idiopathic pulmonary fibrosis in US Medicare beneficiaries aged 65 years and older: incidence, prevalence, and survival, 2001-11. Lancet Respir Med. 2014;2(7):566–72.
7. Raghu G, et al. Incidence and prevalence of idiopathic pulmonary fibrosis in US adults 18-64 years old. Eur Respir J. 2016;48(1):179–86.
8. Collard HR, et al. Health care utilization and costs of idiopathic pulmonary fibrosis in U.S. Medicare beneficiaries aged 65 years and older. Ann Am Thorac Soc. 2015;12(7):981–7.
9. Collard HR, et al. Changes in clinical and physiologic variables predict survival in idiopathic pulmonary fibrosis. Am J Respir Crit Care Med. 2003;168(5):538–42.
10. King TE Jr, et al. A phase 3 trial of pirfenidone in patients with idiopathic pulmonary fibrosis. N Engl J Med. 2014;370(22):2083–92.
11. Richeldi L, et al. Efficacy and safety of nintedanib in idiopathic pulmonary fibrosis. N Engl J Med. 2014;370(22):2071–82.
12. Collard HR, et al. Combined corticosteroid and cyclophosphamide therapy does not alter survival in idiopathic pulmonary fibrosis. Chest. 2004;125(6):2169–74.
13. Idiopathic Pulmonary Fibrosis Clinical Research Network, et al. Prednisone, azathioprine, and N-acetylcysteine for pulmonary fibrosis. N Engl J Med. 2012;366(21):1968–77.
14. Ley B, et al. A multidimensional index and staging system for idiopathic pulmonary fibrosis. Ann Intern Med. 2012;156(10):684–91.
15. Ryerson CJ, et al. Predicting survival across chronic interstitial lung disease: the ILD-GAP model. Chest. 2014;145(4):723–8.
16. Stuart BD, et al. Effect of telomere length on survival in patients with idiopathic pulmonary fibrosis: an observational cohort study with independent validation. Lancet Respir Med. 2014;2(7):557–65.
17. Newton CA, et al. Telomere-related lung fibrosis is diagnostically heterogeneous but uniformly progressive. Eur Respir J. 2016;48(6):1710–20.
18. Johannson KA, Balmes JR, Collard HR. Air pollution exposure: a novel environmental risk factor for interstitial lung disease? Chest. 2015;147(4):1161–7.
19. Johannson KA, et al. Acute exacerbation of idiopathic pulmonary fibrosis associated with air pollution exposure. Eur Respir J. 2014;43(4):1124–31.
20. Kaul B, et al. Epidemiology of idiopathic pulmonary fibrosis among U.S. veterans, 2010-2019. Ann Am Thorac Soc. 2022;19(2):196–203.
21. Kaul B, et al. Agent Orange exposure and risk of idiopathic pulmonary fibrosis among U.S. veterans. Am J Respir Crit Care Med. 2022;206(6):750–7.
22. Abramson MJ, et al. Occupational and environmental risk factors for idiopathic pulmonary fibrosis in Australia: case-control study. Thorax. 2020;75:864.
23. Barber CM, Fishwick D. Importance of past occupational exposures in the rising incidence of idiopathic pulmonary fibrosis in the U.K. Thorax. 2012;67(3):264.
24. Baumgartner KB, et al. Cigarette smoking: a risk factor for idiopathic pulmonary fibrosis. Am J Respir Crit Care Med. 1997;155(1):242–8.

25. Blanc PD, et al. The occupational burden of nonmalignant respiratory diseases. An official American Thoracic Society and European Respiratory Society statement. Am J Respir Crit Care Med. 2019;199(11):1312–34.
26. Fingerlin TE, et al. Genome-wide association study identifies multiple susceptibility loci for pulmonary fibrosis. Nat Genet. 2013;45(6):613–20.
27. Zhang D, et al. Utility of whole genome sequencing in assessing risk and clinically relevant outcomes for pulmonary fibrosis. Eur Respir J. 2022;60(6):2200577.
28. Kim JS, et al. MUC5B, telomere length and longitudinal quantitative interstitial lung changes: the MESA lung study. Thorax. 2023;78(6):566–73.
29. Moll M, et al. A polygenic risk score for idiopathic pulmonary fibrosis and interstitial lung abnormalities. Am J Respir Crit Care Med. 2023;208(7):791–801.
30. Zhang D, et al. Telomere length and immunosuppression in non-idiopathic pulmonary fibrosis interstitial lung disease. Eur Respir J. 2023;62(5):2300441.
31. Podolanczuk AJ, et al. Design and rationale for the prospective treatment efficacy in IPF using genotype for NAC selection (PRECISIONS) clinical trial. BMC Pulm Med. 2022;22(1):475.
32. Oldham JM, et al. Proteomic biomarkers of survival in idiopathic pulmonary fibrosis. Am J Respir Crit Care Med. 2024;209(9):1111–20.
33. Bowman WS, et al. Proteomic biomarkers of progressive fibrosing interstitial lung disease: a multicentre cohort analysis. Lancet Respir Med. 2022;10(6):593–602.
34. Koo CW, et al. Quantitative CT and machine learning classification of fibrotic interstitial lung diseases. Eur Radiol. 2022;32(12):8152–61.
35. Chung JH, et al. A deep learning-based Radiomic classifier for usual interstitial pneumonia. Chest. 2024;165(2):371–80.
36. Walsh SLF, et al. Deep learning for classifying fibrotic lung disease on high-resolution computed tomography: a case-cohort study. Lancet Respir Med. 2018;6(11):837–45.
37. Christe A, et al. Computer-aided diagnosis of pulmonary fibrosis using deep learning and CT images. Investig Radiol. 2019;54(10):627–32.
38. Jacob J, et al. Mortality prediction in idiopathic pulmonary fibrosis: evaluation of computer-based CT analysis with conventional severity measures. Eur Respir J. 2017;49(1):1601011.
39. Thillai M, et al. Deep learning-based segmentation of computed tomography scans predicts disease progression and mortality in idiopathic pulmonary fibrosis. Am J Respir Crit Care Med. 2024;210(4):465–72.
40. Pan J, et al. Unsupervised machine learning identifies predictive progression markers of IPF. Eur Radiol. 2023;33(2):925–35.
41. Morris ZS, Wooding S, Grant J. The answer is 17 years, what is the question: understanding time lags in translational research. J R Soc Med. 2011;104(12):510–20.
42. Kaul B, et al. Variability in global prevalence of interstitial lung disease. Front Med (Lausanne). 2021;8:751181.

# Chapter 11
# The Future of Precision Medicine in Interstitial Lung Disease

**Traci N. Adams, Chandni Patel, and Mridu Gulati**

## Introduction

Interstitial lung disease (ILD) is a heterogeneous group of conditions characterized by inflammation and/or fibrosis of the lung [1]. Within the umbrella term of ILD are more than 100 distinct diagnoses, including but not limited to idiopathic pulmonary fibrosis (IPF), connective tissue disease-related ILD (CTD-ILD), and fibrotic hypersensitivity pneumonitis (fHP). In patients presenting with ILD, current guidelines recommend a thorough history and physical examination, serologic testing for autoimmune conditions, high-resolution computed tomography (HRCT), and, in some cases, histopathology to identify a particular diagnosis [1].

Historically, obtaining an accurate diagnosis was critical, because ILD treatment has been driven by diagnosis [1]. Clinical decisions and trial design had previously targeted immunosuppressive therapies for more inflammatory phenotypes (i.e., mycophenolate for scleroderma-associated ILD in Scleroderma Lung Study) [2] and antifibrotic therapies for IPF [3–5]. Yet even within such categorizations, considerable heterogeneity in natural history and treatment responses remain. CTD-ILD patients often demonstrate partial or no responses to immunosuppressive therapy, often experiencing the same inexorable decline in lung function presumed to be seen only in IPF patients. The clinical course of IPF) also varies considerably, with some patients progressing more slowly than others. Ultimately, the current

T. N. Adams (✉) · C. Patel
Division of Pulmonary and Critical Care Medicine, University of Texas Southwestern Medical Center, Dallas, TX, USA
e-mail: traci.adams@utsouthwestern.edu; Chandni.Patel@UTSouthwestern.edu

M. Gulati
Yale Occupational Medicine and Environmental Medicine, Yale School of Medicine, New Haven, CT, USA
e-mail: mridu.gulati@yale.edu



B. F. Collins, S. B. Montesi (eds.), *Precision Medicine in Interstitial Lung Disease*, Respiratory Medicine, https://doi.org/10.1007/978-3-031-87183-2_11

diagnosis-driven approach remains woefully inadequate, leaving clinicians and investigators limited in their ability to tailor management decisions for an individual patient or design clinical studies for specific patient populations [6–8].

Attempts to refine prognostication and treatment decisions have incorporated phenotypes based on the trajectory of the patient over time [1]. Patients with a progressive fibrotic phenotype (PF-ILD), defined by fibrotic ILD of any cause with a worsening of physiologic and/or radiographic studies over the prior 2 years, are more likely to continue to progress and may have a higher mortality than patients without a progressive fibrotic phenotype [9]. A randomized clinical trial evaluating nintedanib in PF-ILD found that nintedanib slowed progression of disease compared to placebo [10]. In 2022, clinical guidelines were issued defining progressive pulmonary fibrosis (PPF) as a phenotype that describes patients with fibrotic lung diseases other than IPF that demonstrated progression in at least two of the three following domains: respiratory symptoms, physiology, and/or radiographic evidence of fibrosis [1].

The limitation of an approach to treatment that relies on a PF-ILD phenotype is that clinicians must wait until their patients progress in order to determine their risk of future progression; this phenotype cannot be determined at the patient's initial clinic visit if no prior data is available.

Given the limitations in both diagnosis- and phenotype-based treatment algorithms, the decision between observation and early initiation of treatment is unclear at many patients' initial visit [6]. Miscalculations in this decision may lead to progression off therapy or overtreatment of patients who may have been stable off therapy. We envision that the future of diagnostic evaluation of ILD will integrate multi-omic data in order to accurately predict a patient's disease behavior, optimal baseline treatment strategy, and expected rate of progression. In this chapter, we discuss the future roles of genetic biomarkers, exhaled breath analysis, bronchoscopy, molecular biomarkers, big data, and artificial intelligence (AI) in a precision medicine approach to screening, diagnosing, and treating ILD.

## Future of Precision Medicine in Preclinical Research

Preclinical research plays a crucial role in the field of precision medicine. Mouse models with knock-in mutations in either misfolding or trafficking of surfactant protein C (SP-C) enable the study of early events in the initiation of pulmonary fibrosis; as these models spontaneously develop fibrosis, they secrete cytokines and biomarkers that may also be detected in humans with pulmonary fibrosis [11, 12]. Moreover, murine models allow for genetic manipulation or deletion of cell lines, allowing researchers to delineate the role of certain cell types in pulmonary fibrosis [13].

Precision-cut lung slices (PCLSs) are 300–500 μm thick sections of lung tissue that can be generated from explanted or resected lung tissue [14]. They allow for live imaging of cell-cell and cell-extracellular matrix (ECM) interaction ex vivo.

Early stages of fibrosis can be induced in this model [15], but limiting factors include limited culture time, the absence of ventilation or perfusion, and the absence of nonresident cells [16].

Hydrogel biomaterials are engineered to study cell-matrix interactions in real time [17]. These materials allow for controlled biological studies to understand cell-matrix interactions and ECM remodeling [17]. This model is limited in its ability to mimic in vivo ECM and lacks an air-liquid interface [16].

Organoids are 3D structures that mimic that organ's microenvironment and enable the study of cell-cell interactions [18, 19]. They can incorporate disease-specific pluripotent stem cells (PSCs). An IPF phenotype was created using combinations of PSC-derived cell types and ECM [18, 19]. Organoids may be useful in drug screening, but limitations include the absence of vascular and air flow and the lack of standardization of differentiation procedures for PSCs from any lung cell type [16].

Preclinical research can rapidly facilitate a more detailed understanding of the functional significance of findings from omics-based human studies as well as study the impact of environmental interactions [16]. Further, with improved collaboration between basic and translational researchers as well as drug developers, these models may serve as an avenue to a platform for drug discovery and validation and may help with selection of the most promising agents for subsequent evaluation in clinical trials [16].

## The Future of Precision Medicine in Early Detection, Diagnosis, and Prognostication

### *Interstitial Lung Abnormalities*

Because IPF and PPF treatments are unable to reverse fibrosis, researchers have considerable interest in early detection of disease. Interstitial lung abnormalities (ILAs) are CT findings that are potentially compatible with ILD in patients without clinical suspicion of ILD [20]. ILAs are a purely radiographic finding, often defined by an arbitrary cutoff of over 5% lung zone involvement. One study reported an overall pooled prevalence of ILAs of 10%, including 7%, 7%, and 26% in lung cancer screening, general population at risk, and familial subgroups [21]. Differentiation between ILAs and early ILD requires clinical evaluation and longitudinal follow-up [20]. ILAs are frequently found in patients undergoing lung cancer screening [20]. Risk factors for progression to ILD include fibrotic ILAs, short leukocyte telomere length (LTL), MUC5B promoter variant, and probable or definite usual interstitial pneumonia pattern (UIP) [20].

Precision medicine approaches seek to better define and characterize risk factors for ILAs. A genome-wide association study (GWAS) of subjects with ILAs reaffirmed the presence of 5 of 12 previously reported IPF GWAS foci and identified 2 novel loci [22]. A recent study described a polygenic risk score derived from a GWAS of common variants, noting the observed heritability of IPF to be 28% [23]. AI and deep learning algorithms can assist with detection of ILAs as well as define features that predict progression [24, 25].

Further development and refinement of risk models that integrate genetic, demographic, and radiographic data to predict progression are needed to guide management decisions in patients with ILAs and to enrich clinical trials aimed at slowing the progression of ILA to early ILD in higher-risk individuals [20].

## *The Role of Genetics in ILD Risk Assessment, Diagnosis, and Management*

A significant unmet need in the field of pulmonary fibrosis is the identification of populations for screening and prevention [16]. IPF is a polygenic disease with a variety of genetic variants contributing to disease risk. Genetic variants are predominantly classified by allele frequency. Common variants, or single-nucleotide polymorphisms (SNPs), have a minor allele frequency (MAF) > 5% and confer only a mildly increased risk of disease. An example of a common variant in ILD is the rs35705950 in the promoter region of *MUC5B*, which carries less than a 1% risk of development of ILD [8]. Paradoxically, this polymorphism in MUC5B was also associated with a decreased risk of IPF mortality.

Twenty common variants have been associated with development of IPF in genome-wide association studies [8]. Because each common variant itself carries a low risk of disease, a genetic panel will likely be needed to determine an individual's risk of ILD and guide risk/benefit discussion regarding screening and management.

Rare variants, in contrast, generally have a MAF < 0.1% and confer a greater risk of developing ILD than common variants. Rare variants causing ILD include mutations in genes encoding surfactant protein and in genes encoding proteins in the telomerase complex, such as *TERT*, *TERC*, *RTEL1*, *PARN*, *NAF1*, *DKC1*, *TINF2*, *ZCCHC8*, and *NOP10*. These variants in telomerase complex genes typically result in short LTL [26]. Individuals with these rare variants would ideally have HRCT for ILD screening due to the high prevalence of ILD in this population. A pathogenic *TERT* variant, for example, leads to pulmonary fibrosis in 50–60% of individuals by age 60 [27]. That said, there are not yet evidence-based guidelines regarding timing of initial screening or appropriate intervals. Insurance coverage may also be a barrier in some countries.

While rare in the general population, telomerase gene mutations are found in approximately 25% of patients with familial ILD [26]. Genetic testing for rare variants in telomerase-related genes is recommended in ILD patients with a family history of pulmonary fibrosis or a personal or family history of conditions associated with disorders of telomere biology, including cirrhosis, leukemia, lymphoma, and early graying [26, 28]. Patients with rare variants in telomerase-related genes may have differing specific ILD diagnoses, including IPF, fHP, or undifferentiated ILD (U-ILD), but their ILD is uniformly progressive regardless of underlying diagnosis and associated with a poor prognosis [29]. This finding suggests that the genetic diagnosis may be more important than the specific ILD diagnosis (IPF vs. fHP) [26].

Short LTL can also be seen in adult-onset sporadic ILD patients without a rare variant in telomerase-related genes [30], and short LTL is potentially causative of ILD [31]. Even for patients without a rare variant in telomerase-related genes, LTL may also be an important prognostic marker [26]. Studies across cohorts and across ILD diagnoses have shown that short LTL is associated with higher mortality [32, 33].

In addition to its impact on prognosis, short LTL may also impact treatment [26]. A major breakthrough in the clinical implications of telomere length came in the evaluation of the effect of immunosuppression in patients with short LTL. Multiple studies have demonstrated an increase in mortality among patients with short LTL when exposed to immunosuppression [34, 35]. While we lack randomized controlled trials to assess the outcomes of patients with short LTL on immunosuppression, existing data suggests immunosuppression is harmful in these patients and should be avoided [34, 35].

We suggest that LTL testing be considered in patients with fibrotic ILD in whom immunosuppression is being offered, particularly in patients with a personal or family history of conditions associated with short LTL who do not have an identified telomerase mutation [26, 35]. For some patients with short LTL, invasive diagnostic procedures could be avoided, as their genetics are likely a more important driver of their disease than their specific diagnosis. Further, in patients with short LTL, immunosuppression should be avoided, and early initiation of antifibrotic therapies should be prioritized [26]. Challenges in the field of precision medicine in ILD include improving the understanding of the biology of telomere-immunosuppression interaction and developing short LTL prediction models that allow for optimal patient selection for LTL testing.

Recent studies have incorporated genetic risk into analysis of treatment response as well as clinical trial design. Unfortunately, despite previous findings that danazol increased telomere length, no treatment effect was seen in a cohort of 50 patients with IPF, including some with telomere syndromes [36]. A retrospective study using patient registry data demonstrated that those with the *G allele in rs2076295 within the DSP gene experienced improved outcomes with nintedanib as compared to those with a TT allele [37]. Single-nucleotide polymorphisms (SNPs) in TOLLIP may confer increased risk of IPF. Post hoc analyses of the PANTHER trial revealed that individuals with rs3750920 TT TOLLIP genotype experienced slower disease progression and reduced mortality in patients treated with NAC. These findings led to the ongoing PRECISIONS (Prospective tReatment EffiCacy in IPF uSing genotype for Nac Selection) clinical trial, a multicenter randomized controlled trial assessing efficacy of N-acetylcysteine among IPF patients with the rs3750920 TT TOLLIP genotype.

## *The Role of Environmental Influences in the Development of ILD*

Environmental influences are important risk factors for the development of ILD including HP, occupational lung diseases (i.e., pneumoconiosis), and even IPF, where exposures occur in 44% of individuals [38–41]. The interaction between repeated exogenous insults and genetic predisposition impact the development and progression of pulmonary fibrosis [39].

Exposures may increase the risk of the development and progression of ILD by contributing to short LTL [42]. Such exposures include traffic-related air pollution (particulate matter, black carbon, benzene, and toluene), polycyclic aromatic hydrocarbons, N-nitrosamines, pesticides, lead, hazardous waste exposure, and tobacco smoke [42].

The impact of air pollution on ILD outcomes has received increasing attention with numerous studies reporting increased incidence, FVC decline, and rates of IPF exacerbations [5]. Air pollution may lead to senescence in inflammatory cells and oxidative stress. In addition to shortened telomeres, air pollution may lead to epigenetic alterations such as DNA methylation in regions linked with pulmonary fibrosis [43]. One study demonstrated that the highest IPF incidence occurred in individuals with the highest polygenic risk scores (13 SNPs) exposed to air pollution [23].

Genetic risks modify outcomes and treatment responses in exposure-related disease. Short LTL is associated with increased mortality in fHP. Further studies have suggested that while immunosuppression with MMF may benefit fHP patients, those with fHP and short telomeres experience poorer transplant free survival when treated with MMF.

In the future of precision medicine, environmental exposures will need to be integrated into multi-omic data to define an individual's risk for developing ILD.

## *The Role of Molecular Biomarkers for ILD Diagnosis and Prognosis*

Biomarkers have been used to distinguish between IPF and non-IPF ILDs. Matrix metalloprotein-7, surfactant protein-D, and osteopontin can help to distinguish IPF from other idiopathic interstitial pneumonias [44], but additional research is needed to determine an optimal panel of peripheral blood biomarkers. An ideal biomarker would provide a diagnosis but even more importantly predict disease course and treatment responsiveness.

Although numerous biomarkers have been associated with disease progression in ILD, there is no clinically used blood-based biomarker that predicts an individual's disease progression [16]. Plasma omega-3 fatty acids were found to be associated with DLCO progression in one study and are a possible biomarker [45]. Other biomarkers that have been associated with ILD prognosis include but are not limited to CA-125, CA 19–9, CCL 18, CXCL-13, KL-6, and MMP-7 [8, 46, 47]. A panel of 17 biomarkers has been associated with near-term disease progression, defined as at least 10% decline in FVC, death, or transplant over 1 year in patients with non-IPF ILD [48]. A 52-gene signature in peripheral blood was also able to predict IPF mortality [49]. Additional research is needed to identify blood-based biomarkers or combinations of biomarkers that can predict near- and long-term disease progression and guide management decisions [16].

## *Future of Precision Medicine in Exhaled Breath Analysis*

The composite of exhaled breath analysis includes evaluation of volatile compounds found in exhaled air as well as of nonvolatile organic compounds and water-soluble molecules found in exhaled breath condensate (EBC) [50]. EBC is of particular importance as the organic acids, proteins, and cytokines isolated from EBC may function as biomarkers in enhancing our ability to understand, diagnose, prognosticate, and treat fibrotic ILD.

Obtaining accurate EBC samples is an intricate multistep process that involves collection of patient condensate from tidal breathing followed by subsequent cooling, storage, and processing of each sample. The coating within collection devices, patient's respiratory variables (tidal volume and minute ventilation), rate and degree of cooling, methods of storage that limit sample interaction with ambient air, and further processing protocols must be intentionally prespecified, as each can have independent and unique impacts on the final concentration of individual biomarkers in the EBC [51]. Lyophilization of the EBC sample improves the accuracy of resultant EBC pH by removing volatile acids and acids from oral contamination. However, investigators may not routinely choose to process samples via lyophilization as it is time-consuming and introduces potential for further processing errors [51].

Recent studies have investigated the value of reactive oxygen species, vascular endothelial growth factor (VEGF), and lysophosphatidic acid (LPA) from the EBC of patients with fibrotic ILD. While all three are hypothesized to contribute to fibrosis in ILD, VEGF and LPA are of special interest as both are associated with treatment options. Nintedanib has been shown to have anti-VEGF activity, and an experimental drug for fibrotic ILD inhibits the enzyme that produces LPA [52]. Studies investigating the concentration of VEGF and LPA in EBC show negative correlations between VEGF and pulmonary function tests as well as potentially elevated levels of certain LPA species in patients with IPF [53, 54].

Data obtained from EBC analysis remains preliminary, however. Without standardized EBC collection techniques and verified normal ranges of EBC biomarker concentrations, conclusions from EBC data are not comparable or reproducible across studies. Future developments in the field of exhaled breath analysis will strive to standardize collection techniques, increase the sensitivity of collection devices to detect lower concentrations of molecules, as well as determine normal ranges of molecule concentrations in EBC. Once these parameters are achieved, data obtained from EBC may become integral in diagnosing, treating, and prognosticating fibrotic ILD.

## *The Future of Minimally Invasive Diagnostic Procedures in ILD*

The field of precision medicine in ILD remains in its infancy, and at this time, treatment decisions typically rely on both specific ILD diagnosis and the PF-ILD phenotype [1]. Identification of a specific ILD diagnosis in many cases can be done noninvasively through a thorough history and physical examination, serologies, and imaging [1]. However, in some patients, the diagnosis remains unclear after completion of the noninvasive evaluation [1]. Historically, patients with an unclear diagnosis after noninvasive evaluation underwent surgical lung biopsy (SLB) for diagnosis, followed by a multidisciplinary discussion [55]. SLB has a diagnostic yield of approximately 90% but is complicated by a 1–2% mortality rate [56–59]. Many patients have prohibitively high risk for SLB due to age, severity of underlying ILD, and/or significant comorbidities, and emergent SLB carries a mortality rate of 25% [57, 60].

The recognition of the high morbidity and mortality of SLB led to efforts to obtain lung biopsy through bronchoscopic techniques [61]. The yield of standard transbronchial lung biopsy (TBLB) in ILD is only 20–30% [62, 63]. Genomic classifiers have been developed to distinguish between UIP and non-UIP patterns [1]. Genomic classifier testing predicts histopathologic UIP in patients with ILD with a specificity of 92% and improves diagnostic confidence [64]; however, sensitivity is only 68%, testing is not widely available, and the test is unable to differentiate between non-UIP patterns [64]. Given these limitations, current IPF guidelines do not recommend for or against the use of genomic classifiers [1].

Transbronchial lung cryobiopsy (TBLC) was developed to obtain tissue samples larger than those obtained via TBLB with lower complication rates than SLB [29]. TBLC has a diagnostic yield of 70–80% [65, 66], and while it is safer than SLB, complication rates of TBLC are as high as 23% (9% pneumothorax and 14% moderate-severe bleeding) [65–67]. Guidelines from the American Thoracic Society (ATS) suggest that TBLC is an acceptable alternative to SLB for making a histopathological diagnosis of ILD in experienced centers [1], while the European Respiratory Society guidelines recommend TBLC as a replacement for SLB [61]. Research is needed to evaluate TBLC techniques that have lower complication rates and higher yield.

Recent advances in TBLC include decreasing the size of the probe to reduce complication rates. Prior studies of TBLC have evaluated a 1.9 mm and 2.4 mm probe [66, 68], but a 1.1 mm probe is now available [69]. The larger probes require removal of the bronchoscope after a sample has been obtained and thus contribute to uncontrolled bleeding that often requires insertion of a bronchial blocker [70].

The 1.1 mm probes have reduced rates of major bleeding compared to the larger probes due to both the smaller sample sizes and the ability to leave the bronchoscope in the airway while removing the probe with the sample [70]. Safety data for the 1.1 mm probe size comes from studies of TBLC for pulmonary nodules [69], and additional data is needed in ILD patients. The reduction in complication rates of TBLC may lead to wider uptake of TBLC and a subsequent reduction in the number of SLBs performed in the diagnostic evaluation of ILD.

Additional developments in the field of bronchoscopic diagnosis of ILD include optical coherence tomography (OCT) and confocal laser endomicroscopy (CLE) [71, 72]. Endobronchial OCT is an imaging technique that employs near-infrared light to visualize structures with a 2-μm resolution of microscopy [71]. A proof-of-concept study evaluating endobronchial OCT demonstrated excellent sensitivity and specificity in distinguishing UIP from non-UIP ILDs compared to the gold standard of surgical lung biopsy [73]. Additional research is needed to elucidate this technique's interobserver reliability, applicability in diverse populations, and ability to predict more specific histopathologic patterns [71].

Confocal laser endomicroscopy (CLE) is a minimally invasive technique that combines high-resolution and real-time microscopic analysis of tissue architecture [72]. In studies of ILD patients, CLE may be able to distinguish between inflammatory and fibrotic ILDs [72]. Additional research is needed to define specific CLE patterns in ILD and its role in the diagnostic evaluation of ILD [72].

## The Future of Big Data and Technology in ILD

"Big data" accompanied by sophisticated computational technologies have provided rich sources of data and the tools needed for investigators to study. In the clinical arena, rapid developments in computational technologies and the field of artificial intelligence have had and will likely continue to have the most immediate impact on the field of radiology. Visual analyses of HRCTs require specialized expertise and are all notoriously plagued by interobserver variability [74]. Subtle abnormalities characteristic of ILAs remain a challenge with radiologists sometimes even struggling to differentiate such findings from dependent atelectasis. Quantitative CT (QCT) analyses, a method derived from measuring attenuation values, can be quite informative with respect to ILAs and have been shown to correlate with patient outcomes [75]. QCT, however, fails to identify more complex patterns and features of fibrosis that are so critical to distinguishing more clinically relevant progressive disease [75].

Each HRCT consists of large quantities of metadata and individual pixels stored in unstructured ways [75]. Analyses can occur at the individual pixel level, segmented regions, or over the whole lung to describe texture and shape; such analyses can be then translated into numerical values and subsequently validated against clinical measures of disease, disease severity, and prognostic markers, ultimately leading to the establishment of digital biomarkers. Such vast datasets are ideal targets to apply machine learning and deep learning methodologies. Machine learning, unsupervised and supervised, refers to a branch of artificial intelligence in which computer systems are trained on a specific data file, with unsupervised learning models applied to unlabeled datasets [76]. Deep learning (such as convoluted neural networks), is a type of machine learning using multilayered artificial neural networks; deep learning models allow for automatic extraction and learning from large datasets [76, 77].

Machine and deep learning classifiers have begun to emerge in the field of ILD [76, 78]. Data texture analysis (DTA) is a deep learning tool that quantifies fibrosis and predicts lung function declines [79]. CALIPER, a post processing software derived from machine learning applications, has been used to identify a novel digital biomarker, pulmonary vessel volume, which in turn has been shown to correlate with lung function decline. Machine learning classifiers for UIP have also been described [80]. SOFIA is an example of a convolutional neural network capable of classifying fibrotic lung disease and identifying a UIP probability score [81]. More recently, lung, vascular, and fibrosis volumes derived from deep learning-based segmentation of CT scans has been associated with reduced progression-free survival, while decreasing lung volume and increasing fibrosis over time have also been associated with worsened survival [77]. Radiomics refers to the field where high-throughput extraction quantitative features from images are compared with clinical and biologic characteristics. Correlations between radiomics-based models and cellular infiltration on biopsy specimens have been reported [82]. Radiomics has also been used to predict mortality in rapidly progressive ILD patients and dermatomyositis-related ILD [83]. Radiomics can also be used to classify patients; for example, radiomic profiling has been used to identify two distinct groups of SSc-ILD patients correlating with differential progression-free survival [84].

Investigators continue to confront a number of obstacles with respect to clinical research and the application of AI tools in the field of radiology. Such challenges include the need for large quantities of high-quality data sets, lack of standardization of image acquisition, data privacy, and generalizability of resultant models. Human involvement in research design and application of findings remains essential.

Large quantities of clinical data can be mined from a number of sources: patient registries, administrative claims data, and electronic health records. ILD registries have proliferated worldwide in recent decades, often accompanied by biorepositories [85]. Older studies regarding natural history of disease relied on single-center designs or data derived from highly selected patients enrolled in clinical trials. Registries reflect real-world clinical practice and provide longitudinal data on patient-reported outcomes, physiologic and radiologic testing, as well as clinical events such as hospitalizations, acute exacerbations, transplantation, and death. National and international registries allow for analyses of regional practices. While the power provided by combining such large datasets is enticing, investigators must remain cautious regarding the quality and completeness of data. Significant heterogeneity may exist in how and where clinical data is collected with some centers requiring a rigorous review of data at a specialized center and others obtaining information from more local community practices. Missing data is a prevalent limitation to most registries, with many patients with progressive disease dropping out of registries. Registry data can be combined with other administrative datasets such as insurance claims to provide a more complete picture regarding healthcare utilization [85].

Claims data, similar to patient registries, provide large geographically diverse samples sizes as well as insight into real-world practices and associated healthcare costs. These datasets have been used to estimate disease incidence and prevalence [86–89], identify risk factors [90], and describe healthcare utilization and outcomes [91–93] across diverse ILD subgroups including CTD -ILD, fHP, PPF, and IPF. Unlike registry data, clinical details such as symptomatology and the actual results of objective physiologic, laboratory, and radiologic testing are lacking. Validation of case finding algorithms, ostensibly using medical record review, is vital and may be particularly challenging with respect to identifying patients with progressive pulmonary fibrosis [94, 95].

Electronic health records provide vast amounts of longitudinal clinical detail but require time-consuming review and manual abstraction of unstructured information. Automated data extraction and natural language processing offer methodologies to streamline data collection [96]. Machine learning algorithms and modeling strategies offer opportunities to enhance cohort identification and subsequent analyses [97]. Ultimately, the integration of multi-omics and clinical datasets using advanced strategies to analyze and interpret information will transform the future of pulmonary fibrosis clinical care and research.

## Economics and Equity in Precision Medicine

As advances continue to flourish on the precision medicine landscape, the scientific and clinical community should proceed with caution while working to transition applications of these breakthroughs into the clinical realm.

Many novel findings are derived from studies that lack racial and ethnic diversity, with minorities and disadvantaged populations generally underrepresented in scientific research. A multitude of factors account for such gaps ranging from socioeconomic disparities that often coexist with environmental and occupational exposures to reduced access to care. The incorporation of diverse populations into various biologic and clinical datasets used for research is essential to ensure that newly identified biomarkers are representative and predictive across broad populations. As an example, genetic factors may differ by race. Black race is associated with longer telomere length, while the MUC5B variant is less common. Hence, it is significant that investigators have confirmed that age- and sex-adjusted leukocyte telomere length below the median is associated with pulmonary fibrosis across all racial groups—Black, Hispanic, Asian, and White [98]. Further, limited studies exist to characterize risk factors, disease course, and treatment responses among various ethnic groups. While Black patients represent more than three times the population of patients with autoimmune disease, racial and ethnic minorities are significantly underrepresented in clinical studies and registries [99].

In the clinical arena, biomarkers have the potential to enhance or supplant existing approaches to diagnostic algorithms and clinical trial design. The ideal biomarker, whether used to diagnose, prognosticate, or identify/assess potential treatment response to specific therapeutics, must not only be sensitive and specific but readily accessible and cost-effective. Peripheral blood biomarkers, for example, are easily attained as compared to lung tissue or bronchoalveolar lavage fluid which requires invasive procedures. The application of machine learning and convolutional neural networks to identify patterns and quantify disease involvement in CT scans has shown great promise; yet, researchers and clinicians should continue to monitor the potential cumulative radiation exposure incurred by repeated studies. Biomarkers should be developed not from single-center studies but from multicenter well-characterized cohorts. Finally, validation of novel biomarkers in longitudinal studies should be conducted to affirm a positive impact on clinical care [6, 100].

## The Future of Clinical Trial Design in Fibrotic ILD

Randomized controlled trials (RCTs) are currently the gold standard to assess for the safety and efficacy of investigational drugs but are limited by cost, duration, and inefficiency of patient selection [8]. Precision medicine can help determine which existing drugs may be most useful for a particular patient and inform clinical trial design for investigational drugs in three ways: (1) appropriate selection of patients for a clinical trial may reduce the number of patients who need to be enrolled; (2) inclusion of biomarkers as primary endpoints in clinical trials may reduce the duration of clinical trials; and (3) creation of novel trial designs such as adaptive clinical trials [8].

Most RCTs in ILD use a diagnosis-driven or phenotype-driven approach to patient selection [3, 10]. Genetic and proteomic data may predict which pathways are upregulated in a particular patient and may allow studies to select for a patient population most likely to respond to a given drug [8]. Careful patient selection could reduce the number of patients enrolled and therefore reduce the cost of clinical trials. One example of a genotype-driven study is the PRECISIONS trial, in which patients with a diagnosis of IPF and a particular TOLLIP SNP were randomized to N-acetylcysteine or placebo [101]. Whereas N-acetylcysteine did not show a benefit in all patients with IPF [102], the PRECISIONS study may identify a subset of patients who benefit [101].

Furthermore, RCTs in ILD typically require a 1-year follow period for relevant clinical outcomes, including FVC decline, death, or transplant. If a change in biomarkers in the short term can predict long-term clinical outcomes, clinical trial duration, and therefore cost, may be reduced [6, 8].

Finally, precision medicine may allow for adaptive clinical trial design [103]. In adaptive clinical trials, multiple therapies can be studied in an ongoing manner [103]. Interventions may be added to or removed from the study on the basis of a predefined decision algorithm, and the algorithm can be refined based on real-time data [103]. This trial design can increase the number of drugs tested, allow for more inclusive patient enrollment, and more quickly identify beneficial drugs than existing RCT design [103]. REMAP-ILD is a published protocol for the global delivery of adaptive trial design in ILD [104].

## Conclusion

While precision medicine in ILD is in its infancy, exciting developments are likely to revolutionize the diagnosis and treatment landscape of ILD in coming years. We propose that data is sufficient to recommend LTL testing in the evaluation of patients with fibrotic ILD who have clinical evidence to suggest a disorder of telomere biology. We suggest that integration of genomic, transcriptomic, epigenomic, proteomic, metabolomic, and radiomic data will help clinicians determine whether observation or early initiation of treatment is appropriate for an individual patient, select treatment, and obtain information on the efficacy of treatment before adverse outcomes such as FVC decline develop. Abraham Lincoln said, "The best way to predict the future is to create it." We eagerly look forward to creating and integrating multi-omic data sets for the future of precision medicine in ILD.

**Conflict of Interest Statement** The authors have no conflicts of interest to report.

**Funding** None.

## References

1. Raghu G, Remy-Jardin M, Richeldi L, et al. Idiopathic pulmonary fibrosis (an update) and progressive pulmonary fibrosis in adults: an official ATS/ERS/JRS/ALAT clinical practice guideline. Am J Respir Crit Care Med. 2022;205(9):e18–47.
2. Tashkin DP, Roth MD, Clements PJ, et al. Mycophenolate mofetil versus oral cyclophosphamide in scleroderma-related interstitial lung disease (SLS II): a randomised controlled, double-blind, parallel group trial. Lancet Respir Med. 2016;4(9):708–19.
3. King TE Jr, Bradford WZ, Castro-Bernardini S, et al. A phase 3 trial of pirfenidone in patients with idiopathic pulmonary fibrosis. N Engl J Med. 2014;370(22):2083–92.
4. Richeldi L, du Bois RM, Raghu G, et al. Efficacy and safety of nintedanib in idiopathic pulmonary fibrosis. N Engl J Med. 2014;370(22):2071–82.
5. Antoniu SA. Cyclophosphamide for scleroderma interstitial lung disease. Expert Opin Investig Drugs. 2007;16(3):393–395; Tashkin DP, Elashoff R, Clements PJ et al. Cyclophosphamide versus placebo in scleroderma lung disease. N Engl J Med. 2006;354(25):2655–2666.

6. Maher TM, Nambiar AM, Wells AU. The role of precision medicine in interstitial lung disease. Eur Respir J. 2022;60(3):2102146.
7. Glenn LM, Troy LK, Corte TJ. Novel diagnostic techniques in interstitial lung disease. Front Med (Lausanne). 2023;10:1174443.
8. Karampitsakos T, Juan-Guardela BM, Tzouvelekis A, Herazo-Maya JD. Precision medicine advances in idiopathic pulmonary fibrosis. EBioMedicine. 2023;95:104766.
9. Oldham JM, Lee CT, Wu Z, et al. Lung function trajectory in progressive fibrosing interstitial lung disease. Eur Respir J. 2022;59(6):2101396.
10. Flaherty KR, Wells AU, Cottin V, et al. Nintedanib in progressive Fibrosing interstitial lung diseases. N Engl J Med. 2019;381(18):1718–27.
11. Nureki SI, Tomer Y, Venosa A, et al. Expression of mutant Sftpc in murine alveolar epithelia drives spontaneous lung fibrosis. J Clin Invest. 2018;128(9):4008–24.
12. Katzen J, Wagner BD, Venosa A, et al. An SFTPC BRICHOS mutant links epithelial ER stress and spontaneous lung fibrosis. JCI Insight. 2019;4(6)
13. Moore BB, Lawson WE, Oury TD, Sisson TH, Raghavendran K, Hogaboam CM. Animal models of fibrotic lung disease. Am J Respir Cell Mol Biol. 2013;49(2):167–79.
14. Gerckens M, Alsafadi HN, Wagner DE, Lindner M, Burgstaller G, Konigshoff M. Generation of human 3D lung tissue cultures (3D-LTCs) for disease modeling. J Vis Exp. 2019;144
15. Alsafadi HN, Staab-Weijnitz CA, Lehmann M, et al. An ex vivo model to induce early fibrosis-like changes in human precision-cut lung slices. Am J Physiol Lung Cell Mol Physiol. 2017;312(6):L896–902.
16. Montesi SB, Gomez CR, Beers M, et al. Pulmonary fibrosis stakeholder summit: a joint NHLBI, three lakes foundation, and Pulmonary Fibrosis Foundation workshop report. Am J Respir Crit Care Med. 2024;209(4):362–73.
17. Saleh KS, Hewawasam R, Serbedzija P, et al. Engineering hybrid-hydrogels comprised of healthy or diseased decellularized extracellular matrix to study pulmonary fibrosis. Cell Mol Bioeng. 2022;15(5):505–19.
18. Wilkinson DC, Alva-Ornelas JA, Sucre JM, et al. Development of a three-dimensional bioengineering technology to generate lung tissue for personalized disease modeling. Stem Cells Transl Med. 2017;6(2):622–33.
19. Wilkinson DC, Mellody M, Meneses LK, Hope AC, Dunn B, Gomperts BN. Development of a three-dimensional bioengineering technology to generate lung tissue for personalized disease modeling. Curr Protoc Stem Cell Biol. 2018;46(1):e56.
20. Hatabu H, Hunninghake GM, Richeldi L, et al. Interstitial lung abnormalities detected incidentally on CT: a position paper from the Fleischner society. Lancet Respir Med. 2020;8(7):726–37.
21. Luo F, Zhu M, Wilson KC. Adult interstitial lung abnormalities: the new frontier of pulmonary fibrosis. Am J Respir Crit Care Med. 2023;208(6):651–2.
22. Hobbs BD, Putman RK, Araki T, et al. Overlap of genetic risk between interstitial lung abnormalities and idiopathic pulmonary fibrosis. Am J Resp Crit Care. 2019;200(11):1402–13.
23. Moll M, Peljto AL, Kim JS, et al. A polygenic risk score for idiopathic pulmonary fibrosis and interstitial lung abnormalities. Am J Respir Crit Care Med. 2023;208(7):791–801.
24. Shiraishi Y, Tanabe N, Sakamoto R, et al. Longitudinal assessment of interstitial lung abnormalities on CT in patients with COPD using artificial intelligence-based segmentation: a prospective observational study. BMC Pulm Med. 2024;24(1):200.
25. Bermejo-Pelaez D, Ash SY, Washko GR, San Jose Estepar R, Ledesma-Carbayo MJ. Classification of interstitial lung abnormality patterns with an Ensemble of Deep Convolutional Neural Networks. Sci Rep. 2020;10(1):338.
26. Zhang D, Newton CA. Familial pulmonary fibrosis: genetic features and clinical implications. Chest. 2021;160(5):1764–73.
27. Diaz de Leon A, Cronkhite JT, Yilmaz C, et al. Subclinical lung disease, macrocytosis, and premature graying in kindreds with telomerase (TERT) mutations. Chest. 2011;140(3):753–63.

28. Newton CA, Oldham JM, Applegate C, et al. The role of genetic testing in pulmonary fibrosis: a perspective from the Pulmonary Fibrosis Foundation genetic testing work group. Chest. 2022;162(2):394–405.
29. Newton CA, Batra K, Torrealba J, et al. Telomere-related lung fibrosis is diagnostically heterogeneous but uniformly progressive. Eur Respir J. 2016;48(6):1710–20.
30. Cronkhite JT, Xing C, Raghu G, et al. Telomere shortening in familial and sporadic pulmonary fibrosis. Am J Respir Crit Care Med. 2008;178(7):729–37.
31. Duckworth A, Gibbons MA, Allen RJ, et al. Telomere length and risk of idiopathic pulmonary fibrosis and chronic obstructive pulmonary disease: a Mendelian randomisation study. Lancet Respir Med. 2021;9(3):285–94.
32. Stuart BD, Lee JS, Kozlitina J, et al. Effect of telomere length on survival in patients with idiopathic pulmonary fibrosis: an observational cohort study with independent validation. Lancet Respir Med. 2014;2(7):557–65.
33. Ley B, Newton CA, Arnould I, et al. The MUC5B promoter polymorphism and telomere length in patients with chronic hypersensitivity pneumonitis: an observational cohort-control study. Lancet Respir Med. 2017;5(8):639–47.
34. Newton CA, Zhang D, Oldham JM, et al. Telomere length and use of immunosuppressive medications in idiopathic pulmonary fibrosis. Am J Respir Crit Care Med. 2019;200(3):336–47.
35. Zhang D, Adegunsoye A, Oldham JM, et al. Telomere length and immunosuppression in non-idiopathic pulmonary fibrosis interstitial lung disease. Eur Respir J. 2023;62(5):2300441.
36. Hoffman TW, van Moorsel CHM, van der Vis JJ, Biesma DH, Grutters JC. No effect of danazol treatment in patients with advanced idiopathic pulmonary fibrosis. ERJ Open Res. 2023;9(5):00131.
37. Doubkova M, Kriegova E, Littnerova S, et al. DSP rs2076295 variants influence nintedanib and pirfenidone outcomes in idiopathic pulmonary fibrosis: a pilot study. Ther Adv Respir Dis. 2021;15:17534666211042529.
38. Raghu G, Remy-Jardin M, Ryerson CJ, et al. Diagnosis of hypersensitivity pneumonitis in adults. An official ATS/JRS/ALAT clinical practice guideline. Am J Respir Crit Care Med. 2020;202(3):e36–69.
39. Stanel SC, Callum J, Rivera-Ortega P. Genetic and environmental factors in interstitial lung diseases: current and future perspectives on early diagnosis of high-risk cohorts. Front Med (Lausanne). 2023;10:1232655.
40. Jumat MI, Hayati F, Syed Abdul Rahim SS, et al. Occupational lung disease: a narrative review of lung conditions from the workplace. Ann Med Surg (Lond). 2021;64:102245.
41. Gandhi SA, Min B, Fazio JC, et al. The impact of occupational exposures on the risk of idiopathic pulmonary fibrosis: a systematic review and meta-analysis. Ann Am Thorac Soc. 2024;21(3):486–98.
42. Zhang X, Lin S, Funk WE, Hou L. Environmental and occupational exposure to chemicals and telomere length in human studies. Occup Environ Med. 2013;70(10):743–9.
43. Yang IV, Pedersen BS, Rabinovich E, et al. Relationship of DNA methylation and gene expression in idiopathic pulmonary fibrosis. Am J Respir Crit Care Med. 2014;190(11):1263–72.
44. White ES, Xia M, Murray S, et al. Plasma surfactant protein-D, matrix metalloproteinase-7, and osteopontin index distinguishes idiopathic pulmonary fibrosis from other idiopathic interstitial pneumonias. Am J Respir Crit Care Med. 2016;194(10):1242–51.
45. Kim JS, Ma SF, Ma JZ, et al. Associations of plasma Omega-3 fatty acids with progression and survival in pulmonary fibrosis. Chest. 2024;165(3):621–31.
46. Clynick B, Corte TJ, Jo HE, et al. Biomarker signatures for progressive idiopathic pulmonary fibrosis. Eur Respir J. 2022;59(3):2101181.
47. Organ LA, Duggan AR, Oballa E, et al. Biomarkers of collagen synthesis predict progression in the PROFILE idiopathic pulmonary fibrosis cohort. Respir Res. 2019;20(1):148.
48. Bowman WS, Newton CA, Linderholm AL, et al. Proteomic biomarkers of progressive fibrosing interstitial lung disease: a multicentre cohort analysis. Lancet Respir Med. 2022;10(6):593–602.

49. Herazo-Maya JD, Sun J, Molyneaux PL, et al. Validation of a 52-gene risk profile for outcome prediction in patients with idiopathic pulmonary fibrosis: an international, multicentre, cohort study. Lancet Respir Med. 2017;5(11):857–68.
50. van der Sar IGWM, Moor CC. Exhaled breath analysis in interstitial lung disease. Curr Opin Pulm Med. 2023:443–50.
51. Ahmadzai HHS, Hettiarachchi R, Lin J-L, Thomas PS, Zhang Q. Exhaled breath condensate: a comprehensive update. Clin Chem Lab Med. 2013;51:1343–61.
52. Maher TM, et al. Safety, tolerability, pharmacokinetics, and pharmacodynamics of GLPG1690, a novel autotaxin inhibitor, to treat idiopathic pulmonary fibrosis (FLORA): a phase 2a randomised placebo-controlled trial. Lancet Respir Med. 2018;6:627–35.
53. Jaskiewicz KMK, Maskey-Warzechowska M, Paralusz K, Siemiez N, Nejman-Gryz P, Barnas M, Krenke R, Gorska K. Exhaled biomarkers in idiopathic pulmonary fibrosis-a six-month follow-up study in patients treated with Pirfenidone. J Clin Med. 2020;9
54. Montesi SBMS, Brenner LN, Gorshkova IA, Berdyshev EV, Tager AM, Shea BS. Docosatetraenoyl LPA is elevated in exhaled breath condensate in idiopathic pulmonary fibrosis. BMC Pulm Med. 2014;14
55. Raghu G, Collard HR, Egan JJ, et al. An official ATS/ERS/JRS/ALAT statement: idiopathic pulmonary fibrosis: evidence-based guidelines for diagnosis and management. Am J Respir Crit Care Med. 2011;183(6):788–824.
56. Otsuka H, Sano A, Azuma Y, et al. Surgical lung biopsy for interstitial lung diseases-a single center study of 129 patients. J Thorac Dis. 2022;14(6):1972–9.
57. Fisher JH, Shapera S, To T, Marras TK, Gershon A, Dell S. Procedure volume and mortality after surgical lung biopsy in interstitial lung disease. Eur Respir J. 2019;53(2):1801164.
58. Ambrogi V, Mineo TC. VATS biopsy for undetermined interstitial lung disease under non-general anesthesia: comparison between uniportal approach under intercostal block vs. three-ports in epidural anesthesia. J Thorac Dis. 2014;6(7):888–95.
59. Ayed AK, Raghunathan R. Thoracoscopy versus open lung biopsy in the diagnosis of interstitial lung disease: a randomised controlled trial. J R Coll Surg Edinb. 2000;45(3):159–63.
60. Bando M, Ohno S, Hosono T, et al. Risk of acute exacerbation after video-assisted thoracoscopic lung biopsy for interstitial lung disease. J Bronchol Interv Pulmonol. 2009;16(4):229–35.
61. Korevaar DA, Colella S, Fally M, et al. European respiratory society guidelines on transbronchial lung cryobiopsy in the diagnosis of interstitial lung diseases. Eur Respir J. 2022;60(5):2200425.
62. Adams TN, Batra K, Silhan L, et al. Utility of bronchoalveolar lavage and transbronchial biopsy in patients with interstitial lung disease. Lung. 2020;198(5):803–10.
63. Sheth JS, Belperio JA, Fishbein MC, et al. Utility of transbronchial vs surgical lung biopsy in the diagnosis of suspected fibrotic interstitial lung disease. Chest. 2017;151(2):389–99.
64. Kheir F, Uribe Becerra JP, Bissell B, et al. Use of a genomic classifier in patients with interstitial lung disease: a systematic review and meta-analysis. Ann Am Thorac Soc. 2022;19(5):827–32.
65. Kheir F, Uribe Becerra JP, Bissell B, et al. Transbronchial lung cryobiopsy in patients with interstitial lung disease: a systematic review. Ann Am Thorac Soc. 2022;19(7):1193–202.
66. Sethi J, Ali MS, Mohananey D, Nanchal R, Maldonado F, Musani A. Are transbronchial cryobiopsies ready for prime time?: a systematic review and meta-analysis. J Bronchol Interv Pulmonol. 2019;26(1):22–32.
67. Fortin M, Liberman M, Delage A, et al. Transbronchial lung cryobiopsy and surgical lung biopsy: a prospective multi-centre agreement clinical trial (CAN-ICE). Am J Respir Crit Care Med. 2023;207(12):1612–9.
68. Zhou G, Ren Y, Li J, et al. The effect of 1.9-mm versus 2.4-mm probes in transbronchial cryobiopsies for interstitial lung diseases: a prospective analysis. Ann Transl Med. 2021;9(1):20.
69. Kim SH, Mok J, Kim S, et al. Clinical outcomes of transbronchial cryobiopsy using a 1.1-mm diameter cryoprobe for peripheral lung lesions – a prospective pilot study. Respir Med. 2023;217:107338.

70. Herath S. Use of the 1.1 mm cryoprobe through the radial EBUS GS (without the need for a bronchial blocker) to obtain samples safely in diagnosing PPL. Respirol Case Rep. 2023;11(4):e01128.
71. Marinescu DC, Ryerson CJ. Endobronchial optical coherence tomography for the diagnosis of fibrotic interstitial lung disease: a light at the end of the tunnel? Am J Respir Crit Care Med. 2021;204(10):1122–4.
72. Tian S, Huang H, Zhang Y, et al. The role of confocal laser endomicroscopy in pulmonary medicine. Eur Respir Rev. 2023;32(167):220185.
73. Nandy S, Raphaely RA, Muniappan A, et al. Diagnostic accuracy of endobronchial optical coherence tomography for the microscopic diagnosis of usual interstitial pneumonia. Am J Respir Crit Care Med. 2021;204(10):1164–79.
74. Walsh SLF, Wells AU, Desai SR, et al. Multicentre evaluation of multidisciplinary team meeting agreement on diagnosis in diffuse parenchymal lung disease: a case-cohort study. Lancet Respir Med. 2016;4(7):557–65.
75. Choe J, Hwang HJ, Lee SM, Yoon J, Kim N, Seo JB. CT quantification of interstitial lung abnormality and interstitial lung disease: from technical challenges to future directions. Investig Radiol. 2024;60:43.
76. Barnes H, Humphries SM, George PM, et al. Machine learning in radiology: the new frontier in interstitial lung diseases. Lancet Digit Health. 2023;5(1):e41–50.
77. Thillai M, Oldham JM, Ruggiero A, et al. Deep learning-based segmentation of CT scans predicts disease progression and mortality in IPF. Am J Respir Crit Care Med. 2024;210:465.
78. Rea G, Sverzellati N, Bocchino M, et al. Beyond visual interpretation: quantitative analysis and artificial intelligence in interstitial lung disease diagnosis "expanding horizons in radiology". Diagnostics (Basel). 2023;13(14)
79. Humphries SM, Mackintosh JA, Jo HE, et al. Quantitative computed tomography predicts outcomes in idiopathic pulmonary fibrosis. Respirology. 2022;27(12):1045–53.
80. Jacob J, Bartholmai BJ, Rajagopalan S, et al. Automated quantitative computed tomography versus visual computed tomography scoring in idiopathic pulmonary fibrosis: validation against pulmonary function. J Thorac Imaging. 2016;31(5):304–11.
81. Humphries SM, Yagihashi K, Huckleberry J, et al. Idiopathic pulmonary fibrosis: data-driven textural analysis of extent of fibrosis at baseline and 15-month follow-up. Radiology. 2017;285(1):270–8.
82. Haga A, Iwasawa T, Misumi T, et al. Correlation of CT-based radiomics analysis with pathological cellular infiltration in fibrosing interstitial lung diseases. Jpn J Radiol. 2024;42:1157.
83. He W, Cui B, Chu Z, et al. Radiomics based on HRCT can predict RP-ILD and mortality in anti-MDA5 + dermatomyositis patients: a multi-center retrospective study. Respir Res. 2024;25(1):252.
84. Schniering J, Maciukiewicz M, Gabrys HS, et al. Computed tomography-based radiomics decodes prognostic and molecular differences in interstitial lung disease related to systemic sclerosis. Eur Respir J. 2022;59(5):2004503.
85. Culver DA, Behr J, Belperio JA, et al. Patient registries in idiopathic pulmonary fibrosis. Am J Respir Crit Care Med. 2019;200(2):160–7.
86. Fernandez Perez ER, Kong AM, Raimundo K, Koelsch TL, Kulkarni R, Cole AL. Epidemiology of hypersensitivity pneumonitis among an insured population in the United States: a claims-based cohort analysis. Ann Am Thorac Soc. 2018;15(4):460–9.
87. Olson AL, Patnaik P, Hartmann N, Bohn RL, Garry EM, Wallace L. Prevalence and incidence of chronic fibrosing interstitial lung diseases with a progressive phenotype in the United States estimated in a large claims database analysis. Adv Ther. 2021;38(7):4100–14.
88. Singer D, Bengtson LGS, Conoscenti CS, et al. Claims-based prevalence of disease progression among patients with fibrosing interstitial lung disease other than idiopathic pulmonary fibrosis in the United States. Ann Am Thorac Soc. 2022;19(7):1112–21.
89. Sparks JA, Jin Y, Cho SK, et al. Prevalence, incidence and cause-specific mortality of rheumatoid arthritis-associated interstitial lung disease among older rheumatoid arthritis patients. Rheumatology (Oxford). 2021;60(8):3689–98.

90. Raghu G, Chen SY, Hou Q, Yeh WS, Collard HR. Incidence and prevalence of idiopathic pulmonary fibrosis in US adults 18-64 years old. Eur Respir J. 2016;48(1):179–86.
91. Nasser M, Larrieu S, Boussel L, et al. Estimates of epidemiology, mortality and disease burden associated with progressive fibrosing interstitial lung disease in France (the PROGRESS study). Respir Res. 2021;22(1):162.
92. Olson AL, Hartmann N, Patnaik P, et al. Healthcare resource utilization and related costs in chronic fibrosing interstitial lung diseases with a progressive phenotype: a US claims database analysis. Adv Ther. 2022;39(4):1794–809.
93. Olson AL, Maher TM, Acciai V, et al. Healthcare resources utilization and costs of patients with non-IPF progressive fibrosing interstitial lung disease based on insurance claims in the USA. Adv Ther. 2020;37(7):3292–8.
94. Cho SK, Doyle TJ, Lee H, et al. Validation of claims-based algorithms to identify interstitial lung disease in patients with rheumatoid arthritis. Semin Arthritis Rheum. 2020;50(4):592–7.
95. Esposito DB, Lanes S, Donneyong M, et al. Idiopathic pulmonary fibrosis in United States automated claims. Incidence, prevalence, and algorithm validation. Am J Respir Crit Care Med. 2015;192(10):1200–7.
96. Farrand E, Collard HR, Guarnieri M, et al. Extracting patient-level data from the electronic health record: expanding opportunities for health system research. PLoS One. 2023;18(3):e0280342.
97. Farrand E, Gologorskaya O, Mills H, Radhakrishnan L, Collard HR, Butte AJ. Machine-learning algorithm to improve cohort identification in interstitial lung disease. Am J Respir Crit Care Med. 2023;207(10):1398–401.
98. Adegunsoye A, Newton CA, Oldham JM, et al. Telomere length associates with chronological age and mortality across racially diverse pulmonary fibrosis cohorts. Nat Commun. 2023;14(1):1489.
99. Jalbert AC, Siafa L, Ramanakumar AV, Assayag D. Gender and racial equity in clinical research for idiopathic pulmonary fibrosis: a systematic review and meta-analysis. Eur Respir J. 2022;59(3):2102969.
100. Newton CA, Herzog EL. Molecular markers and the promise of precision medicine for interstitial lung disease. Clin Chest Med. 2021;42(2):357–64.
101. Podolanczuk AJ, Kim JS, Cooper CB, et al. Design and rationale for the prospective treatment efficacy in IPF using genotype for NAC selection (PRECISIONS) clinical trial. BMC Pulm Med. 2022;22(1):475.
102. Idiopathic Pulmonary Fibrosis Clinical Research N, Raghu G, Anstrom KJ, King TE Jr, Lasky JA, Martinez FJ. Prednisone, azathioprine, and N-acetylcysteine for pulmonary fibrosis. N Engl J Med. 2012;366(21):1968–77.
103. Pallmann P, Bedding AW, Choodari-Oskooei B, et al. Adaptive designs in clinical trials: why use them, and how to run and report them. BMC Med. 2018;16(1):29.
104. Kulkarni T, Kawano-Dourado L, Johannson K, et al. A randomized, embedded, multifactorial adaptive platform trial for ILD (REMAP-ILD): the conceptual design. Eur Respir J. 2023;62(suppl 67):OA2588.

# Correction to: All in the Family: Role for Precision Medicine in Screening and Disease Course Prediction

**Laurence Pearmain, Jack Callum, Stefan Stanel, and Pilar Rivera-Ortega**

## Correction to:
## Chapter 2 in: B. F. Collins, S. B. Montesi (eds.), *Precision Medicine in Interstitial Lung Disease*, Respiratory Medicine, https://doi.org/10.1007/978-3-031-87183-2_2

This title was recently published. The authorship of the chapter was updated incorrectly and has been corrected as below in the revised publication.

Current Author Order
Laurence Pearmain and Pilar Rivera Ortega

Updated Author Order with Affiliations
Laurence Pearmain, Jack Callum, Stefan Stanel, and Pilar Rivera-Ortega

Laurence Pearmain
Respiratory NIHR Clinical Lecturer, University of Manchester, Manchester, UK

Respiratory Specialist Registrar, Wythenshawe Hospital, Manchester University NHS Foundation Trust, Manchester, UK

Jack Callum
Respiratory Consultant, Homerton University Hospital NHS Foundation Trust, London, UK

Stefan Stanel
Interstitial Lung Disease Unit, Wythenshawe Hospital, Manchester University NHS Foundation Trust, Manchester, UK

Pilar Rivera-Ortega
Interstitial Lung Disease Unit, Wythenshawe Hospital, Manchester University NHS Foundation Trust, Manchester, UK

---

The updated version of this chapter can be found at
https://doi.org/10.1007/978-3-031-87183-2_2



B. F. Collins, S. B. Montesi (eds.), *Precision Medicine in Interstitial Lung Disease*, Respiratory Medicine, https://doi.org/10.1007/978-3-031-87183-2_12

# Index




B. F. Collins, S. B. Montesi (eds.), *Precision Medicine in Interstitial Lung Disease*, Respiratory Medicine, https://doi.org/10.1007/978-3-031-87183-2

GPSR Compliance

*The European Union's (EU) General Product Safety Regulation (GPSR) is a set of rules that requires consumer products to be safe and our obligations to ensure this.*

*If you have any concerns about our products, you can contact us on ProductSafety@springernature.com*

In case Publisher is established outside the EU, the EU authorized representative is:

Springer Nature Customer Service Center GmbH
Europaplatz 3
69115 Heidelberg, Germany

**Batch number: 10732090**

Printed by Printforce, the Netherlands